REPRODUCTION, CHILDBEARING AND MOTHERHOOD: A CROSS-CULTURAL PERSPECTIVE

REPRODUCTION, CHILDBEARING AND MOTHERHOOD: A CROSS-CULTURAL PERSPECTIVE

PRANEE LIAMPUTTONG
EDITOR

Nova Science Publishers, Inc.
New York

NOTICE TO THE READER

LIBRARY OF CONGRESS CATALOGING-IN-PUBLICATION DATA

Reproduction, childbearing, and motherhood : a cross-cultural perspective / [edited by] Pranee Liamputtong.
   p. ; cm.
 Includes bibliographical references and index.
 ISBN-13: 978-1-60021-606-0 (hardcover)
 ISBN-10: 1-60021-606-4 (hardcover)
 1. Childbirth--Cross-cultural studies. 2. Human reproduction--Cross-cultural studies. 3. Motherhood--Cross-cultural studies. I. Liamputtong, Pranee, 1955-
 [DNLM: 1. Parturition--ethnology. 2. Cross-Cultural Comparison. 3. Maternal Behavior--ethnology. 4. Pregnancy--ethnology. WQ 300 R425 2007]
 RG652.R444 2007
 362.198--dc22
  2007007646

Published by Nova Science Publishers, Inc. ✦ *New York*

DEDICATION

To my mother, Yindee Liamputtong,
who gave birth to eight children and raised us amidst poverty;
and
To all of the women in my family who have become, or choose not to become, mothers:
Prapaporn, Somsri, Chalita, Araya, Pattanee, Kalaya, Piriya & Kristin

CONTENTS

PREFACE

Although reproduction including infertility, abortion, childbearing and motherhood is a significant human experience, its social meaning is shaped by the culture in which women live. Reproduction and its management, therefore, occur within the social and cultural context of the event. As such, reproductive beliefs and practices differ across social and cultural settings.

This volume focuses on reproduction, childbearing and motherhood. I bring together a number of researchers who carry out their research regarding reproduction, childbearing and motherhood from diverse cultural settings. In this volume, I will show that despite the modernization of the society and advanced medical technology and knowledge in reproduction, traditions continue to exert influence on how the women and their families manage their reproduction, childbearing and motherhood in their societies.

Readers may question why this book is needed? Culture has played a significant role in reproductive lives of women in most parts of the world. The social context of reproduction also plays an essential part in how women give birth and manage their reproduction. These issues are crucial for health and social care providers not only in any social group but in multicultural societies where people are drawn from diverse cultural backgrounds. I contend that by taking cultural issues into account can culturally sensitive care be achieved in health services in any society. This book intends to assist health and social care providers and policies makers to make changes in their health and social settings to be more culturally sensitive and meaningful to women who become mothers and those who choose not, or are unable, to become mothers.

The book will be of interest to those who have their interests in working with women and reproduction from a cross-cultural perspective. It will be useful for students and lecturers in courses like midwifery, anthropology, sociology, social work, nursing, and medicine. It will also be of interest to many lay readers who are interested in cross-cultural issues regarding reproduction and procreation.

In constructing this book, I owe my gratitude to many people. First, to all contributors in this volume, who work hard in order to get their chapters to me on schedule, and who are patient with my constant emails to remind them of their dead line. I also wish to thank Rosemary Oaks who helped reading and making comments on some chapters in the book. I wish to thank Liz Hoban and Chimaraoke Izugbara who pointed me to many potential contributors, many of whom I would not have found without their assistance. Lastly, I wish to thank Maya Columbus of Nova Science Publishers who provided me a contract to write the book.

Pranee Liamputtong
Melbourne, Australia
August 2006

ABOUT THIS BOOK

This book comprises 16 chapters, and I put them into four parts. Chapter 1 aims to set the scene of the book. As such, I intend to provide readers with empirical research regarding reproduction, childbearing and motherhood from a cross-cultural perspective. I will discuss salient issues regarding procreation, reproduction and motherhood in different societies. I will show that women are seen as the markers of reproduction; they are responsible for procreation and reproduction. If they fail to do so, or worse, if they deny doing so, often blame falls upon them. For those who become mothers, these norms function to protect not only the women but also their newborn infants. This can be seen clearly with cultural beliefs and practices regarding the postpartum period as I have outlined in this chapter. But, in many societies cultural norms tend to be replaced by medicalization of childbirth. I do not deny that modern birth can be beneficial to many women, but all too often, the overmedicalized birth has made other types of birth (such as births assisted by TBAs) irrelevant.

Becoming a mother brings joy to women, and most women would attest to this. But, under certain circumstances, it can be distressful for women, particularly those who do not have a support network, like those who are immigrant women. They often have to deal with the double transition of their lives, not only as mothers but also as displaced people. I contend that culture still plays a vital role in women's reproduction and procreation. We must acknowledge the importance of culture and incorporate it in the provision of health care for women in all societies.

Part One is about reproduction and procreation. In Chapter 2, Tatjana Alvadj writes about the changed perceptions of fertility as a result of migration amongst immigrant women in Edmonton, Canada. Women, she suggests, conceptualize their reproductive role based on social, political and economical expectations of the society in which they live. In many cultures, fertility is understood, not only as a way to secure procreation within a family, but also as a responsibility for the broader collective welfare. The idea of family prestige, economic well-being, and/or political enhancement plays a significant role in shaping the concept of female fertility. For its importance for the collective, fertility is established as the basic criterion in measuring female accomplishments, and as such, exists at the heart of social interest. In a process of migration, change, and integration into a different, modern state society, the women face expectations based on different criteria. Instead of a holistic mélange of private and public affairs, they find that the social life is highly compartmentalized. The matter of childbearing is transferred from the center of social interest into the realm of privacy and 'personal' choices. The programmed integration for immigrant women, mostly gender blind and operating from the mainstream prospective, do not take the important element of female fertility into serious consideration. As a result, immigrant women often struggle with identity crisis, as well as marital and health problems caused by the overwhelming responsibilities of bearing the children, taking care of the family and fitting into the new society by attending school or working. The research project "Immigrant Women and Fertility: Rights and Responsibilities" explores the change of the concept of fertility as a result of migration from one cultural environment to another. This research demonstrates that reproductive rights and responsibilities of immigrant women is a challenging issue that is often perceived as a private matter, and as such rarely addressed in public. It indicates that the importance of fertility in the process of integration of immigrant women exceeds the private domain and becomes a political issue that needs adequate attention and action.

In Chapter 3, Suzanne Belton discusses unwanted pregnancy and Burmese women. She suggests that motherhood is immensely popular and the majority of women experience at least one pregnancy in their lifetime. But not all pregnancies are desired or the circumstances of conception joyful. Pregnancies can be mistimed or completely rejected. We still live in a world where it is not possible to plan or control fertility completely. For Burmese women who have limited access to modern contraceptive technology, or whose socio-political environment precludes their ability to regulate their own fertility, unplanned and unwanted pregnancy is a common experience. Abortion is one method a woman may choose to end a pregnancy. Burmese women in Tak Province Thailand have no access to safe abortion and use traditional methods of fertility regulation which while effective at ending pregnancy often cause serious complications. Traditional 'menstrual regulation' can be done without direct acknowledgement of pregnancy as abortion is socially taboo and religiously vetoed. This chapter explains Burmese ways of 'bringing down the blood' and women's narratives of a liminal state of fecundity in the borderlands of Burma and Thailand.

Lakshmi Ramachandar and Pertti Pelto look at decisions about abortion and women's roles and strategies, a result of their community-based study in a rural district of Tamil Nadu, India, in Chapter 4. This paper examines the complex of economic, cultural and other reasons underlying the choices for pregnancy termination (MTP) among rural Indian women. Their aim is to explore the complexities of motivation that lie beneath the (often) superficial explanations reported in the literature. The extensive abortion research literature in India is quite unanimous in noting that married women are the overwhelming majority of abortion seekers, and that "the majority of women opt for abortion because of 'already many children'". Their data show, however, that women and their families have many different explanations and motives for keeping their families small.

The data for this chapter are from a community-based study in 2001-2002 in a rural district of Tamil Nadu, in south India, in which they interviewed 97 married women who had had recent abortions. Although economic reasons (unable to support and feed any more children) were often the initial answer during interviews, additional, often complex, other motives emerged. The strong desire to support much expanded education for both sons and daughters is a new pattern, that has spread into practically all rural areas. In addition to the much increased investment in education, families are also wanting to have money for consumer goods that were not central in the motivations of the past generation.

Unusual cultural motives for abortion sometimes arise because of pregnancies that occur at "inauspicious times", or in "inauspicious circumstances". The cultural belief that pregnancy and childbirth in "older women" is shameful was cited by several women. Sex selective abortion is another well-known, culturally driven pattern that is particularly important in south Asia, as in other strongly "patrilineal" societies. The choice of abortion as a means for limiting family size must also be seen in relation to complex beliefs and concerns about the alternative strategies of contraception. These cultural ideas are, in turn, related to concepts about women's bodies and physiological functioning.

In Chapter 5, Hoa Ngan Nguyen and Pranee Liamputtong examine the lived experiences of abortion among young women in Ho Chi Minh City, Viet Nam. They find that facing unwanted pregnancy before marriage was stressful for both the women and the men. Their feelings ranged from fear, sadness, anxiety, and silence. However, confronting this event was more stressful for women than men. Difficulties or uncertainty about getting married, such as getting approval from the boyfriends' family, a moral reputation of women and their parents, warded off a marriage solution. Consequently, the choice of abortion was unavoidable in this context. Abortion is not only an inevitable consequence of social constraints, but is also a doubled stressful experience when young women suffer it in silence. The task of improving sexual lives of Vietnamese young people, particularly women, involves a long road to travel. In this study, Hoa Ngan Nguyen and Pranee Liamputtong have at least started this long journey. It is hoped that further research will be undertaken to fulfill this goal. Only then, they contend, will many sexually active young people in Vietnam no longer suffer in silence.

Childbearing issues are presented in Part Two of the book. In this Part, I begin with celebrating safe childbirth in Cambodia, by Elizabeth Hoban in Chapter 6. In this chapter, Elizabeth Hoban contends that pregnancy, childbirth and post-parturition are natural, biosocial, life-crisis events. In order to deal with the dangers and the existential uncertainty associated of birth, people tend to produce a set of internally consistent and mutually dependent practices and beliefs to manage physiologically and socially problematic aspects of parturition in a way that makes sense in the particular cultural context. In rural Cambodia the time-honored and universal practice of *ang pleen* (mother roasting) is one such example. Mother roasting begins immediately after childbirth and is terminated 5-10 days post-birth and it forms part of a suite of postpartum practices, which include drinking Khmer herbs and eating hot food such as *bor bor* (rice soup), to ensure women's humoral balance is returned immediately post-birth and throughout the postpartum period thereby preventing life threatening conditions such as *chiem chok* (stuck blood), *toah* (relapse) or a weak and aching body in old age.

At the cessation of mother roasting when a woman leaves the roasting bed, her family celebrates the woman's safety and the end of her confinement by holding a *tumleak cɔ̆ɔŋ kraɲcɔ̆ɔ* ceremony. There are two components to the ceremony and they include, a *saen doon taa* which is a ritual to thank ancestral spirits for their part in the safe birth, and the second component is specifically for the grandmother midwife and her spirit teacher who are thanked and publicly acknowledged for heir role in ensuring the woman *claan tonle* (crossed the river), the Khmer metaphor for childbirth. These traditional knowledges and practices are widespread in rural Cambodia, including for women who give birth in a health facility in the care of a trained midwife.

This chapter draws on ethnographic research that Hoban carried out in 2000-2001 in rural Cambodia that explored the role of grandmother midwives in Safe Motherhood initiatives in a modernizing health system in Cambodia. During this study, she participated in and documented more thank twenty *tumleak cɔ̄ɔŋ krañcɔ̄ɔ* ceremonies and all were remarkably similar, including for women who birthed in health facilities, for young and well-off women. These ceremonies are religious in meaning and context. They do not translate into the secular and Westernized ways of doing birth in rural Cambodia, however, they do co-exist and are complimented by modern medicine and therapies and as such maintain their spiritual significance and practical application, both of which guarantee women's physical and cultural safety.

In Chapter 7, Margaret Chesney presents childbirth and the Dai in Pakistan. As a UK midwife, she has made nine field trips to work in a Red Crescent Maternity hospital in the interior of the Punjab, Pakistan. Following the first four field trips, an evaluation study was carried out, thereafter research was undertaken on women's experience of birth in Pakistan. The objective of her research was to increase awareness of birth in Pakistan. She utilzed ethnographic method and worked with a gatekeeper to gain access to Pakistani women's group in the North of England, from which ten women agreed to be interviewed. A further six women were interviewed during a field trip to Pakistan in 2000. In this chapter, Chesney discusses some themes emerging from her data: Birth practices in a Red Crescent Hospital in Pakistan; The Dai, a family thing; and East and West time. The chapter concludes with 3 short stories that became parables; as the messages within may serve as guides to the reader to more understanding of women's lives in a developing country.

Naomi McPherson, in Chapter 8, discusses changing conceptions of childbirth in West New Britain, Papua New Guinea. Drawing on five periods of ethnographic research in the Bariai, West New Britain, Papua New Guinea over the past 23 years, this chapter explores Bariai women's changing experiences of pregnancy and childbirth. As context to these changes, she begins with a brief overview of Bariai beliefs and values pertaining to women's bodies, conception theory, women's knowledge of childbearing and village birthing. She shows how colonialism, Catholicism, and the state have contributed to the Bariai traditional reproductive care system. Women's lives and their health have been affected by breakdown of traditional sexual taboos, increased family size, hard manual labour, and the necessity for a cash income. Rather than government and non-government agency time and funds continually being invested in under-funded and under-used western-style clinics and birthing practices, she concludes that time and funds should be directed to disease eradication. It is diseases such as malaria and tuberculosis that compromise women's reproductive health and their quality of life and which contribute to under-five mortality rates.

Chimaraoke Otutubikey Izugbara and Joseph Kinuabeye Ukwayi write about a continuing challenge of unsafe childbearing in rural Nigeria in chapter 9. They ask: How do hospitals feature as birthing sites in the imaginaries of local southern women? Current debates surrounding the uptake of hospitals for obstetric services by women in the global south have yet to engage with this urgent question. Relying on data elicited from ethnographic research among rural Nigerian women, including TBAs (Traditional Birth Attendants), they analyze local women's narratives surrounding the hospital as a site for birthing, in the search, among other things, for the patterns of obstetric care seeking which these constructions authorize. Although recognized as a popular birthing site used by women, the hospital was not spoken of as a space where women's need for risk-free birthing could be actualized. Hospital-based deliveries were also surrounded by stories and folklores which framed the hospital as a setting where women experienced unfavorable treatments and where maternal risks can be exacerbated. All in all, rural Nigerian women's narratives surrounding the hospital reinforce, with details, the significance of making formal hospital-based obstetric services more responsive to local women's cultural needs and sensitivities, adding validity to the need for a more public, academic-oriented discourse about the narrative production of health in local southern societies

In Part Three of this volume, issues regarding immigrant women who are now living in Canada and Australia are also included. Denise Spitzer, in chapter 10, discusses what she terms a "hard labour" and it refers to the childbirth experience that involves minority women and nurses in Canada. In this chapter, she examines the experiences of South Asian, Vietnamese and Aboriginal Canadian women giving birth in hospital during a period of health care restructuring. These perspectives were complemented by an investigation of the attitudes of nursing staff who served, for these women, as the most obvious face of the health care institution. Importantly, relations between nursing staff and labouring women were contextualized by historical developments and circulating stereotypes often producing misunderstandings that had the potential to create tensions between patients and staff. The reduction in time allotted for hospital stays following delivery further exacerbated the situation as potentially time-consuming encounters with minority women were avoided in favour of less troublesome interactions. For many women who battled for attention, for options and for information while undergoing childbirth, the result was hard labour. Hard labour was also characterized by a distinctive sense of loss of control. While all individuals who enter into the institutional setting of the hospital as patients are compelled to relinquish control as they are subjected to the discipline of hospital regimens, minority women reported a heightened sense of this loss due to greater cultural distance from the dominant middle-class, Euro-Canadian values that imbued hospital policies, procedures and expectations. Minority women, however, were not completely bereft and women from each minority community managed to find culturally consonant paths of resistance to ease their transition into motherhood in the hospital environment. While some women found ways to circumvent interactions and unwanted interventions by avoiding staff, most used both support-seeking and support-giving strategies to shore up their sense of identity and of strength to assert control over their circumstances. Both groups of informants, however, agreed that the presence of cultural health brokers could positively alter the power imbalances between minority patients and hospital staff and help mitigate the experience of hard labour.

In Chapter 11, Lina Abboud and Pranee Liamputtong point to the experiences of having a baby in a new home from the accounts of Lebanese immigrant women who are living in Melbourne, Australia. Pregnancy, birth and motherhood have different meanings and significance to women and the community from the "Arab world", and share the values and beliefs of the Arab culture. The focus of this chapter is on the women from societies where Arabic is the official language. The Arab world is made up of twenty-two countries who are members of the Arab League of Nations. This includes the countries of Algeria, Bahrain, Comoros, Djibouti, Egypt, Iraq, Jordan, Kuwait, Lebanon, Libya, Mauritania, Morocco, Oman, Palestine, Qatar, Saudi Arabia, Somalia, Sudan, Syria, Tunisia, United Arab Emirates and Yemen. In defining the Arabic-speaking community, it is a cultural group sharing a common language, heritage, values and beliefs of an Arab culture. The main countries of origin of Arabic-speaking immigrants to Australia include Lebanon, Egypt, Syria, Iraq, Jordan, and Palestine. Both Christianity and Islam are important faiths for Arabic speakers in Australia.

In their study, Abboud and Liamputtong conducted a study to gain an insight into the experiences of pregnancy, birth and the postnatal period of women from an Arabic-speaking background who have given birth in Melbourne, Australia. They examined women's accounts of the pregnancy period, the labor, the hospital stay, and the time immediately after the birth. This study is an important research project because there are only a few studies conducted in Australia that explore some aspect of the birthing experiences of women from an Arabic-speaking background. There are also a small number of studies worldwide which target Arabic-speaking women and examine their experiences of birth either in their home country or after migrating to another country. Their study enables the investigation and exploration of the experiences and perceptions of the women as well as the variations of the experiences of the group of women form Arabic backgrounds.

In Chapter 12, Paola Hernandez writes about childbirth and Somali refugee women in Australia. Drawing on fieldwork undertaken over the last three years, the chapter examines the way in which the experience of resettlement has impacted on women's lives during these times. Paola Hernandez argues that for many of the women interviewed, pregnancy and birth in the Australian context has significantly altered women's sense of self. While medical care is welcomed by the women and is able to be freely accessed during pregnancy and birth, women's experiences during these times often highlight the way in which the refugee experience, including resettlement, continues to impact on women's lives. This is particularly visible in the way in which women interpret and make sense of what is often considered to be 'normal' or 'natural' practices encountered during pregnancy and birth in Australia. For example, there appears to be concern about antenatal appointment and resistance to cesarean sections. There have also been significant changes to customs such as the 40-day confinement period. As a result, women often face pregnancy and birth with some trepidation and anxiety rather than the sense of security one might expect because of women's greater access to health care and material security found in Australia. On the other hand, it is also evident from women's responses that while the social setting impacts on women's experiences and lives, these forces are not all encompassing. Within the context of reproduction and the medicalization of birth women's agency does play a role. Drawing on specific social and cultural understandings and knowledge women are able to challenge and contest certain procedures in their hospital care as well as the way in which certain practices are understood.

Part Four of this book dedicates to motherhood. In Chapter 13, Jamileh Abu-Duhou writes about the motherhood experience of Palestinian women. In Palestine, the discussion of Palestinian women's motherhood experience must be placed within both the cultural context and the context of the Palestinian National Struggle, as women came to signify the nation, and those who bear and nurture children for the national struggle. Based on ethnographic research conducted in Palestine from October 2000 to May 2001, this chapter will examine the ways in which the cultural construction of motherhood, and the ways in which the political and national pressure to preserve and reproduce the Palestinian National Collective have represented Palestinian women as reproducers of the nation, as such controlling their reproductive rights by encouraging them to have children who will become members of the national struggle and reproduce the boundaries of the symbolic identity of their nation. In short, in this chapter, Jamileh Abu-Duhou attempts to highlight the interconnection between the cultural construction of mother hood and that of being a mere reproducer of the national boundaries.

In Chapter 14, Pranee Liamputtong and Denise Spitzer present motherhood from the Hmong immigrant women perspective. They suggest in this chapter that Hmong women bear the primary responsibility for both the social and biological reproduction of a culture. Motherhood and the attendant expectations of mothers as socializing agents of their offspring are particularly charged responsibilities for migrant women as these roles are vital to maintaining the reputed integrity of ethnic boundaries. The efforts of Hmong mothers in Australia to fulfil these duties are challenged by the disparate context in which our informants find themselves. Thus, truncated familial networks and different patterns in economic activities, labour market participation, and domestic labour, have inevitably altered mothering and childrearing roles and practices. Moreover, the response of dominant Anglo-Australian society to the size of Hmong families can be troubling to mothers. These perceptions may further engender Us/Other distinctions contributing to the perceived need to stabilize the borders of Hmong ethnicity.

Investing in children may be an important way of ensuring the continuity of Hmong culture, yet, our informants were also aware that the integrity of the borders they, as other migrant women, have been charged with upholding are in fact more fluid than are often acknowledged. While they may anticipate that their Australian-born children will forge new identities, Hmong mothers, too, negotiate multiple hybrid identities commonly emerge from the unsettling nature of migration and the fractured nature of diasporic cultures.

Ruth de Souza has her discussion on motherhood masala in Chapter 15. Migration, she suggests, leads to transformation, willingly or unwillingly, for both the migrant and the receiving society. The changes that result can be superficial or visible; for example, cuisine or more subtle and private, such as identities. In considering motherhood in a new country, women are challenged with an opportunity to reshape their identity, from viewing their culture as static with fixed boundaries and members to fluid, pliable, negotiated and renegotiated through interactions with others. The pluralising of identities that accompanies migrant motherhood is brought to the fore with migrant women having to sift and reclaim aspects of culture that may have been lost, preserve memories of cultural practices, transmit, maintain or discard traditional perinatal practices and choose new practices. In addition, there may be old and new authority figures in the shape of midwives or mothers to appease. This chapter provides an overview of how women originating from Goa, India who had babies in New Zealand actively considered their past, present and future in terms of cultural maintenance and reclamation during the perinatal period. The history of Goan colonisation as a catalyst for dispersal had already led to the modification of cultural practices. The development of plural identities and the strategic utilization of cultural resources new and old are examined, as is the potential to apply notions of cultural safety to migrant health. The chapter concludes with a discussion of the implications of plural identities for health services and workforce development in New Zealand.

Alexandra Gartrell writes about accessing marriage and motherhood from the experience of women with disability in rural Cambodia in Chapter 16. In this chapter, Gartrell examines how disability disrupts women's access to their greatest source of status in Cambodia – marriage and motherhood. Disability disrupts women's access to their greatest source of status in Cambodia – marriage and motherhood. Women with disability are less likely than women without disability or men with disability to marry and have children, if they wish. Not only does this negatively impact on women with disability's socio-cultural status, self-esteem and dignity, but it also shapes their livelihood security. Disability reinforces women's weak structural position and the impact of the multiple sources of vulnerability they face. Excluded from participation in the 'male' productive sphere and the 'female' reproductive and nurturing role, it has been argued that women with disability are doubly oppressed - or 'freer' to be non-traditional. Her research found both typologies to be true in rural Cambodia.

Without husbands and children the capacity of women with disability to conform to traditional Cambodian gender ideals and gain status is greatly reduced; women face considerable difficulties finding a partner relationship because of cultural attitudes toward gender and disability. With limited choices, some women with disability seek to acquire status in non-traditional ways, such as via employment, whilst others depend on the labour power of kin for their livelihood. One woman with disability in her study described herself as 'waiting at home like a pig to be fed': idioms such as this reveal feelings of dependency and uselessness, but also vulnerability and loss of dignity. The paths taken by women with disability are not determined by choice alone, in fact, they may be considered as shaped by default rather than preference.

ABOUT THE EDITOR

Pranee Liamputtong is Personal Chair in Public Health at the School of Public Health, La Trobe University, Melbourne, Australia. Pranee was born in Thailand and now living in Australia. She has two daughters. Pranee has previously taught in the School of Sociology and Anthropology and worked as a public health research fellow at the Centre for the Study of Mothers' and Children's Health, La Trobe University. Pranee has her particular interests on issues related to cultural and social influences on childbearing, childrearing and women's reproductive and sexual health. She has published several books and a large number of papers in these areas.

Her three books on these issues have been used widely in health area: *My 40 days: A cross-cultural resource book for health care professionals in birthing services* (The Vietnamese Antenatal/Postnatal Support Project, 1993); *Asian mothers, Australian birth* (Ausmed Publications, 1994); *Maternity and reproductive health in Asian societies* (with Lenore Manderson, Harwood Academic Press, 1996).

Her more recent books include: *Asian mothers, Western birth* (new edition of Asian mothers, Australian birth, Ausmed Publications, 1999); *Living in a new country: Understanding migrants' health* (Ausmed Publications, 1999); *Hmong women and reproduction* (Bergin & Garvey, 2000); *Coming of age in South and Southeast Asia: Youth, courtship and sexuality* (with Lenore Manderson, Curzon Press and Nordic Institute of Asian Studies (NIAS), 2002); and *Health, social change and communities* (with Heather Gardner, Oxford University Press, 2003). The most recent book on *Mae: Becoming a mother among Thai women in Northern Thailand* will be published by Lexington Books, Lanham in 2007.

Her first research method book is titled *Qualitative research methods: A health focus* (with Douglas Ezzy, Oxford University Press, 1999, reprinted in 2000, 2001, 2003, 2004); and the second edition of this book is titled *Qualitative research methods* (2005). Her recent books include: *Health research in cyberspace: Methodological, practical and personal issues* (Nova Science Publishers, 2006), and *Researching the vulnerable: A guide to sensitive research methods* (Sage Publications, 2006). She is completing a book on *Knowing differently: An introduction to experiential and art-based research methods* (with Jean Rumbold, which will be published by Nova Science Publishers, New York, 2007). She is now working on *Doing Cross-Cultural Research: Methodological and Ethical Perspectives.*

ABOUT THE CONTRIBUTORS

Lina Abboud has qualifications in teaching and experience in research. She has completed her master degree by research at the School of Public Health, La Trobe University. She has an interest in women's health and well-being and learning for children through different methods. With several publications, Lina's research mainly focuses on recounts from women and her partner of miscarriage and of women's experiences with childbearing and childrearing. Her research has a particular focus on women from an Arabic-speaking background with a further interest in experiences of childbirth among women of non-English speaking backgrounds. Currently, she is involved in community development projects and programs for children and students in schools focusing on personal development and being a facilitating coach of learning.

Jamileh Abu-Duhou is a Research Fellow at the Menzies School of Health Research in Darwin, Australia. She is a Medical Anthropologist with over fifteen years research and community development experience working in the Middle East. Her research focused on issues of gender and social equity and the provision of equitable health care across gender, cultural, social, and economic status. Her research has focused on linking research to policy and practice and on the development of models which link all three to improve the delivery of health and other related services. Her doctoral research covered an analysis of gender-based violence in the Palestinian society. In this, she attempted to situate gender-based violence within the cultural, legal, religious and family and kinship practices which perpetuate violence against women. The research drew on findings from research conducted in other conflict-affected communities.

Tatjana Alvadj is an anthropologist working for Planned Parenthood Edmonton, Canada as a Sexual Health Educator for Ethno-cultural Communities. She conducts community-based research focused on immigration, gender and sexuality. Her work also includes activism and advocacy for immigrant women and youth.

Suzanne Belton is a research associate in the Institute of Advanced Studies at Charles Darwin University. Her current research examines minority people's birth practices and traditions in Southern China. She completed her doctoral thesis in 2005 from the University of Melbourne, Faculty of Medicine in the Key Centre for Women's Health in Society. Her thesis examines Burmese women's reproductive health in the context of forced migration with a particular focus on fertility regulation and unsafe abortion. During 1997 to 1999 she spent two and a half years living in Thailand as an Australian Overseas Volunteer where she worked with hill-tribe (Hmong and Yeo) women and girls in northern Thailand who were at risk of being trafficked into prostitution, and later with refugees from Burma. She worked closely with Dr Cynthia Maung, winner of several human rights awards, to deliver health education to 'barefoot doctors', traditional birth attendants and women in brothels on the Thai-Burma border. She is a registered midwife with qualifications in community development and family planning. Most of her career has been in the area of women's community health. For three years she had a home-birth practice in South Australia. She is very happy that her family migrated to Australia from Britain. Suzanne has worked in Australia, Thailand, Germany and China.

Margaret Chesney is currently the Director of Midwifery in the Faculty of Health University of Salford. She has over 30 years experience as a nurse and midwife. Her main area of study has been with women from Pakistan. She studied Birth experiences of women in Pakistan after undertaking nine field trips to work in a Red Crescent Maternity Hospital in the Punjab. Further research has been undertaken through the British Council whereby midwives trained in Pakistan were facilitated to study at Salford and work in an NHS Trust in the North West. Margaret is also a QAA Reviewer and has recently been external advisor for Bournemouth and Cardiff Universities for validation events. She is an external examiner for Paisley University and the RCN International MSc. Margaret has been on the RCM Council for the past 5 years. Currently a PhD Supervisor for 3 students plus MSc MPhil student (3 students) Margaret also hold the prestigious position of Lead Midwife for Midwifery Education UKCC, NMC 1999 to date for the University of Salford.

Ruth De Souza is a Senior Research Fellow and Coordinator of Auckland University of Technology's Centre for Asian and Migrant Health Research. She has worked as a nurse-therapist, clinician, educator and researcher. Ruth is actively involved in activities that assist in the inclusion of immigrants and people facing mental health problems in her roles in governance, as columnist and web designer and list owner. Ruth originates from Goa, India but was born in East Africa and is now resident of Laingholm on the fringes of the Waitakere ranges.

Alexandra Gartrell is a human geographer working in the area of disability, social justice and wellbeing. She graduated with her doctorate from the University of Melbourne in 2004. Her thesis was an ethnographic study which examined the lived experience of disability in rural Cambodia. It explored the place based determinants of quality of life, in particular the cultural and socio-economic processes curtailing access to opportunities and socially valued identities. Since completing her doctorate she has conducted research on the social determinants of depress on, access to care and employment pathways of refugees and asylum seekers. She is now at the School of Geography and Environmental Science, Monash University.

Paola Hernandez is currently a doctoral student at La Trobe University in the School of Social Sciences. Her research project explores the experiences of Somali women living in Melbourne during pregnancy and birth. It draws on the social and cultural aspects of birthing and of becoming a mother within the Somali context with a focus on the way in which the refugee experience might shape and influence women's experiences. The project also explores women's perceptions of and encounters with the medical model of care found in Australia. She completed a Bachelor of Arts with Honours in 2000 at La Trobe University with a major in Anthropology. She is married and has two children, aged three and half years and four months. Her research interests include the anthropology of birth, feminist and women studies as well as Latin American politics and social issues.

Elizabeth Hoban is a medical anthropologist and Lecturer in Public Health at Deakin University in Melbourne, Australia, and is a health advocate for marginalized women and their families. Elizabeth has worked in public health research and practice as an aid/development worker, international health adviser, academic and community-based worker in the area of women's health for twenty years in indigenous Australia, the Middle East and Southeast Asia, in particular Cambodia, where she conducted her doctoral and subsequent research in the area of Safe Motherhood. Her research and practice is advocacy based. She has conducted research in partnership with community-based, local and international non-government organizations to raise awareness and inform legislation and policy makers about marginalized women's health and human rights issues with the goal of bringing about structural change in the form of policy and programs, especially women whose legal and migration status is being challenged by the state.

Chimaraoke Otutubikey Izugbara holds a doctorate in medical anthropology. In the fall of 2006, Dr Izugbara was a Fellow of the African Scholars Program at the University of Massachusetts, USA. Currently, he is a visiting scholar at the African Population and Research Center, Nairobi, Kenya and also teaches at the University of Uyo, Nigeria. Izugbara has published widely in the area of reproductive health and African women.

Naomi McPherson is Associate Professor and Head of the Unit for Community, Culture and Global Studies at the University of British Columbia Okanagan, in Kelowna, British Columbia, Canada. She has conducted 30 months of fieldwork (1981, 1982-83, 1985, 2003 and 2005) among the Bariai in northwest New Britain, Papua New Guinea. She has published articles on the ceremonial cycle pertaining to the firstborn child (1985, *Primogeniture and Primogenitor*) birthing (1986, *Childbirth: A Case History from West New Britain, Papua New Guinea*), women, childbirth and development (1994, *Modern Obstetrics in a Rural Setting: Women and Reproduction in Northwest New Britain*). An aspect of her current research, upon which this paper is based, explores the effects of their changing world view on Bariai women's lives, including women's experiences of pregnancy, childbirth and issues of childrearing.

Hoa Ngan Nguyen is a senior researcher at the Southern Institute of Social Sciences in Ho Chi Minh city, Vietnam. She completed her Master of Public Health at La Trobe University, Australia in 2003. She is interested in a range of issues in contemporary Vietnam, including female workers in export processing zones, domestic migration, and reproductive health. Some of her papers have been published in the Journal of Women's Studies, the Review of Social Sciences, and in some books. Her most recent work is on reproductive health of young people in urban areas in Vietnam.

Pertti J. Pelto received his doctorate in anthropology at the University of California (Berkeley) in 1960. Pertti joined the University of Connecticut in 1969, where he helped to establish the Program in Medical Anthropology, which he headed until his retirement in 1993. Since his retirement, Pertti has spent the past 11 years in India, where he is active in giving research training and technical support for a variety of NGOs and other groups involved in HIV/AIDS programmes, reproductive health, and other community health activities. He has consulted for a variety of projects in Bangladesh, Sri Lanka, Pakistan and Nepal, and a wide range of researchers all over India. His best known publication is a book on research methodology, *Anthropological Research, The Structure of Inquiry*, first published in 1970. Since retiring from the University of Connecticut, Pertti has held adjunct academic appointments in Finland (University of Joensuu), Australia (University of Melbourne), India

(M. S University in Baroda) and Johns Hopkins University (USA). Recently, he has co-authored a series of papers on abortion with Lakshmi Ramachandar.

Lakshmi Ramachandar is a freelance medical anthropologist and recently completed her PhD, University of Melbourne, 2004. For the past decade, she has been doing community-based research on sensitive issues such as male sexual health problems, quality of care at government facilities, decision-making, women's empowerment, medical abortion, abortion providers and safety of abortion in rural South India. She provides technical assistance and training to local NGOs in qualitative methods and data analysis using Anthropac and Atlas ti programs. Currently she is continuing her research on medical abortion in Tamil Nadu Southern India.

Denise L. Spitzer holds the Canada Research Chair in Gender, Migration and Health at the University of Ottawa where she is also an associate professor at the Institute of Women's Studies and principal scientist in the Institute of Population Health. A medical anthropologist by training, her work focuses primarily on the impact of marginalization on the health of immigrant and refugee women.

Joseph Kinuabeye Ukwayi is a Nigerian Sociologist. He has longstanding teaching and research interests in health, criminality, and gender issues. Widely published, Joseph's research has primarily focused on the health and wellbeing of marginal groups in the Nigerian Post colony. Currently involved in a nationwide programme to streamline the responses of faith based organizations to the HIV/AIDS pandemic in Nigeria, Joseph has also researched many aspects of health in Nigeria, including the lives of HIV-infected inmates in Nigerian prisons. Joseph currently teaches in the Department of Sociology, Faculty of Social Sciences, University of Calabar, Cross River State, Nigeria, and is working on his doctoral degree at the Department of Sociology and Anthropology, University of Uyo, Uyo, Nigeria.

PART ONE: REPRODUCTION AND PROCREATION

In: Reproduction, Childbearing and Motherhood
Editor: Pranee Liamputtong, pp. 3-34

ISBN: 978-1-60021-606-0
© 2007 Nova Science Publishers, Inc.

Chapter 1

SITUATING REPRODUCTION, PROCREATION AND MOTHERHOOD WITHIN A CROSS-CULTURAL CONTEXT: AN INTRODUCTION

Pranee Liamputtong

By using reproduction as an entry point to the study of social life, we can see how cultures are produced (or contested) as people imagine and enable the creation of the next generation, most directly through the nurturance of children. (Ginsburg and Rapp, 1995: 1-2)

I believe that by subjugated knowledges one should understand something else [...], namely, a whole set of knowledges that have been disqualified as inadequate to their task or insufficiently elaborated: naïve knowledges, located low down on the hierarchy, beneath the required level of cognition or scientificity. (Foucault, 1980: 82)

INTRODUCTION

This chapter aims to set the scene of this book. As such, I intend to provide readers with empirical research regarding reproduction, childbearing and motherhood from a cross-cultural perspective. I shall introduce the following issues: fertility, procreation and infertility, the thorny issue of abortion, childbearing, motherhood, and childbearing experiences of immigrant mothers. In constructing this chapter, I rely heavily on my research with Thai and Hmong women, but I also incorporate relevant literature throughout the chapter.

FERTILITY, PROCREATION AND INFERTILITY

Fertility and procreation play a major role in women's health and well-being in most societies (Sciarra, 1994; Inhorn, 1994a, b; Bhatti et al., 1999; Bentley and Mascie-Taylor, 2000; Boerma and Mgalla, 2001; Feldman-Savelsberg, 2001; Inhorn and Van Balen, 2001; Gerrits, 2001; Jenkins, 2001; Leonard, 2001; Inhorn, 2003a, b; see also Chapters 1 and 14 in this volume). In the Hmong world, for example, having children is essential for parents' well-being, not only in this world but also for the next (Liamputtong Rice, 2000a; see also Chapter 14 in this volume). Children, particularly sons, carry on the family lineage, look after the elderly parents when they are alive, and worship them when they die. Without sons, deceased parents will not be reincarnated. Furthermore, without children in the lineage and clans, Hmong society will cease its existence. Fertility is, therefore, a most crucial part of Hmong life. The failure to be fertile, then, has a profound effect on Hmong lineages, clans and society (Liamputtong Rice, 2000a; cf. Than 2003, for similar perceptions in Myanmar; see also Chapter 15 in this volume).

Although infertility is a biological problem, the experience of infertility is often mediated by cultural practices from within a society. And despite the fact that infertility can occur in both male and female bodies, cross-cultural research reveals that women generally bear the burden (McGilvray, 1982; Feldman-Savelsberg, 1994; Inhorn, 1994a, b; Neff, 1994; Kielmann, 1998; Inhorn, 2002, 2003a, b). Because of the expectation that all women should be fertile, failure to conceive is usually seen as a problem inherent in a woman's body. For example, McGilvray (1982: 62) points out that among Tamil in Batticaloa, Sri Lanka, infertility is primarily seen as a woman's problem, although a supernatural agency may be thought to contribute to her childlessness. The fertility of the husband is rarely questioned, and a woman without children is seen as both "personality unfulfilled and ritually inauspicious". Similarly, Neff (1994: 477) points out that for the Nayars in South India, the woman is most often blamed for her childlessness. The unfortunate woman will be an "inauspicious guest at weddings and sacred rituals" and she is "cut off from networks of sustenance and support". That infertility is a "woman's problem" is clearly evident in Inhorn's study (1994a: 3) among poor urban Egyptian women. Women are blamed for their failure to reproduce, and they bear the burden of overcoming it through "a therapeutic quest that is sometimes traumatic and often unfruitful" (see also Inhorn, 2003a, b).

In many other societies, infertility is seen as unnatural and, as I have suggested, it is the woman who bears the blame. In Hmong culture, an infertility problem is perceived to be located within the woman's body. Infertility also taints women's moral identities. In Hmong culture, it is Hmong women, not men, who are blamed for being infertile, either because of the malfunctioning of the woman's body, her own bad behavior, or her supernatural misfortune. Her "afflicted body" provides legitimate grounds for the husband to bring in a second wife to bear children for him, and the childless woman has no say in this matter. Indeed, she has proven to him and his family that she may endanger the continuity of the family line, which in turn threatens the reproduction of Hmong society (Liamputtong Rice, 2000a).

Indeed, male infertility is rarely acknowledged in many societies, and perhaps particularly in patrilineal ones (Sciarra, 1994; Inhorn, 1996; Hamberger and Janson, 1997; Boerma and Mgalla, 2001; Gerrits, 2001; Van Balen and Inhorn, 2001; Inhorn, 2002, 2003a, b). As Greer (1984: 34) argues, "the reason why male sterility is seldom recognized is precisely because the recognition would strike at the heart of morality: all order and coherence would be put in jeopardy". Similarly, in Hmong culture, men are thought to govern the Hmong world. Only men can perform important tasks and only men can carry on the clan name (Liamputtong Rice, 2000a). The notion that men are infertile and, therefore, are unable to have their own sons (in particular) to continue their duties is seen as unacceptable, even immoral. Inhorn (1994a, b) too argues that infertility challenges men's procreative power.

Women, through their "faulty bodies", are nearly always blamed for not being able to bring men's children into the world. Therefore, male infertility is seldom recognized in many cultures, although the women believe that the male can also contribute to their infertility.

In other words, infertility in many societies is seen as the woman's problem. Infertility is an affliction of her body, her identity and on the "local moral worlds" (Kleinman, 1992) in which she lives. That her "infertile body" in some ways reflects the patrilineal, patriarchal "social body" is clear when blame is assigned and control on the woman's body exercised (Douglas, 1970). Among the Hmong, at both the individual and societal levels, being fertile is a crucial part of Hmong life, for fertility ensures the continuation of the clan, lineage group, and family - the three important pillars of Hmong society (Yang, 1992). Infertility, therefore, has profound implications for Hmong societal life. Women are seen as bearers of children, and must have as many children as they can. Failure to do so results in suffering both in this life and the next.

It seems clear that infertile women carry not only heavy personal cost but also social stigma (Whiteford and Gonzalez, 1995; Van Balen and Inhorn, 2001). This social stigma can have an extensive impact on the life of infertile women, and as Sciarra (1994: 155-156) contends, it can "affect a woman for the remainder of her life, preventing subsequent marriage, and making her economically vulnerable". And this has led to "profound social suffering" for infertile women in many parts of the world (Inhorn, 2003b: 1838; Than 2003). An infertile woman in Myanmar is referred to as "*amjoum*". The social stigma that these infertile women carry with them is so great that there is still a belief that even Buddhist monks would not accept the offering from these women (Than, 2003).

ON NOT BECOMING A MOTHER: THE THORNY ISSUE OF ABORTION

Throughout history, women have had to deal not only with their ability to become pregnant and give birth, but also their desire to limit or control their own reproduction. Abortion has been one means that women have used to control their reproduction in many societies (Devereux, 1955; Casey, 1960; Jochle, 1974; Conway and Slocumb, 1979; Oylebola, 1981; Tiwari et al., 1982; Weniger et al., 1982; Newman, 1985; Kong et al., 1986; LaFleur, 1992; Riddle, 1992; Hardacre, 1997; Moskowitz, 2001; Rozario, 2002; Juarez et al., 2004; Whittaker, 2004). Cross-cultural exploration of abortion has begun to receive more attention since the publication in 1955 of "A study of Abortion in Primitive Society" by Devereux. Three decades later, Newman (1985) published her book on the fertility regulations among women in different cultures, including Malaysia, Afghanistan, Egypt, Colombia, Peru, Costa Rica and Jamaica. In this publication, abortion is discussed in relation to family planning and international health. Ginsburg (1989, 1998) linked abortion with the cultural construction of gender, motherhood and social responsibility in American society. More recent publications on abortion about women in different cultures are in a special issue of "Reproductive Health Matters" (Berer, 1997) and "Social Science and Medicine" (Rylko-Bauer, 1996) journals, in edited collections by Githens and Stetson (1996) and Mundigo and Indriso (1999), and an authored book by Whittaker (2004). In these publications, abortion is examined from social, cultural, political and public health perspectives.

Recent works of Sobo in Jamaica (1996), Renne in Nigeria (1996), Johnson et al. in Romania (1996), Ba-Thike in Myanmar (1997) and Andrea Whittaker in Thailand (2004) also confirm the work of social researchers in Newman's book on the ways in which women have managed their fertility: contraceptives, emmenagogues, fertility enhances, and abortifacients. And my work (Liamputtong, 2003) on the cultural beliefs and practices of fertility control methods including abortion in Hmong culture reflects those of women in other parts of the world.

Although abortion has been one among a continuum of fertility regulation options for women in many parts of the world, it is also perceived with ambiguity (Cannold, 1998; Shrage, 2003). As Hadley (1996: 30) argues:

> Abortion is probably the oldest, most common and universal method by which women have controlled their fertility, long before the law regulated it. Women determined to end their pregnancies have always known a wide variety of ways to do so. Until relatively recently it has certainly not attracted the shame or stigma which clings to it today.

Hadley (1996: 162) also suggests that there is a "culture of shame" attached to abortion, and this encourages abortion to be seen differently to other fertility regulation methods such as birth control. In this light, abortion has tended to be seen as a moral issue and condemned by people in most parts of the world (Luker, 1984; Ginsburg, 1989, 1998; Shrage, 2003; Whittaker, 2004).

In my study with Hmong women, to some extent, the women also condemn those who abort their babies, but this condemnation is largely dependent on what groups these women belong to (Liamputtong, 2003). Hmong women believe that certain groups of women, including older women and women who have had several children, have the right to abort their babies. These women are seen as having the privilege of terminating their pregnancies if they do not wish to have more children. Those who are still young and have not produced "enough" children do not have this privilege. If they abort their babies, they are condemned by their society.

Why do women belief that older women or women with several children have the right for abortion? Nichter and Nichter (1996) and Bledsoe et al. (1994) have noted in their studies of fertility regulation, that fertility control methods are weighed differently at different points in the reproductive life span and in relation to both a woman's reproductive and productive capacity. In Hmong culture, this is partly related to the need for producing many children. Children in Hmong culture are important for Hmong lineage, which in turn is essential for the survival of Hmong society (Liamputtong Rice, 2000a). As Symonds (1996: 121) contends,

> A woman who desires to control her own reproduction ... is socially discouraged from doing so, through the influence of a pervasive cultural discourse which suggests that in so doing she would also be upsetting the state of cosmological equilibrium that must be maintained through the continued and prolific reproduction of her husband's (and, in effect, her own) lineage.

After having produced several children, however, women may not be under as much pressure as when they were young. Since most Hmong women are married when they are relatively young, by the time they are over the age 40 they may have already given birth to several children (Liamputtong Rice, 1995, 2000a; Liamputtong, 2003). This has ensured that they have produced children for the continuation of Hmong society. Within the context of Hmong culture, the women's belief is, thus, logical.

Women may wish to control their fertility by means of abortion, but their wishes may be constrained by a societal norm which places a great deal of pressure on women to continue producing children (see Nguyen and Liamputtong, this volume). In a culture that values having many children, abortion will not be easily accepted because it stops women from having children, which upsets the cosmological balance of the society. Precisely, this is what Susanna Rance (2000: 78) unashamedly remarks:

> Abortion is constructed as socially dangerous for reasons far removed from any concern for public health. Rather, it is represented as risky because it puts at risk patriarchal control of women's sexuality and fertility, a system of beliefs which fears rejection of maternity by a woman-mother.

This has implications for women who may wish to terminate their pregnancies. If women are constrained by their cultural expectations, they may not be able to fulfill their personal needs and hence are denied their wishes to control their own reproduction. Therefore, the right to abortion, which has been an emerging agenda for women in many parts of the world (Luker, 1984; Condit, 1990; Petchesky, 1990; Correa, 1994; Rance, 2000; De Bruyn, 2001; Liamputtong, 2003), may not be accessible to many women in more traditional societies due to their cultural restriction. See also Chapters 3, 4, and 5 in this volume for women's decisions against becoming a mother and how they deal with the thorny issue of abortion in different societies.

ON BECOMING A MOTHER: CHILDBEARING

Childbirth, from the biomedical perspective, is focused on the physiological aspects of the event. As such, childbirth is seen as an illness requiring medical attention (Rothman, 1989; Martin, 1992; Liamputtong, 2005; Liamputtong and Watson, 2006). In Western societies, childbirth, therefore, takes place in hospitals and women are under the control of medical management from pregnancy to the postpartum period (Martin, 1992; Davis-Floyd, 1992, 1994; Davis-Floyd and Sargent, 1997; Possamai-Inesedy 2005). However, from the social science perspective, it is argued that although childbirth is a significant human experience, its social meaning is "shaped by the culture in which birthing women live" (Lefkarites, 1992: 385). As Jordan (1993: 1) succinctly puts, "birth is everywhere socially marked and shaped". Childbirth and its management, therefore, occur within the social and cultural context of the event (Raphael-Leff, 1991; Lefkarites, 1992; Jordan, 1993; Liamputtong Rice and Manderson, 1996; Davis-Floyd and Sargent, 1997; Hoban, 2002, in press). As social scientists have found, childbirth practices differ across social and cultural settings.

> Cultures throughout the world express the meaning of childbirth through different beliefs, customs and practices. These diverse cultural interpretations are part of a larger integrated system of beliefs concerning men, women, family, community, nature, [and] religion (Lefkarites, 1992: 385).

Pregnancy and Birth

As I have suggested, childbearing in any society is a biological event, but the birth experience is also socially constructed and it takes place within a cultural context and is shaped by the perceptions and practices of that culture. Therefore, there are many beliefs and practices relating to the childbearing process that the woman and her family must observe to ensure the health and well-being of not only herself but also that of her newborn infant (MacCormack, 1982; Laderman, 1984, 1987; Sich, 1988; O'Dempsey, 1988; Steinberg, 1996; Jordan, 1997; Liamputtong Rice, 2000a, b; Samuel, 2002; Liamputtong, 2005a, b; Liamputtong et al., 2005).

Childbirth, according to Laderman (1984: 549), "is the most significant of all rites of passage, conferring new status of the parents and changing a nonentity, the unknown fetus in the womb, into an individual with kinship ties, functions and potentialities within a society". Although conception occurs within a woman's body (her womb), pregnancy is given "meaning by the dialogue between empirical perceptions and a system of symbols that takes place in every culture. They are elaborated and accompanied by behavioural changes that define the roles of the actors and are intended to protect those who, by virtue of their liminality, are especially vulnerable to harm". In this sense, both mothers and their fetuses/babies are vulnerable entities which need to be protected by rituals.

In discussing childbirth in Malay women, Laderman (1987: 124) argues that childbirth is "not only a physiological event", but also "a stage in a rite of passage requiring spiritual prophylaxis and ritual expertise". In a normal birth, a woman separates from others by retreating into her bedroom and giving birth with a minimum of assistance. However, in certain circumstances, such as a long and difficult labour, a woman may require not only physical support but also spiritual and ritual aid from traditional healers and there are people around her who can help.

In most traditional societies, a labouring woman is usually assisted by other women or birth attendants (WHO, 1978; Sargent, 1982; Goldsmith, 1990; Kitzinger, 1997; Hoban, 2002, in press; Samuel, 2002; Chapters 6, 7, 8, and 9 in this volume). As Goldsmith (1990: 25) suggests, in most traditional societies, women do not give birth among strangers. Women carry out their "intimate act" among those whom they "know well and trust". Most often, women give birth with the assistance of their mothers-in-law and their husbands. Even the healers, who are called in when complications occur, are those whom the women know. Goldsmith (1990) argues that familiarity with the people around her helps a woman in traditional societies have "a positive attitude toward the birth process". This argument may also be applicable to women who give birth among those whom they know well and trust. Although birth is seen as a woman's affair, it is also related to the family, the community, the society and the supernatural world. This can be clearly seen in the case of a difficult birth with the healing processes involving many people and supernatural beings. These "helpers" relieve the woman's difficulties in bringing another life into society. In many cultures, birth has social meanings which are a part of the larger social system which involves not only the woman, but also her family, the community, the society and the supernatural world, as Lefkarites (1992: 385) points out:

> Childbirth is a significant human experience, its social meaning shaped by culture in which birthing women live. Cultures throughout the world express the meaning of childbirth through

different beliefs, customs and practices. These diverse cultural interpretations are part of a larger integrated system of beliefs concerning men, women, family, community, nature, religion, and supernatural powers.

It appears that traditional childbirth practices have not totally disappeared in many societies, but they have also gradually diminished. Why has this happened? Birth in most societies has been medicalized, hence, it management is controlled by doctors, nurses and it occurs in hospital settings. In these societies, the medicalization of childbirth, like childbirth in many western societies, makes medical knowledge "supersede" other kinds of relevant sources of knowledge such as cultural beliefs and practices (Jordan, 1994; Davis-Floyd and Jordan, 1997; Whittaker, 2002a, b; Liamputtong, in press; see also Chapter 9 in this volume). As such, traditions may no longer be relevant, or at worse, must be relinquished. Cultural knowledge has become structurally inferior to Western biomedicine (Lee, 1982; Whittaker, 2002b). In addition, modernization of the society may also contribute to this and results in the neglect of many traditional practices of pregnancy and birth in hospitals (Whittaker, 2000, 2002a, b; Hoban, 2002, in press; Liamputtong, 2005a, b).

The Medicalization of Childbirth

Due to the modernization or westernization of many more traditional societies, childbirth, as I have suggested, has become medicalized. In turn, the medicalization of childbirth has resulted in a highly technological approach with routine hospital procedures (Muecke, 1976; Rothman, 1989; Martin, 1992; Jordan, 1994; Lazarus, 1994; Ram, 1994: Davis-Floyd, 1993; Lane, 1995; Campero et al., 1998; Zadoroznyj, 1999; Stein and Inhorn, 2002; Possamai-Inesedy 2005). Childbirth within this medicalized framework is seen as a medical problem which can only be handled by medical professionals such as doctors, and nurses in a hospital setting. Defining birth as such, it comes "an event controlled by more or less anonymous specialists carrying out standardized techniques on a woman's body" (Muecke, 1976: 379). In most industralized countries, childbirth is seen as a diseased state, a physical bodily disturbance (Cosminsky, 1982: 225); the women's body is the subject of control by medical professionals and technology (Martin, 1992; Davis-Floyd, 1993, 1994; Lane, 1995; Zadoroznyj, 1999; Stein and Inhorn, 2002; Possamai-Inesedy 2005). A woman is required not only to give birth in hospital where she may have little or no control, but she is also given the message, as Davis-Floyd (1987: 497) contends, about her powerlessness, "defectiveness", and her dependence on science and technology (Liamputtong Rice and Manderson, 1996: 5; Fox and Worts, 1999; Possamai-Inesedy 2005; Fisher et al., 2006). Very often too, traditional knowledge and practices are ignored or dismissed by the medicalized birthing system. Hoban (2002: 30) speaks clearly about this.

> Medicalization and modernization has shown no respect for the integrity of the indigenous systems, and disregards the internally consistent knowledge and practices that have ensured parturient womens' safety, often in difficult and hostile political, economic and physical circumstances.

Ironically, what we have seen too is that women may see modern birth as safer for themselves and their babies. As Muecke (1976: 381) found several decades ago that Thai women in Chiang Mai adopted the Western model of birth because they "perceive it as much safer, as reducing the risk of death during delivery". Women also believed that doctors can help in time of difficulty with birth due to their "esoteric knowledge", western medications, and modern equipment used in hospital (Muecke, 1976: 381). To the women, hospital birth then provides them and their newborn babies with extra protection. I have also found this in my recent work with Thai women in northern Thailand (Liamputtong, 2005), as I shall outline in the following section.

Giving Birth in Hospital

Childbirth in many developing countries has become medicalized and professional delivery in a medical environment is increasingly being promoted (Kabakian-Khasholian et al., 2000; see also Chapters 7, and 9 in this volume). Under the medicalization of childbirth, care provided to women, as Campero and colleagues (1998: 396) put it, is undertaken "exclusively by doctors and nurses who generally consider labor and childbirth as potentially pathological conditions for which the mother and/or child require specialized and technological care". Within this framework, health care providers stand out as key players in childbirth. Some writers maintain that the focus on medicalized birth all too often leads to problems associated with medical dominance, poor communication between health care providers and the women, and impersonal treatment in hospital births (Kabakian-Khasholian et al., 2000: 111; Phillips, 1996, Liamputtong Rice, 1999a). Due to this, feminist writers have demanded the right for women to make choices about childbirth and at the same time criticize "overmedicalization" of childbirth in the West (Arney, 1982; Martin, 1992; Cunningham, 1993; Davis-Floyd, 1993, 1994; Lane, 1995; Fox and Worts, 1999; Zadoroznyj, 1999; Possamai-Inesedy 2005).

As a result of modernization or westernization of Thai society, childbirth in Thailand has also become medicalized (Muecke, 1976; Whittaker, 2000; Liamputtong, 2003a, b; Liamputtong, in press). As in other societies, childbirth in Thailand has increasingly moved from a familial and social domain to that of hospital-based medicine, which for many, is an unfamiliar institutional setting and knowledge base (Liamputtong Rice and Manderson, 1996). The medicalization of childbirth, in turn, has resulted in a highly technological approach with routine hospital procedures (Muecke, 1976).

In my study (Liamputtong, 2003a, b; Liamputtong, in press), the Thai women's narratives reveal that childbirth was managed within the medical system. Contrary to what Muecke (1976) found several decades ago that just over half (51.7%) of northern Thai women gave birth in hospital, all women (except one) in this study had their babies in hospital. In fact, I have found that the women in my study wished to have professional deliveries in the hospital setting. The Thai women in this study, similar to women in other parts of the world (Kempe et al., 1994; Kahakian-Khasholian et al., 2000), gave safety as the primary reason for their choices of births in hospitals. For example, Johnson and others (1992) point out in their study of pregnant women in England that women chose hospital-based births because of their fear of the risk of unforeseen complications that may occur during the birthing process. Recently, Kahakian-Khasholian and colleagues (2000) also show that women in Lebanon seek hospital births because they believed it was safer than homebirths. Whittaker (2000) also found in her study that women in northeastern Thailand chose to give birth in hospitals due to their beliefs that childbirth is dangerous and that hospital birth is safer and modern.

Noticeably too, women's embodied experiences with hospital births tend to reveal the "passivity" discourse (Szasz and Hollenger, 1956; Liamputtong, 2005b; Liamputtong, in press). As Kabakian-Khasholian and colleagues (2000) have shown in their study, women accord total trust in their doctors and very rarely question the many routine procedures in hospitals. Why is this so? Straten and others (2002: 227) point to the importance of "public trust" in health care. Accordingly, public trust in health care is "defined as being confident that you will be adequately treated when you are in need of health care; this means confidence in the agency relation between patients and health care providers" (see also Mooney and Ryan, 1993; Bluff and Holloway, 1994; Gray, 1997; Gilbert, 1998; Mechanic, 1998; Mechanic and Meyer, 2000). As patients, Gilson (2003: 1457) contends, public trust in health care "provides the basis for our judgment that health care providers will act in our best interests". Straten and colleagues (2002: 228) suggest, public trust in health care can be perceived as "a way of enabling people to deal with the uncertainties and risks associated with handing their fate over to health care providers" (see also Misztal, 1996; Gilbert, 1998). As childbirth is seen as critical life event and individual women do not know beforehand the outcomes of their pregnancies, women may hand over control of their situation to health care providers. Gilson (2003: 1459) suggests that, "trust in providers may matter more to vulnerable patients with higher risks", such as women in childbirth. As childbirth is a life crisis event, women giving birth may have a higher level of trust in their caregivers than other users of the health care system. Muecke (1976: 381) too points out that Thai women in the North would leave the close support of their families to give birth in a lonely place in hospital and tolerate the invasion of their bodily privacy because they believe that "doctors know best" (see also Liamputtong, in press).

However, the passivity of the women may be due to, as Campero and colleagues (1998: 396) suggest, the medicalization of childbirth. Under the medicalized birth, the medical staff have authority due to their esoteric knowledge (Muecke, 1976: 381; Bluff and Holloway, 1994; Jordan, 1994; Davis-Floyd and Sargent, 1997; Zadoroznyj, 1999). As Bluff and Holloway (1994: 163) succinctly put, it may be that women have been encouraged to hand over responsibility for childbirth to health professionals, and hence, "this unquestioning acceptance may lead to a model of passivity in which the women accept passively what is done on their behalf". Additionally, within the medicalized birth, "the encounter takes place in an environment which is unfamiliar to the patient; the patient must adopt physical positions which are uncomfortable, passive, and dependent; and the communication is either scant or very complicated due to the jargon used". Women do not feel that they have the right to express their concerns or doubts. Rather, women enter hospital "feeling that they must be obedient and cooperative". See also Chapters, 7, 8 and 9 in this volume.

Adaptation of Traditional Practices in Modern Hospital

Despite the fact that most hospitals in underdeveloped societies have operated under the biomedical framework, there appears to be in-corporation of traditional practices in some places. Here, I wish to point to the practice in hospitals in northern Thailand. Among postpartum care provided in Thai hospitals in the north is the use of spotlight to help heal the episiotomy wound. Muecke (1976) argues that this is an adaptation of traditional practices of *yu duan* in the era of modernity (see Liamputtong, 2005a, b). Muecke (1976: 381) also suggests that one of the primary goals of the postpartum ritual *yu duan* practices is to dry out the uterus. It has to be noted here that in other parts of Thailand, a traditional practice of *yu fai* (staying-by-the-fire) ritual is observed by a new mother during the first 30 days after birth (Jirojwong, 1996; Liamputtong Rice et al., 1999; Whittaker, 2000, 2002; Liamputtong, 2005a, b; Liamputtong, in press). While observing this ritual, she must keep her body warm, by wrapping herself in a blanket, wearing a long sleeved top and sarong or pants, wrapping a piece of cloth around her head, ears and neck. This ritual has been referred to as a "mother roasting" ritual, a common practice in a number of Southeast Asian cultures (see also Manderson, 1981; Townsend and Liamputtong Rice, 1996; Liamputtong Rice, 2000a, b; Liamputtong Rice et al., 1999; Whittaker, 2000, 2002; Hoban, 2002, in press and Chapter 6 in this volume) and is regarded as vital to the well-being of a new mother. It helps to restore "heat" lost in childbirth, to flush out retained blood and placenta from the uterus, to make the uterus shrink to its normal size and to dry out the tear of the perineum. However, *yu fai* ritual is not observed in the northern part of Thailand (Liamputtong, 2004a; Liamputtong, in press). A new mother only observes *yu duan* ritual. *Yu duan* ritual requires all other aspects as in *yu fai*, except for the stay-by-the-fire aspect.

The adoption of spotlights in hospital may be due the fact that, as Muecke (1976: 381) contends, there is "some syncretism" between Thai tradition and Western models of childbirth in Thai hospitals. Health professionals in Thai hospitals appreciate the benefits of some Thai traditional practices, but often adapt the practice to suit the hospital equipment. As a spotlight is accessible in hospitals and elsewhere, the use of it to replace an elaborate ritual of *yu duan* is easily accepted. Although the women might continue to practice *yu duan* rituals upon returning home, the attempt by the hospital to incorporate a Thai traditional practice is warmly welcomed by Thai women, particularly the women in my study. I contend that the practice of spotlight in hospital may not only practically assist them in the healing process but also provides the women with symbolic ritual (Liamputtong, 2004a).

Postpartum Practices as Rites of Passage

Ginsburg and Rapp (1995: 2) contend that reproduction, including childbirth, is "inextricably bound up with the production of culture". Childbirth including the period immediately following birth is an event in which traditions are deeply involved (Symonds, 1991, Liamputtong Rice 2000b, 2004). It is seen as "a dangerous and liminal period when a new mother and her newborn are in an 'in-between' world" (Symonds, 1991: 265). The childbirth process is often characterized by unpredictability, tension and danger (Symonds, 1991). Hence, there are many rules that women and their families must adhere to in order to avoid negative consequences. In this liminal stage, women must be segregated from the society at large (Turner, 1979).

Postpartum beliefs and practices are pervasive. The majority of women in more traditional societies observe postpartum beliefs and practices strictly, although we have also seen some changes in more educated and urbanized women (see Pillsbury, 1982; Laderman, 1983; Chu, 1996; Townsend and Liamputtong Rice, 1996; Hundt et al., 2000; Liamputtong,

2000a, b; Whittaker, 2000, 2002; Hoban, 2002, in press; Hunter, 2002; Liamputtong, 2005a, b; Tsianakas and Liamputtong, 2006). There are strict rules which govern what a new mother can or cannot do during the 30 or 40 days period after birth.

Existing empirical findings point to conceptualizing postpartum practices as rites of passage (van Gennep, 1966). The postpartum period in many societies is seen as a dangerous, powerful or polluting stage (Kitzinger, 1982). Following Turner's (1967, 1979) theory, Davis-Floyd (1992: 18) argues that this liminality is the "stage of being betwixt and between, neither here nor there - no longer part of the old and not yet part of the new". The liminal states are often connected with birth and death, the theory offers illuminating patterns of childbirth in many traditional societies (Turner, 1979; Davis-Floyd, 1992).

In rites of passage, people are separated from ordinary society. This can be seen clearly with women during the postpartum period. In most societies, parturient women are usually separated from normal social activities. A woman who has just given birth is vulnerable to dangers and illnesses due to her physical and emotional weakness caused by the act of giving birth. She is also capable of causing danger to others due to her perceived polluted nature of childbirth and its blood. The seclusion of rites of passage is, therefore, an attempt to safeguard the woman from danger as well as to protect others around her from her "liminal and polluted state" of health. Within this seclusion period, a new mother is cared for by her close female kin in a separate room, or part of the house, where she does not have contacts with outsiders. Her diet and behavior are monitored and modified throughout the seclusion period. The postpartum practice is seen as beneficial to women's health and well-being (see Chapters 6, 8 and 13 in this volume).

Despite changes in the women's lives, postpartum beliefs and practices remain an essential part for postnatal care for women and have important consequences for women's health and well-being. In Thai culture (Boonmongkon et al., 2001, 2002; Whittaker, 2000, 2002; Liamputtong and Naksook, 2003a), for example, many women see their reproductive health problems as the consequence of inadequate postpartum practices (Boonmongkon et al., 2001, 2002; Whittaker, 2000, 2002; Liamputtong and Naksook, 2003). Thai women also believed that the effects of postpartum taboos would continue for the rest of their lives. It is imperative that postpartum care for women incorporates local traditions so that women's health can be optimized at the time when they are in the most vulnerable stage of their lives. See Chapters 6, 7, 8 and 9 in this volume.

TRADITIONAL BIRTH ATTENDANTS (TBAS)

Traditional... birth attendants are found in most societies. They are often part of the local community, culture and traditions, and continue to have high social standing in many places, exerting considerable influence on local health practices. (WHO, 1978: 63)

Traditional birth attendants (TBAs) have played a vital role in pregnancy and birth in many societies (Laderman, 1983; Ityavyar, 1984; Mangay Maglacas and Simons, 1986; Anuman Rajadhon, 1987; McConville, 1988; Daly and Pollard, 1990; Jeffery and Jeffery, 1993; Jordan, 1993; Camey et al., 1996; Jirojwong, 1996; Manderson, 1996; Kitzinger, 1997; Whittaker, 2000, 2002a, b; Harris, 2002, Hoban, 2002, in press; Rozario and Samuel, 2002; Than, 2003; Izugbara and Ukmayi, 2004; Liamputtong et al., 2005; see also Chapters 6, 7, 8 and 9 in this volume). Newar women in Nepal, for example, give birth with the assistance of *aji*; Grandmother in local term, as Johnson (2002: 39) tells us:

> Giving birth is a women's affair, and men are not usually present. In addition to her mother-in-law, and when possible her own mother and other relatives, a woman giving birth is assisted by a traditional birth attendant, called *aji*, or Grandmother, who is an experienced older relative or neighbour. Each family has a relationship with a particular *aji*, and she is called whenever they have a birth.

Lefeber and Voorhoever (1997: 1175) suggest that a traditional birth attendant does "more than just deliver babies. As part of the local community she is acquainted with the woman and her family with whom she shares the cultural ideas about how the birth has to be prepared for and performed. She knows the local medicines and rituals which are used before, during and after birth. The work of traditional midwife is adapted and bound to the social and cultural matrix to which she belongs, her beliefs and practices being in accordance with the needs of the local community" (see also Camay et al., 1996; Allotey, 2000; Johnson, 2002; Than, 2003; Izugbara and Ukmayi, 2004). Despite this, the number of TBAs has reduced dramatically in many traditional societies (Harris, 2002; Whittaker, 2002b). But, there are still TBAs delivering infants, particularly in remote areas where modern health care is not accessible by many poor women. This pattern is emerged in other societies (see Jeffery and Jeffery, 1993; Camey et al., 1996; Cosminsky, 2001; Davis-Floyd, 2001; Davis-Floyd et al., 2001; Hsu, 2001, Geurts, 2001, Jenkins, 2001; Chawla, 2002; Hoban, 2002, in press; Jeffery et al., 2002; Rozario and Samuel, 2002; Whittaker, 2002b; Than, 2003). Chawla (2002) contends that among poor women and those living in rural areas in India, around 90 percent of them continue to give birth with the help of *dais*, local TBAs. *Dais*, Chawla (2002: 150) points out, "share the cultural and ethno-medical orientations of the women they serve. *Dais* are also often the only affordable and accessible practitioners available to poor urban and rural women". Indeed, recent studies have pointed to the existence and persistence of TBAs in different societies (See Consminsky, 2001; Davis-Floyd, 2001; Jenkins, 2001; Geurts, 2001; Hsu, 2001; Hoban, 2002, in press; Than, 2003; Izugbara and Ukmayi, 2004). Hoban's work in Cambodia confirms this. Hoban (2002: 18) puts it clearly that these studies:

> Testify that indigenous birth attendants' ethno-obstetric practices have not been overtaken by modern obstetrics. Instead, birth attendants have developed practices and strategies of negotiation and accommodation in diverse and complex environments.

Here, I wish to focus on a TBA in Thai culture. A traditional birth attendant or an old granny midwife (Muecke, 1976: 380), known as *mor tamyae* in Thailand (Anuman Rajdhon, 1968; Jirojwong 1996, Whittaker 2000, 2002a, b), but called *mae jang* in the North, is a caregiver for women (Liamputtong et al., 2005; cf. Kitzinger 1982, Laderman 1987; Camey et al., 1996; Lefeber and Voorhoever 1997, Liamputtong Rice 2000a; Hoban, 2002, in press; Paul and Rumsey 2002; Rozario and Samuel, 2002; Than, 2003). *Mae jang* deliveries birth in the villages, and assists women with postpartum practices during the first month after birth.

When the labour begins, *mae jang* will be summoned to the woman's home. A husband is expected to assist *mae jang* and the labouring woman. The birth mostly takes place in a kitchen where hot water can be prepared. Mattresses are folded up for the woman to prop her back up against when pushing. A husband provides physical support to a labouring woman. He sits behind her with his legs astride her shoulders so that when contractions are intense she holds on to his muscled thighs, which give her strength to push. A piece of strong wood or bamboo is tied to a post or a wall where the woman can push her feet against. If there is no husband assisting a woman at birth, a piece of long cloth or rope is hung onto the rafters of the room. This is for the woman to cling onto when contractions are intense. The traditional birth attendant squats at the woman's thighs and wait to catch the baby when it emerges so that the baby will not drop. After the birth, the husband boils the water for the midwife to wash the placenta, clean the body of the new mother and the newborn. He also cleans up remnants of birth and the floor and prepares a bed for his wife who must observe a postpartum ritual for the whole month and he buries the placenta of his newborn infant (Liamputtong et al., 2005).

Mae jang may also help a woman to have an easy birth by manipulating her abdomen and uterus during pregnancy. This is known as "*klang tong*" or "*kwag tong*" in northern Thai. Essentially, the midwife massages and pushes the uterus upward to make it "loosened up". This will create enough space within the uterus to make the baby move easier in the womb, and hence, make it easy to emerge, but also it can ensure that the baby is not squashed and deformed inside the womb. This ritual is done two to three times per week from the sixth month onward (Liamputtong et al., 2005.

In my study (Liamputtong et al., 2005), several women from rural area mentioned that they were themselves delivered by *mae jang* which was some twenty years ago. One woman was delivered by *mae jang* in her village home prior to moving into Chiang Mai metropolitan area, and she explained:

> My mother told me that I was born with the help of *mae jang* at home. My mother could not get to hospital in time so my grandfather had to summon *mae jang* in the village.

One urban educated woman in my study said she was the fourth child in the family of ten children and she and her older siblings were born at home with the assistance of *mae jang*. Some other women said that their siblings were also born with the assistance of *mae jang* and this occurred only six years ago. Most rural women are knowledgeable about traditional birth and the role of traditional midwives. But, women in Chiang Mai city tend to lack this knowledge. It seems, then, that *mae jang* in some rural parts of Thailand still exists despite the fact that childbirth in Thailand has been medicalized. Muecke (1976: 377), in her study in early 1970s, also points out that, two systems of childbirth existed in Chiang Mai: "the indigenous tradition-honoring and domestic North Thai system of delivery and postnatal care, and the imported medical and institutionalized Western system of obstetrics". Whittaker (2000, 2002a, b) and Jirojwong and Manderson (1999) have also observed in their studies in northeast Thailand and in far north Queensland respectively.

The Safe Motherhood Initiative has advocated the increase in the number of skilled birth attendants including TBAs, so that women in rural areas and resource-poor settings who have limited access to modern maternal health services and care may have safe births and hence maternal mortality may be reduced (Walraven and Weeks, 1999; Allotey, 2000; Hoban, 2002; Izugbara and Ukmayi, 2004). Although we have seen attempts from many societies, it seems that there are still many obstacles to achieve this (Stephens, 1992; Hoban, 2002; see Chapters 6 and 8 in this volume). Births assisted by TBAs are still largely seen as unsafe (Mangay-

Angara, 1981; Manderson, 1996; Harris, 2002). In societies where discourses of modernity are pervasive (such as in South and Southeast Asia), Samuel (2002: 7) suggests, the TBAs would still be seen as "ignorant, dirty and dangerous". It seems that an attempt to bring back TBAs in many societies still has a long way to go.

MOTHERHOOD

Research concerning motherhood in the past decade has taken a social constructionist or feminist standpoint (Oakley, 1980; Boulton, 1983; Wearing, 1984; Ussher, 1990; Phoenix and Woollett, 1991; Richardson, 1993; Brown et al., 1994; Ribbens, 1994; Brown et al., 1997; Weaver and Ussher, 1997; Gross, 1998; Lupton, 2000; Liamputtong, 2001, 2006; Liamputtong et al., 2000, 2004; Rendina and Liamputtong, 2006; Buultjens and Liamputtong, 2007). An interesting pattern emerging from these studies is that motherhood is seen "as an area of ambivalence for women" (Weaver and Ussher, 1997: 51; see also Oakley, 1980; Wearing, 1984; Rendina and Liamputtong, 2006; Buultjens and Liamputtong, 2006). In Boulton's work (1983) with mothers from middle and working class backgrounds about motherhood and daily lives, the women in her study expressed contradictory feelings about being a mother. Motherhood was burdensome but it also provided enjoyment and pleasure. Despite negative aspects of motherhood, women described being a mother as rewarding. Similar patterns have also been found in studies with Australian-born women in Melbourne (Brown et al., 1994; Rendina and Liamputtong, 2006; Buultjens and Liamputtong, 2007).

Weaver and Ussher (1997) examine the expectations, experiences and motherhood changes among mothers of young children in North London. Similarly, they find that "societal myths were implicated for giving a false impression of motherhood" (p. 51). When this is combined with the high demands of childcare, it leads to "disillusionment and a sense of lost identity". The reality of being a mother is contrary to the idealized image of motherhood normally presented in the media. This makes many women feel inadequate. Some women say that they are seen as "just a mother" implying that motherhood is a normal mundane part of womanhood and mothers are people without intelligence and status. This reinforces the image of "lost self" (p. 64) among women in this study. Despite this image, women try to find ways which they can use to counteract negative aspects of motherhood by emphasising the positive emotional aspects of motherhood. They affirm themselves that even though their lives are changed after becoming a mother, their inner selves are not affected by motherhood. Women also point to the positive side of motherhood, particularly the joys of seeing their children grow and their deep emotional warmth and love for their children.

Although existing literature about motherhood has provided a rich understanding of motherhood and women's personal experiences of becoming a mother, it has largely been examined from a western cultural perspective. As Bhopal (1998: 485) argues, "motherhood has often been examined from a white, western perspective, neglecting divisions based upon 'race' and ethnicity." Similarly, Squire (1989) suggests that there is a tendency for most research with women on motherhood is undertaken on white and middle class females. Current social constructions of motherhood do not reflect the realities of non-Western mothers. Hence, they are socially constructed as "other" (Bhopal, 1998: 486; Phoenix and Woollett, 1991: 18). It is possible that women from different cultural backgrounds may have different perceptions and experiences of motherhood. In Bhopal's study (1998), for example, she demonstrates that South Asian women living in East London see motherhood as a natural result of an arranged marriage linking to the importance of bearing male children in order to continue the ancestral line and to enhance the family pride and honour. Bhopal (1998: 492) argues that it is through this "social construction of motherhood that women are judged as a good or a bad mother".

Thai women in my study, for example, see motherhood in a variety of ways (Liamputtong et al., 2000, 2004; Liamputtong, in press). Common to all women, however, is the perception that motherhood is not an easy task; endless childcare and energy put into mothering is continuous and tiring. Some women believe that motherhood means self-sacrifice and endless concern. But, others say that motherhood brings joy and pleasure to their lives. This overpowering sense of love and involvement with the child makes the negative aspects worthwhile (Boulton, 1983; Weaver and Ussher, 1997; Liamputtong, 2006; Rendina and Liamputtong, 2006; Liamputtong, in press). In their study, Weaver and Ussher (1997: 65) also find that the discourses around the theme of overwhelming love highlight "the positive emotional aspects of motherhood".

Previous research undertaken with Western women tends to, or at least partially, interprets motherhood as a negative aspect of women's lives (Antonis, 1981; Ussher, 1990; Phoenix and Woollett, 1991; Woollett and Phoenix, 1991; Weaver and Ussher, 1997; Brown et al., 1997; Thurtle, 2003; Rendina and Liamputtong, 2006; Buultjens and Liamputtong, 2007). Weaver and Ussher (1997), for example, point out in their study that women see motherhood as mandatory and women must not be selfish by putting themselves before their children. Because of this belief, many women feel frustrated and, at times, motherhood has "led to a feeling of hopelessness" (p. 59). But, this pattern is not observed in my study with Thai women (see Liamputtong et al., 2000, 2004). Although women see their role as "a selfless Madonna" who is prepared to sacrifice everything for their children, motherhood does not contain the negative image as presented in Weaver and Ussher's study (1997).

Weaver and Ussher (1997) suggest that the most overwhelming part of becoming a mother is the change that it brings to a woman's life, particularly to her perception of herself. This is also true with the Thai women in my study (Liamputtong et al., 2000, 2004; Liamputtong, 2006, in press). However, changes tend to be positive. These include motherhood making women to be more responsible toward everything including their own well-being and it makes themselves and their spouses more mature. This is, however, not to say in this study that there are no negative aspects of motherhood among Thai women. Women mention several negative perspectives including putting the child before themselves and the continuation of worry and concern about the well-being and health of their child. Motherhood, to some women, also means worse health for them (see also Liamputtong and Naksook, 2003a; Liamputtong, 2006, in press).

In Thai culture, family members including their spouses and others play a significant role in the way women become mothers and mother their children. This also affects their perceptions of motherhood. For the women who live with their extended families, the support they receive during the postpartum period and thereafter helps them to cope with the demands of childcare. As mentioned, for the whole month after giving birth women are required to rest. All household chores including taking care of a newborn infant are undertaken by other family members, particularly their mothers and sisters: they are "other mothers" who provide support to mothers. Husbands also play a significant role in this. The support women receive helps them not to feel isolated as they are surrounded by their kin. This is contrary to the findings of previous studies with western women (see Rendina and Liamputtong, 2006; Buultjens and Liamputtong, 2007). Sharpe (1984), for example, points to the isolation women experience because they spend a large amount of time at home with their young children. In Weaver and Ussher's study (1997) women felt tied to the house in caring for their children. In Brown et al.'s study (1997), they also comment that isolation is real for many of Australian-born women. This is largely, perhaps, because women in these studies do not have "other mothers" on whom they can rely to bring up their young children. These two reasons help to explain why Thai women's perceptions and experiences of motherhood in my study are different from their Western counterparts. See Chapters 13, 14, 15 and 16 for issues regarding motherhood in different societies in this volume.

Motherhood and Childbearing: Stories of Immigrant Mothers

Motherhood

Studies with immigrant women in Australia (Liamputtong, 2000; Liamputtong and Naksook, 2003b; Liamputton, 2006) have shown how migrant women deal with the double transition, or as McMahon (1995) proposes, "multiple identities", of becoming mothers and bringing their children up in a new country. Despite differences between women, they all see that they are now living in an entirely new environment, which is, in many ways, different from the one from which they originally come. This has marked impact on their lives as wives and mothers. Many immigrant mothers feel the double burden of motherhood and of living in their new homeland (see also Chapters 14 and 15 in this volume).

In my study with Thai immigrant women (Liamputtong and Naksook, 2003b), there are several dominant discourses concerning motherhood emerging from the women's accounts. First, cultural upbringing plays a major role in the way new mothers view motherhood and childrearing. Migrant women struggle to find a comfort zone between their cultural traditions and the culture of their new homeland. They attemt to accommodate the differences as best as they can, passing on as much of their cultural traditions as their partners will allow. Often, they are disappointed if they are prevented from doing so. This is similar to what Liam (1991, 1999) has found in her study with first-time Chinese immigrant mothers. Liam (1991: 128) points out that:

> Living in a new land where the basic beliefs and values of mainstream culture are different from one's own upbringing, a migrant mother faces the challenge of reframing her own set of values and beliefs or of developing a new and more appropriate set for herself and her Australian-born children. She may hold on to what she is familiar with as long as possible or she may loosen her grip on her own past and begin to allow new or other perspectives to enter into her life space which is being transformed by virtue of the migration.

Secondly, there are several issues that women express as the main concerns of their lives as wives and mothers in their new homeland. Social isolation is real for many migrant mothers in this study (see also Liamputtong, 2001). Although social isolation is also prevalent among mothers in Western societies (e.g. Boulton, 1983; Sharp, 1984; Wearing, 1984; Richards, 1985; Brown et al., 1994, 1997; Maushart, 1997; Rendina and Liamputtong, 2006; Buultjens and Liamputtong, 2007), the isolation among Thai migrant mothers is more marked. A lack of support is their main difficulty in being a mother and bringing children up in their new homeland. In Thailand, childrearing is a responsibility shared among members of the extended family and others such as neighbours (Potter, 1977; Richter et al., 1992; Naksook, 1994; Segaller, 1995; Liamputtong, in press). However, when being a new mother in Australia women have to single-handedly take up all the responsibilities at home. This is particularly so if their husbands have a full-time job or if they still believe that domestic duties are a woman's job. In Bhopal's study (1998) with South Asian mothers in East London, she demonstrates that support from mothers-in-law and sisters assist the women a great deal with their motherhood and mothering roles. The support also helps to eliminate the feelings of isolation and loneliness among these mothers.

Women in my study (Liamputtong, 2001; Liamputtong and Naksook, 2003b) have a strong feeling about preserving Thai traditions and the Thai language in their new homeland. Despite this, women also realise that this may not be possible with their lives in Australia due to the force of different cultural traditions tending toward the culture of their new homeland. They, however, try their best to maintain Thai traditions. For some women, this can be a difficult task particularly if their spouses oppose their attempts. Many women have difficulties in maintaining Thai language at home with their Australian-born children and husbands. This is largely due to the fact that Australia is still a monolingual society with English used as the official language and medium of exchange in all matters. Australia has the policy of multiculturalism that encourages the acquisition and maintenance of ethnic languages and cultures among the migrant population (Liamputtong Rice, 1997, 1999; Jupp, 2002; Liamputtong et al., 2003). Despite this, as Liam (1991: 156) points out, "the influence of the English language remains overpowering; it is still the language which gives a person access to information and resources". Due to this, mothers adopt an increasing use of English expressions in their daily conversations with their Australian-born children. This is inevitable because the children speak mainly English at school (or even at home).

On the other side of the coin, some women see life in their new homeland better, not only for themselves but particularly for their children. This life chance is expressed more among poor women who come from rural areas and have little education. These women believe that their life may not have been improved had they still lived in Thailand. They see being married to Australian men and living in a new country as a way to give them a chance of having a better life and living standards, and this also greatly assists them with their mothering roles.

In my study (Liamputtong and Naksook, 2003b), the life of motherhood in a new homeland also presents an interesting pattern. A woman in a Thai traditional family is generally encouraged to have more than one child, particularly when the first one is female. Similar to other Asian cultures, the Thais believe that only the male descendent may carry on the name of the family into infinity (Potter, 1977). Living away from Thailand and the strong influence of Thai culture and family influences, would Thai mothers be likely to have more children? In this study it shows that women have mixed feelings about this. Some women want to have more children because they believe that their children need companions. Life is lonely in a new homeland because relatives and friends (if they have some) live far apart. Living in Thailand, a child is usually surrounded by many people and the children can play in the street or front yard, but this does not happen in their new county due to lack of familial support. Some women want more children because they feel obliged to try to give a male child to their husband's family, despite the fact that their husbands are from Anglo-Celtic backgrounds. More importantly, however, the anti-Asian feelings when Pauline Hanson was leading the One Nation party in the Australian politics (Jupp, 2002), which was still prevalent when my study was being conducted, created a sense of fear and insecurity amongst the mothers in this research. This has led many mothers to consider more seriously about having fewer children. This is perhaps why many women in my study desire to maintain the Thai cultural identity because they believe this may equip their children to survive in what they perceive as a hostile environment of their new homeland.

Experiences of Immigrant Mothers in Australian Hospitals

Studies concerning immigrant women and childbearing in western societies have pointed to many difficulties experienced by these women when seeking care during their childbearing period (Liamputtong Rice and Naksook, 1998, 1999; Liamputtong Rice. 2000; Small et al., 1999, 2003, 2004; Yelland et al., 1999; Katbamna, 2000; D'Souza et al., 2002; Tsianakas and Liamputtong, 2002; Liamputtong and Watson, 2002, 2006; Richens, 2003; Jayaweera et al., 2005; see also Chapters10, 11, and 12 in this volume).

In my study with Hmong immigrant women in Melbourne, Australia (Rice, 1999; Liamputtong Rice, 2000), I have found that although in general Hmong women feel satisfied with their childbirth experiences in Australian hospitals, women also report some difficulties with their caregivers and hospital routines. There are at least three important issues contributing to these difficulties in hospital.

Primarily, difficulties are due to differences in cultural beliefs and expectations. As I have previously pointed oufFrom a social science perspective, childbearing is not only a biological event, but is also determined by the social and cultural environments within which it occurs. In different societies, we find different patterns of childbearing. In the case of Hmong women, their childbearing patterns and expectations are different from Western norms. One Hmong woman in my study (see Rice, 1999; Liamputtong Rice, 2000) was told to have her tubes tied. This clearly shows that the Western doctor did not appreciate the value Hmong people place on having many children. Similarly, women were not allowed to put their newborn infants on the bed with them. The women wished to protect their newborn by keeping the baby near them, but their caregivers saw this practice as dangerous by. Due to the different systems of cultural beliefs and practices, Hmong women's views about their childbirth expectations conflict with those of their caregivers, and this contributes to difficulties when they give birth in a new country.

Secondly, difficulties faced by Hmong women are due to the lack of effective communication between health professionals and the women. This is partly due to the lack of English proficiency on the part of the women (Rice, 1999). Similar problems have been documented by researchers working with other groups of immigrant women (Homans, 1982; Liamputtong Rice, 1993, 1994; Small et al., 1999, 2003, 2004; Woollett and Dosanjh-Matwala, 1990; Yelland et al., 1998; Liamputtong Rice and Naksook, 1999; Tsianakas and Liamputtong, 2002; Liamputtong and Watson, 2002, 2006; see also Chapters 11, 12 and 13 in this volume). As mentioned, most Hmong women do not have enough English to communicate with their caregivers. Some have to rely on their husbands who also communicate ineffectively due to their limited English. However, the lack of information and clarification on the part of health caregivers also contributes to misunderstanding and miscommunication. One woman in my study believed that if she did not follow her caregivers' instructions she would not receive any further help. This, clearly, is an example of miscommunication. Is this what her caregivers actually said to her, or is it due to some misunderstanding caused by English expression? Is it perhaps a lack of clear explanation from health professionals about the birth process? The woman received assistance from an interpreter at the time of consultation. What part does this three-way communication contribute to the misunderstanding by the women? In the study conducted by Small and colleagues (1999), communication was found to be essential in providing good care for women of non-English speaking backgrounds. Women not fluent in English had problems in communicating with their caregivers and hence had less positive experiences of their care than those who could speak better English. In addition, women in Small et al.'s study expressed their strong desire to be able to speak English so that they could themselves communicate with their caregivers. Hmong women in my study are no exception.

Difficulties are also due to the fact that women are not being informed and offered choices when having their babies in Australia. This may be because childbirth has been medicalized in Western societies. Due to this, health professionals, particularly doctors, have become experts on childbirth and their decisions are considered more important than those of the women. These issues have been found even among women from Western backgrounds (Romalis, 1981; Oakley, 1986; Martin, 1987; Rothman, 1984, 1991; Lazarus, 1994; Lane, 1996; Possamai-Inesedy, 2005). As illustrated, women feel that when a decision about childbirth is made, they do not have any choices. They are either not informed about birth procedures or are coerced to follow their caregivers' instructions. Women feel that they have no control of their own bodies and feel resentment towards hospital policy and practices. One woman in my study was persuaded to undergo a caesarean operation, and she strongly believed that she was coerced to do so (Rice, 1999).

In Liamputtong and Watson's study with Southeast Asian immigrant women (2006), we found that the women's narratives reveal a voice of passivity; a voice not able to be heard in the health care system. Other studies (Small et al., 1999, 2002; Rice, 1999, 2000; Tsianakas and Liamputtong, 2002; Liamputtong and Watson, 2002) have also documented this pattern. Some passive voices are because of women's trust in authoritative knowledge of their health care providers and medical intervention (Davis-Floyd and Sargent, 1997; Jordan, 1997; Kabakian-Khasholian et al., 2000). This is the product of medicalized births in western societies that work to disempower childbearing women (Zadoroznyj, 1999; Possamai-Inesedy, 2005). But, for others, this is due to the women's lack of sufficient English. Only 11 women who participated in this study said they were confident enough to communicate with their caregivers in English. Although attempts have been made to ensure that women are informed about their health care, there are still women, particularly of ethnic minorities, who do not have an adequate understanding of the implications of services offered to them (Liamputtong and Watson, 2002). This results in a feeling of powerlessness among the women, and this powerlessness may have negative consequences for them. As has been found in Small et al.'s study in Melbourne Australia (2002), women who did not speak English very well, or not at all, were twice as likely to have a cesarean birth as those who did not.

The passivity of the women may also lead to a sense of cultural alienation which is prevalent among ethnic minorities in Australia and elsewhere (Bowes and Domokos, 1997;

Fadiman, 1997; Small et al., 1999; Rice, 1999, 2000; Small et al., 2002; Tsianakas and Liamputtong, 2002). Evidence of misunderstanding and, hence, mismanagement in health care resulting from this cultural alienation abounds (Liamputtong Rice et al., 1994; Fadiman, 1997; Rice, 1999, 2000; Liamputtong and Watson, 2002). In my study (see Liamputtong Rice et al., 1994), for example, we found that a Hmong woman experienced ill health due to a loss of her soul after having a cesarean section. This case occurred due to the lack of cultural knowledge among health care providers and hence they mishandled the birth. These women did not feel empowered enough to ask for culturally appropriate birthing care. In my study with Southeast Asian women (Liamputtong and Watson, 2002), we found a woman who felt pressured by health service providers to accept an abortion after an adverse ultrasound result. This pressure was felt mainly due to the lack of a clear understanding and communication between the woman and her caregiver. In both of these cases, these people experienced alienation and remained silent.

What is important here is that it would be too easy for health professionals to conclude that immigrant women do not wish to adapt to living situations in their new country and that is why most of them maintain their traditions. Due to this, conflict between women and their caregivers occurs. However, the results of many studies indicate that very often women made it very clear that they have tried to change their lifestyle in order to be integrated in this society. Many women had home births in their homeland and although they wish to do so here, they still sought help from hospitals. This is because they realize that this is the Australian norm, and they follow it. Antenatal care is a good example. Women attend antenatal checkups unless they have other commitments because they believe that this is what Australian women do. Similarly, although they have great concerns about the future of their own health because they have to abandon or modify many traditional customs in Australia, they do so because this is the way they can adapt to living situations here. It may be true that some women feel strongly that they have to maintain their traditions. However, this is mainly due to their desire to maintain their good health and for the well-being of their newborn, not because they do not wish to adapt.

CONCLUSION

In this chapter, I have discussed salient issues regarding procreation, reproduction and motherhood in different societies. I have shown that women are seen as the markers of reproduction; they are responsible for procreation and reproduction. If they fail to do so, or worse, if they deny doing so, often blame falls upon them. For those who become mothers, these norms function to protect not only the women but also their newborn infants. This can be seen clearly with cultural beliefs and practices regarding the postpartum period as I have outlined in this chapter. But, in many societies cultural norms tend to be replaced by medicalization of childbirth. I do not deny that modern birth can be beneficial to many women, but all too often, the overmedicalized birth has made other types of birth (such as births assisted by TBAs) irrelevant.

Becoming a mother brings joy to women, and most women would attest to this. But, under certain circumstances, it can be distressful for women, particularly those who do not have a support network, like those who are immigrant women. They often have to deal with the double transition of their lives, not only as mothers but also as displaced people.

In summing up, I contend that culture still plays a vital role in women's reproduction and procreation. We must acknowledge the importance of culture and incorporate it in the provision of health care for women in all societies, and as Lefkarites (1992: 410) writes:

> It is respectful of cultural diversity and supportive of policies that are truly concerned with a healthier outcome for mother, baby, and other significant family members.

REFERENCES

Allotey, P., 2000, 'Where There's No Tradition of Traditional Birth Attendants: Kassena Kankana District, Northen Ghana', in M. Berer and T.K. Sundari Ravindran (eds.), *Safe Motherhood Initiatives: Critical Issues*, pp. 147-154. Reproductive Health Matters: London.

Anuman Rajadhon, Phya, 1987, *Some Traditions of the Thai and Other Translation of Phya Anuman Rajadhon's Articles on Thai Customs*, Thai Inter-Religious Commission for Developmen and Sathirakoses Nagapradipa Foundation: Bangkok.

Arney, W.R., 1982, *Power and the Profession of Obstetrics*, University of Chicago Press: Chicago.

Ba-Thike, K., 1997, 'Abortion: A Public Health Problem in Myanmar', *Reproductive Health Matters,* 9: 94-100.

Bentley, G.R., & Mascie-Taylor, C.G.N., (eds.) 2000, *Infertility in the Modern World: Present and Future Prospects*, Cambridge University Press: Cambridge.

Berer, M., 1988, 'Whatever Happened to 'A Women's Right to Choose'?', *Feminist Review*, 29: 24-37.

Berer, M., 1997, 'Abortion: Unfinished Business', *Reproductive Health Matters*, 9: 6-9.

Bhatti, L.I., Fikree, F.F., & Khan, A., 1999, 'The Quest of Infertile Women in Squatter Settlement of Karachi, Pakistan: A Qualitative Study', *Social Science and Medicine*, 49: 637-649.

Bhopal, K., 1998, 'South Asian Women in East London: Motherhood and Social Support', *Women's Studies International Forum*, 21, 485-492.

Bledsoe, C.A., Hill, a., D'Alessandro, u., & Langerick, P., 1994, 'Constructing Natural Fertility: The Use of Western Contraceptive Technologies in Rural Gambia', *Population and Development Review,* 20: 81-113.

Bluff, R., & Holloway, I., 1994, ''They Know Best': Women's Perceptions of Midwifery Care During Labour and Childbirth', *Midwifery*, 10: 57-164.

Boerma, J.T., & Mgalla, Z., (eds.) 2001, *Women and Infertility in Sub-Saharan Africa: A Multi-disciplinary Perspective*, KIT Publishers: Amsterdam.

Boonmongkon, P., Nichter, M., & Pylypa, J., 2001, '*Mot Luuk* Problems in Northeast Thailand: Why Women's Own Health Concerns Matter as Much as Disease Rates', *Social Science and Medicine*, 53: 1095-1112.

Boonmongkon, P., Nichter, M., Pylypa, J., Sanhajariya, N., & Saitong, S., 2002, 'Women's Health in Northeast Thailand: Working at the Interface Between the Local and the Global', in A. Whittaker (ed.), *Women's Health in Mainland Southeast Asia*, pp. 59-80. The Haworth Press: New York.

Boulton, M. G., 1983, *On Being a Mother: A Study of Women With Pre-School Children*, Tavistock: London.

Brown, S., Small, R., & Lumley, J., 1997, 'Being a 'Good Mother', *Journal of Reproductive and Infant Psychology*, 15: 185-200.

Brown, S., Small, R., Lumley, J., & Astbury, J., 1994, *Missing Voices: The Experiences of Motherhood*, Oxford University Press: Melbourne.

Buultjens, M., & Liamputtong, P., 2007, When giving life starts to take the life out of you: Women's experiences with postnatal depression following childbirth. *Midwifery*, 23: 77-91.

Cabigon, J.V., 1996, 'Use of Health Services by Filipino Women During Childbearing Episodes', in P. Liamputtong Rice & L. Manderson (eds.), *Maternity and Reproductive Health in Asian Societies*, pp. 83-99. Amsterdam: Harwood Academic Publishers.

Camey, X.C., Barrios, C.G., Guerrero, X.R., Nunez-Urquiza, R.M., Hernandez, D.G., & Glass, A.L., 1996, 'Traditional Birth Attendants in Mexico: Advantage and Inadequacies of Care for Normal Deliveries', *Social Science and Medicine*, 43(2): 199-207.

Campero, L., Garcia, C., DiAz, C., Ortiz, O., Reynoso, S., & Langer, A., 1998, '"Along I Wouldn't Have Known What to Do": A Qualitative Study on Social Support During Labor and Delivery in Mexico', *Social Science and Medicine*, 47(3): 395-403.

Cannold, L., 1998, *The Abortion Myth: Abortion and the Changing Future for Women*, Allen & Unwin, Sydney.

Casey, R.C.D., 1960, 'Alleged Anti-Fertility Plants of India', *Indian Journal of Medical Sciences*, 14: 590-600.

Chawla, J., 2002, '*Hawa, Gola* and Mother-in-Law's Big Toe: On Understanding *Dais'* Imagery of the Female Body', in S. Rozario & G. Samuel (eds.), *Daughters of Hariti: Childbirth and Female Healers in South and Southeast Asia*, pp. 147-162. Routledge: London.

Chu, C., 1996, '"Tso Yyueh-Tzu (Sitting the Month) in Contemporary Taiwan', in P.Liamputtong Rice and L. Manderson (eds.), *Maternity and Reproductive Health in Asian Societies*, pp. 191-204. Harwood Academic Publishers: Amsterdam.

Condit, C.M., 1990, *Decoding Abortion Rhetoric: Communicating Social Change*, University of Illinois Press: Urbana.

Conway, G.A., & Slocumb, J.C., 1979, 'Plants Used as Abortifacients and Emmenagogues by Spanish New Mexicans', *Journal of Ethnopharmacology*, 1: 241-261.

Correa, S., 1994, *Population and Reproductive Rights: Feminist Perspectives from the South*, Zed Books:London.

Cosminsky, S., 1982, 'Childbirth and Change: A Guatemalan Study', in C.P. MacCormack (ed.), *Ethnography of fertility and birth*, pp. 205-229. Academic Press: London.

Cosminsky, S., 2001, 'Midwifery Across the Generations: A Modernizing Midwife in Guatemala', *Medical Anthropology*, 20: 345-378.

D'Souza, L., Turner, A., & Garcia, J., 2002, *Access to Care for Very Disadvantaged Childbearing Women: Report of a Descriptive Survey of Services for Women from Non-English Speaking Backgrounds, Asylum Seekers and Women at Risk from Domestic Violence*, National Perinatal Epidemiology Unit, Oxford.

Daly, C., & Pollard, A.J., 1990, 'Traditional Birth Attendants in the Gambia', *Midwives Chronicle & Nursing Notes*, April: 104-105.

Davis-Floyd, R. E., & Sargent, C.F., eds. 1997, *Childbirth and Authoritative Knowledge: Cross-Cultural Perspectives*, University of California Press: Berkeley.

Davis-Floyd, R. E., 1987, 'The Technological Model of Birth', *Journal of American Folklore*, 100: 479-495.

Davis-Floyd, R.E, 1992, *Birth as An American Rite of Passage*, University of California Press: Berkeley.

Davis-Floyd, R. E., 1994, 'The Technocratic Body: American Childbirth as Cultural Expression', *Social Science and Medicine*, 38(8): 1125-1140.

Davis-Floyd, R.E., 2001, La Partera Professional: Articulaing Identity and Cultural Space for a New Kind of Midwife in Mexico', *Medical Anthropology*, 20: 185-243.

Davis-Floyd, R.E., & Sargent, C.F., 1997, 'Introduction: The Anthropology of Birth', in R.E. Davis-Floyd and C.F. Sargent (eds.), *Childbirth and Authoritative Knowledge: Cross-Cultural Perspectives*, pp. 1-51. University of California Press: Berkeley.

Davis-Floyd, R.E., Pigg, S.L., & Cosminsky, S., 2001, Introduction. Daughters of Time: The Shifting Identities of Contemporary Midwives', *Medical Anthropology*, 20: 105-139.

De Bruyn, M., 2001, *Violence, Pregnancy and Abortion: Issues of Women's Rights and Public Health. A Review of Worldwide Data and Recommendations for Action*, IPAS: Chapel Hill, NC.

Devereux, G., 1955, *A Study of Abortion in Primitive Societies*, International Universities Press: New York.

Douglas, M., 1970, *Natural Symbols*, Pantheon Books: New York.

Fadiman, A., 1997, *The Spirit Catches You and You Fall Down: A Hmong Child, Her American Doctors, and the Collision of Two Cultures*, Farrar, Straus and Giroux: New York.

Feldman-Savelsberg, P., 1994, 'Plundered Kitchens and Empty Wombs: Fear of Infertility in the Cameroonian Grassfields'. *Social Science and Medicine*, 39(4): 463-474.

Feldman-Savelsberg, P., 2001, 'Is Fertility an Unrecognized Public Health and Population Problem? The View from the Cameroon Grassfields', in M.C. Inhorn and F. Van Balen (eds.), *Infertility Around the Globe: New Thinking on Childlessness, Gender, and Reproductive Technologies*, pp. 215-232. University of California Press: Berkeley.

Fisher, C., Hauck, Y., & Fenwick, J., 2006, 'How Social Context Impacts on Women's Fears of Childbirth: A Western Australian Example', *Social Science and Medicine* 63: 64-75.

Foucault, M., 1980, *Power/Knowledge: Selected Interview and Other Writings, 1972-1977*, edited and translated by C. Gordon. Harvester: New York.

Fox, B., & Worts, D., 1999, 'Revisiting the Critique of Medicalized Childbirth: A Contribution to the Sociology of Birth', *Gender & Society*, 13(3): 326-346.

Gerrits, T., 2001, 'Infertility and Matrilineality: The Exceptional Case of Macua of Mozambique', in M.C. Inhorn and F. Van Balen (eds.), *Infertility Around the Globe: New Thinking on Childlessness, Gender, and Reproductive Technologies*, pp. 233-246. University of California Press: Berkeley.

Geurts, K., 2002, 'Childbirth and Pragmatic Midwifery in Rural Ghana', *Medical Anthropology*, 20: 379-408.

Gilson, L., 2003, 'Trust and the Development of Health Care as a Social Institution', *Social Science and Medicine*, 56: 1453-1468.

Ginsburg, F., 1989, 1998, *Contested Lives: The Abortion Debate in an American Community*, University of California Press: Berkeley.

Ginsburg, F.D., & Rapp, R., (eds.) *Conceiving the New World Order: The Global Politics of Reproduction*, Berkeley: University of California Press.

Githens, M., & Stetson, D.M. (eds.) 1996, *Abortion Politics: Public Policy in Cross-Cultural Perspective*, Routledge: London.

Goldsmith, J.,1990, *Childbirth Wisdom from the World's Oldest Societies*, East West Health Books: Brookline, Mass.

Greer, G., 1984, *Sex and Destiny: The Politics of Human Fertility*, Secker and Warburg: London.

Gross, E., 1998, 'Motherhood in Feminist Theory', *Affilia: Journal of Women and Social Work*, 13(3): 269-272.

Hadley, J., 1996, *Abortion: Between Freedom and Necessity*, Virago: London.

Hamberger, L., & Janson, P.O., 1997, 'Global Importance of Infertility and Its Treatment: Role of Infertility Technologies', *International Journal of Gynecology & Obstetrics*, 58: 149-158.

Hardacre, H., 1997, Marketing the Menacing Fetus in Japan, University of California Press: Berkeley.

Harris, A., 2002, 'Beranak and Bekindu: Discourses of Risk and Strength in Childbirth and Post-Partum Practice Among Iban Communities of Pakan', in S. Rozario & G. Samuel (eds.), *Daughters of Hariti: Childbirth and Female Healers in South and Southeast Asia*, pp. 234-255. Routledge: London.

Hoban, E., 2002, *Yeen Sok Sapbaav Haey. We're Sage and Happy Already: Traditional Birth Attendants and Safe Motherhood in a Cambodian Rural Commune*, Unpublished Doctoral Thesis, The Key Centre for Women's Health in Society, the University of Melbourne, Melbourne.

Hoban, E., in press, *Cambodian Women: Childbirth and Maternity in Rural Southeast Asia*, Routledge, Women and Asia Series: London.

Hsu, C., 2001, 'Making Midwives: Postmodern Conditions and Midwifery Training in Saint Lucia', *Medical Anthropology*, 20: 313-344.

Hundt, G.L., Beckerleg, S., Kassem, F., Jafar, A.M.A., Belmaker, I., Saad, K.A., & Shoham-Vardi, I., 2000, 'Women's Health Custom Made: Building on the 40 Days Postpartum for Arab Women', *Health Care for Women International*, 21: 529-542.

Inhorn, M.C., & Van Balen, F., (eds.) 2001, *Infertility Around the Globe: New Thinking on Childlessness, Gender, and Reproductive Technologies*. University of California Press: Berkeley.

Inhorn, M.C., 1994a, '*Kabsa* (A.K.A. Mushahara) and Threatened Fertility in Egypt', *Social Science and Medicine*, 39(4): 487-505.

Inhorn, M.C., 1994b, Quest for Conception: Gender, Infertility, and Egyptian Medical Tradition, University of Pennsylvania Press: Philadelphia.

Inhorn, M.C., 1996, *Infertility and Patriarchy: The Cultural Politics of Gender and Family Life in Egypt*, University of Pennsylvania Press: Philadelphia.

Inhorn, M.C., 2003a, '"The Worms are Weak": Male Infertility and Patriarchal Paradoxes in Egypt', *Men and Masculnities*, 5(3): 236-256.

Inhorn, M.C., 2003b, Global Infertility and the Globalization of New Reproductive Technologies: Illustrations from Egypt', *Social Science and Medicine*, 56: 1837-1851.

Ityavyar, D.A., 1984, 'A Traditional Midwife Practice, Sokoto, Nigeria', *Social Science and Medicine*, 18: 497-501.

Izugbara, C.O., & Ukmayi, J.K., 2004, 'An Intercept Study of Persons Attending Traditional Birth Homes in Rural Southeastern Nigeria', *Culture, Health & Sexuality*, 6(2): 101-114.

Jayaweera, H., D'Souza, L., & Garcia, J., 2005, 'A Local Study of Childbearing Bangladeshi Women in the UK', *Midwifery*, 21: 84-95.

Jeffery, P.M., Jeffery, R., & Lyon, A., 2002, 'Contaminating States: Midwifery, Childbearing and the State in Rural North India', in S. Rozario & G. Samuel (eds.), *Daughters of Hariti: Childbirth and Female Healers in South and Southeast Asia*, pp. 90-108. Routledge: London.

Jeffery, R., & Jeffery, P.M., 1993, 'Traditional Birth Attendants in Rural North India: The Social Organization of Childbearing', in M. Lock & S. Lindenbaum (eds.), *Knowledge, Power and Practice: The Anthropology of Medicine and Everyday Life*, pp. 7-31. University of California Press: Berkeley.

Jenkins, G., 2001, 'Childlessness, Adoption, and *Milagros de dios* in Costa Rica', in M.C. Inhorn and F. Van Balen (eds.), *Infertility Around the Globe: New Thinking on Childlessness, Gender, and Reproductive Technologies*, pp. 171-189. University of California Press: Berkeley.

Jenkins, G.L., 2001, 'Changing Roles and Identities of Midwives in Rural Costa Rica', *Medical Anthropology*, 20: 409-444.

Jirojwong, S., 1996, 'Health Beliefs and the Use of Antenatal Care Among Pregnant Women in Southern Thailand', in P. Liamputtong Rice and L. Manderson (eds.), *Maternity and reproductive health in Asian societies*, pp. 61-82. Harwood Academic Publishers: Amsterdam.

Jochle, W., 1974, 'Menses-Inducing Drugs: Their Role in Antique, Medieval and Renaissance Gynaecology and Birth Control', *Contraception*, 10: 425-432.

Johnson, B.R., Horga, M., & Andronache. L., 1996, 'Women's Perspectives on Abortion in Romania', *Social Science and Medicine*, 42: 521-530

Johnson, M., Smith, J., Haddad, S., Walker, J., & Wong, A., 1992, 'Women Prefer Hospital Births', (Letter), *British Medical Journal*, 305: 255.

Jordan, B., 1993, *Birth in Four Cultures: A Crosscultural Investigation of Childbirth in Yucatan, Holland, Sweden, and the United States*, 4th edn', Waveland Press Inc: Prospect Heights, Illinois.

Jordan, B., 1997, 'Authoritative Knowledge and Its Construction', in R. Davis-Floyd& C.F. Sargent (eds.), *Childbirth and Authoritative Knowledge: Cross-Cultural Perspectives*, pp. 55-79. University of California Press: Berkeley.

Juarez, F., Cabigon, J.V., & Singh, S., 2004, *Changes in the Prevalence of Induced Abortion in the Philippines*, unpublished paper presented at the Population Association of America Annual Meeting, Boston, April 1-3.

Jupp, J., 2002, *From White Australia to Woomera: The story of Australian immigrants*, Cambridge University Press: Cambridge.

Kabakian-Khasholian, T., Campbell, O., Shediac-Rizkallah, M., & Ghorayeb, F., 2000, 'Women's Experiences of Maternity Care: Satisfaction or Passivity?', *Social Science and Medicine*, 51: 103-113.

Katbamna, S., 2000, *'Race' and Childbirth*, Open University Press: Buckingham.

Kempe, A., Stangard, F., Hamman, F., Nooraldin, F.A., Al Atlas, S., Khider, F.S., & Dhman, Z.J., 1994, *The Quality of Maternal and Neonatal Health Services in Yemen: Seen Through Women's Eyes*, Swedish Save the Children (Radda Barnen): Stockholm.

Kitzinger, S., 1997, 'Authoritative Touch in Childbirth: A Cross-Cultural Approach', in R. Davis-Floyd& C.F. Sargent (eds.), *Childbirth and Authoritative Knowledge: Cross-Cultural Perspectives*, pp. 209-232. University of California Press: Berkeley.

Kleinman, A., 1992, 'Local Worlds of Suffering: An Interpersonal Focus for Ethnographies of Illness Experience', *Qualitative Health Research* 2: 127-134.

Kong, Y.C., Xie, J-X., & But, P.P-H., 1986, Fertility Regulating Agents from Traditional Chinese Medicines', *Journal of Ethnopharmacology*, 15: 1-44.

Laderman, C., 1984, 'Food Ideology and Eating Behavior: Contributions from Malay Studies', *Social Science and Medicine*, 19(5): 547-559.

Laderman, C., 1987, *Wives and Midwives: Childbirth and Nutrition in Rural Malaysia*, University of California Press: Berkeley.

Lane, K., 1995, 'The Medical Model of the Body as a Site of Risk: A Case Study of Childbirth', in J, Gabe (ed.), *Medicine, health and risk: Sociological approach*, pp. 53-72. Blackwell: Oxford.

Lazarus, E. S., 1994, 'What Do Women Want?: Issues of Choice, Control, and Class in Pregnancy and Childbirth', *Medical Anthropology Quarterly*, 8(1): 25-46.

Lee, R. L., 1982, 'Comparative Studies of Health Care Systems', *Social Science and Medicine*, 16: 629-42.

Lefkarites, M.P., 1992, 'The Sociocultural Implications of Modernizing Childbirth Among Greek Women on the Island of Rhodes', *Medical Anthropology*, 13: 385-412.

LeFleur, W.R., 1992, *Liquid Life: Abortion and Buddhism in Japan*, Princeton University Press:Princeton.

Leonard, L., 2001, 'Problematizing Fertility: Scientific Accounts and Chadian Women's Narratives', in M.C. Inhorn and F. Van Balen (eds.), *Infertility Around the Globe: New Thinking on Childlessness, Gender, and Reproductive Technologies*, pp. 193-214. University of California Press: Berkeley.

Liam, I.I.L., 1991, *The Challenge of Migrant Motherhood: The Childrearing Practices of Chinese First-Time Mothers in Australia*, unpublished master thesis, Department of Social Work, the University of Melbourne: Melbourne.

Liam, I.I.L., 1999, 'The Challenge of Migrant Motherhood: The Childrearing Practices of Chinese First-Time Mothers in Australia', in P. Liamputtong Rice (ed.), *Asian mothers, Western birth*, pp. 135-160. Ausmed Publications: Melbourne.

Liamputtong, P. 2001, Motherhood and the challenge of immigrant mothers: A personal reflection. *Families in Society*, 82(2), 195-201.

Liamputtong, P., 2003, 'Abortion - Only Some Women Have the Right to Do It? Hmong Women's Perceptions of Abortion', *Health Care for Women International*, 24(3): 230-241.

Liamputtong, P., 2004a, 'Giving Birth in Hospital: Childbirth Experiences of Women in Northern Thailand', *Health Care for Women International*, 25(2): 454-480.

Liamputtong, P., 2004b, '*Yu Duan* Practices as Embodying Tradition, Modernity and Social Change in Chiang Mai, Northern Thailand', *Women & Health*, 40(1): 79-99.

Liamputtong, P., 2005a, 'Birth and Social Class: Northern Thai Women's Lived Experiences of Caesarean and Vaginal Birth', *Sociology of Health & Illness*, 27(1): 243-270.

Liamputtong, P., 2005b, '*Yu Duan* Ritual: The Significance of Traditional Postpartum Beliefs and Practices on Women's Health in Northern Thailand', in R.E. Balin (ed.), *Trends in midwifery research*, pp. 103-118. Nova Science Publishers: New York.

Liamputtong, P., 2006, 'Motherhood and "Moral Career": Discourses of Good Motherhood Among Southeast Asian Immigrant Women in Australia', *Qualitative Sociology*, 29(1): 25-53.

Liamputtong, P., in press, *Mae: The Journey of Becoming a Mother amongst Thai Women in Northern Thailand*, Lexington Books: Lanham, MD

Liamputtong, P., Lin, V., & Bagley, P., 2003, 'Living in a Different Place at a Different Time: Health Policy and Australian Ethnic Communities', in P. Liamputtong and H. Gardner (eds.), *Health, social change and communities*, pp. 257-281. Oxford University Press: Melbourne.

Liamputtong, P., & Naksook, C., 2003a. 'Perceptions and Experiences of Motherhood, Health and the Husband's Roles Among Thai Women in Australia', *Midwifery*, 19(1): 27-36.

Liamputtong, P., & Naksook, C., 2003b, 'Life as Mothers in a New Land: The Experience of Motherhood Among Thai Women in Melbourne', *Health Care for Women International*, 24(7): 650-668.

Liamputtong, P., & Tsianakas, V., 2005, 'Motherhood', in S. Joseph (ed.), *Women, gender and health: Policies in East Asia, Southeast Asia, Australia and the Pacific*, pp. ..... A series in the Encyclopedia of Women and Islamic Cultures. Brill Academic Publishers: Leiden.

Liamputtong, P., & Watson, L., 2002, 'The Voices and Concerns About Prenatal Testing of Cambodian, Lao and Vietnamese Women in Australia', *Midwifery*, 18(4): 304-313.

Liamputtong, P., & Watson, L., 2005, 'Motherhood and health: Narratives of Southeast Asian immigrant women in Australia', in R.E. Balin (ed.), *Trends in midwifery research*, pp. 151-165. Nova Science Publishers: New York.

Liamputtong, P., & Watson, L., 2006, 'The Meanings and Experiences of Cesarean Birth Amongst Cambodian, Lao and Vietnamese Immigrant Women in Australia', *Women & Health*, 43(3): 63-81.

Liamputtong, P., Yimyam, S, Parisunyakul, S., Baosoung, C., & Sansiriphun, N., 2005, 'Traditional Beliefs About Pregnancy and Childbirth Among Women from Chiang Mai, Northern Thailand', *Midwifery*, 12(2): 139-153.

Liamputtong, P., Yimyam, S, Parisunyakul, S., Baosoung, C., & Sansiriphun, N., 2004, 'When I Become a Mother!: Discourses of Motherhood Among Thai Women in Northern Thailand', Women's *Studies International Forum*, 27(5-6): 589-601.

Liamputtong, P., Yimyam, S, Parisunyakul, S., Baosoung, C., & Sansiriphun, N., 2002, 'Women as Mothers: The Case of Thai Women from Northern Thailand', *International Social Work*, 45(4): 497-515.

Liamputtong Rice, P., 1993, *My Forty Days: A Cross-Cultural Resource Book for Health Care Professionals in Birthing Services*, The Vietnamese Antenatal/Postnatal Support Project: Melbourne.

Liamputtong Rice, P., 1995, '*Pog Laus, Tsis Coj Khaub Ncaws Lawm*: The Meaning of Menopause in Hmong Women', *Journal of Reproductive and Infant Psychology*, 13: 79-93.

Liamputtong Rice, P., 1997, 'Multiculturalism Policy and Immigrants' Health: Are We Achieving the Goal?', *Australian and New Zealand Journal of Public Health*, 21: 793-794.

Liamputtong Rice, P., (ed.) 1999, *Asian Mothers, Western Births, New Edition*, Ausmed Publications: Melbourne.

Liamputtong Rice, P., 1999, 'Multiculturalism and the Health of Immigrants: What Public Health Issues Do Immigrants Face When They Move to a New Country?', in P. Liamputtong Rice (ed), *Living in a New Country: Understanding Migrants' Health*, pp. 1-21. Ausmed Publications: Melbourne.

Liamputtong Rice, P., 2000a, *Hmong Women and Reproduction*, Bergin & Garvey: Westport, CT.

Liamputtong Rice, P., 2000b, '*Nyo Dua Hli* – 30 Days Confinement: Traditions and Changed Childbearing Beliefs and Practices Among Hmong Women in Australia', *Midwifery*, 16, 22-34.

Liamputtong Rice, P., Ly, B., & Lumley, J., 1994, 'Soul Loss and Childbirth: The Case of a Hmong Woman', *Medical Journal of Australia*, 160: 577-578.

Liamputtong Rice, P., & Manderson, L., (ed.) 1996, *Maternity and Reproductive Health in Asian Societies*, Harwood Academic Press: Amsterdam.

Liamputtong Rice, P., & Naksook, C., 1998a, 'Caesarean or Vaginal Birth!: Perceptions and Experience of Thai Mothers in Australian Hospitals', *Australian and New Zealand Journal of Public Health*, 22(5), 604-608.

Liamputtong Rice, P., & Naksook, C., 1998b, 'The Experience of Pregnancy, Labour and Birth of Thai Women in Australia', *Midwifery*, 14, 74-84.

Liamputtong Rice, P., Naksook, C., & Watson, L.E., 1999, 'The Experiences of Postpartum Hospital Stay and Returning Home Among Thai Mothers in Australia', *Midwifery*, 15: 47-57.

Liddy, U., 1993, *Abortion: Women's Access and Rights in the Context of the Law*, paper presented at the Law, Medicine and Criminal Justice Conference, 6-8 July 1993, Australian Institute of Criminology: Canberra.

Luker, K., 1984, *Abortion and the politics of motherhood*, University of California Press: Berkeley.

Lupton, D., 2000, ''A Love/Hate Relationship': The Ideals and Experiences of First-Time Mothers', *Journal of Sociology*, 36(1): 50-63.

MacCormack, C. P., (ed.) 1982, *Ethnography of Fertility and Birth*, Academic Press: London.

Manderson, L., 1981, 'Roasting, Smoking and Dieting in Response to Birth: Malay Confinement in Cross-Cultural Perspectives', *Social Science & Medicine*, 15B: 509-529.

Manderson, L., 1996, *Sickness and the State: Health and Illness in Colonial Malaya, 1870-1940*, Cambridge University Press: Cambridge.

Mangay-Maglacas, A., & Simons, J. (eds.) 1986, *The Potential of the Traditional Birth Attendant*, World Health Organization: Geneva.

Martin, E., 1992, *The Woman in the Body: A Cultural Analysis of Reproduction*, Beacon Press: Boston.

Maushart, S., 1997, *The Mask of Motherhood: How Mothering Changes Everything and Why We Pretend It Doesn't*, Vintage: Sydney.

McConville, F., 1988, 'The Birth Attendant in Banglasesh', in S. Kitzinger (ed.), *The Midwife Challenge*, pp. 134-153. Pandora: London.

McGilvray, D.B., 1982, 'Sexual Power and Fertility in Sri Lanka: Batticaloa Tamils and Moors', in C.P. MacCormack (ed.), *Ethnography of Fertility and Birth*, pp. 25-73. Academic Press: London.

McMahon, M., 1995, *Engendering Motherhood: Identity and Self-Transformation in Women's lives*, The Guilford Press: New York.

Moskowitz, M.L., 2001, *The Haunting Foetus: Abortion, Sexuality and the Spirit World in Taiwan*, University of Hawai'i Press: Honolulu.

Muecke, M., 1976, 'Health Care Systems as Socializing Agents: Childbearing the North Thai and Western ways', *Social Science and Medicine*, 10: 337-383.

Mundigo, A.I., & Indriso, C. (eds.) 1999, *Abortion in the Developing World*, World Health Organisation and Zed Books: London.

Neff, D.L., 1994, 'The Social Construction of Infertility: The Case of the Matrilineal Nãyars in South India', *Social Science and Medicine*, 39(4): 475-485.

Newman, L.F., 1985, *Women's Medicine: A Cross-Cultural Study of Indigenous Fertility Regulation*, Rutgers University Press: New Brunswick.

Nichter, M., & M. Nichter, 1996, 'Modern Methods of Fertility Regulation: When and For Whom are They Appropriate?', in M. Nichter and M. Nichter (eds), *Anthropology and international health: Asian case studies*, pp. 71-108. Gordon and Breach Publishers: Amsterdam.

Oakley, A., 1979, *Becoming a Mother*, Martin Roberson: Oxford.

Oakley, A., 1986, *The Captured Womb: A History of the Medical Care in Pregnant Women*, Basel Blackwell: New York.

Oylebola, D.D.O., 1981, 'Yoruba Traditional Healers' Knowledge of Contraception, Abortion, and Infertility', *East African Medical Journal*, 58: 777-748.

Petchesky, R.P., 1986, *Abortion and Women's Choice: The State, Sexuality and Reproductive Freedom*, Verso: London.

Petchesky, R.P., 1990, *Abortion and Woman's Choice: The State, Sexuality and Reproductive Freedom*, Northeastern University Press: Boston.

Phillips, D., 1996, 'Medical Professional Dominance and Client Dissatisfaction: A Study of Doctor-Patient Interaction and Reported Dissatisfaction With Medical Care Among Female Patients at Four Hospitals in Trinidad and Tobago', *Social Science and Medicine*, 42: 1419-1425.

Phoenix, A., & Woollett, A., 1991, 'Motherhood: Social Construction, Politics and Psychology', in A. Phoenix, A. Woollett and E. Lloyd (eds.), *Motherhood: Meanings, practices and ideologies*, pp. 13-27. Sage Publications: London.

Pillsbury, B.L.K. (1978). 'Doing the month': Confinement and convalescence of Chinese women after childbirth. *Social Science & Medicine*, 1978, 12, 11-22.

Ram, K., 1994, 'Medical Management and Giving Birth: Responses of Coastal Women in Tamil Nadu', *Reproductive Health Matters*, 4: 20-26.

Rance, S., 2000, 'Safe Motherhood, Unsafe Abortion: A Reflection on the Impact of Discourse', in M. Berer and T.K. Sundari Ravindran (eds.), *Safe Motherhood Initiatives: Critical Issues*, pp. 73-84. Reproductive Health Matters: London.

Rendina, t., & Liamputtong, P., 2006, 'Prenatal Expectations: The Effects on the Experiences of Motherhood and the Mothering Role Among Australian Women', unpublished manuscript submitted for publication to *Midwifery*.

Renne, E.P., 1996, 'The Pregnancy that Doesn't Stay: The Practice and Perception of Abortion by Ekiti Yoruba Women', *Social Science and Medicine*, 42: 483-494.

Rice, P.L., 2000, 'Rooming-In and Cultural Practices: Choice or Constraint?', *Journal of Reproductive and Infant Psychology*, 18(1): 21-32.

Rice, P.L., 1999, 'What Women Say About Their Childbirth Experience?: The Case of Hmong Women in Australia', *Journal of Reproductive and Infant Psychology*, 17(3): 237-253.

Richardson, D., 1993, *Women, Motherhood and Children*, Macmillan: London.

Richens, Y., 2003, *Exploring the Experiences of Women of Pakistan Origin of UK Maternity Services*, Department of Health, London.

Riddle, J.M., 1992, *Contraception and Abortion From the Ancient World to the Renaissance*, Harvard University Press: Cambridge.

Rothman, B.K., 1989, *Recreating Motherhood*, W.W. Norton: New York.

Rozario, S., & Samuel, G. (eds.), *Daughters of Hariti: Childbirth and Female Healers in South and Southeast Asia*, Routledge: London.

Rozario, S., 2002, 'The Healer on the Margins: The Dai in Rural Bangladesh', in S. Rozario & G. Samuel (eds.), *Daughters of Hariti: Childbirth and Female Healers in South and Southeast Asia*, pp. 130-146. Routledge: London.

Rylko-Bauer, B., 1996, 'Abortion From a Crosscultural Perspective: An Introduction', *Social Science and Medicine*, 42: 479-482.

Sargent, C., 1982, 'Solitary Confinement: Birth Practices Among the Bariba of the People's Republic of Benin', in M.A. Kay (ed.), *Anthropology of human birth*, pp. 193-210. F.A. Davis Company: Philadelphia.

Sciarra, J., 1994, 'Infertility: An International Health Problem', *International Journal of Gynecology & Obstetrics*, 46: 155-163.

Sharpe, S., 1984, *Double Identity: The Lives of Working Mothers*, Penguin Books: Harmondsworth.

Shrage, L., 2003, *Abortion and Social Responsibility: Depolarizing the Debate*, Oxford University Press, New York.

Small, R., Liamputtong Rice, P., Yelland, J., & Lumley, J., 1999, 'Mothers in a New Country: The Role of Culture and Communication in Vietnamese, Turkish and Filipino Women's Experiences of Giving Birth in Australia', *Women & Health*, 22(3): 77-101.

Small, R., Lumley, J., Yelland, J., & Liamputtong Rice, P., 1997, *MINC - Mother in a New Country: Vietnamese, Turkish and Filipino Women's Views of Maternity Care*, Centre for the Study of Mothers' and Children's Health: Melbourne.

Small, R., Yelland, J., Lumley, J., Brown, S., & Liamputtong, P., 2002, 'Immigrant Women's Views About Care During Labor and Birth: An Australian Study of Vietnamese, Turkish and Filipino Women', *Birth*, 29(4): 266-277.

Small, R.; Yelland, J.; Lumley, J., & Liamputtong Rice, P., 1998, 'Is Shared Antenatal Care Really Better for Women of Non-English Speaking Background?: The Mothers in a New Country (MINC) Study', *Medical Journal of Australia*, 168 (1): 15-18.

Sobo, E., 1996, 'Abortion Traditions in Rural Jamaica', *Social Science and Medicine*, 42: 495-508.

Squire, C., 1980, *Significant Differences: Feminism and Psychology*, Sage Publications: London.

Stein, E.A., & Inhorn, M.C., 2002. 'Technologies of Pregnancy and Birth', *Feminist Studies*, 28(3): 611-703.

Steinberg, S., 1996, 'Childbearing Research: A Transcultural Review', *Social Science and Medicine*, 43(2): 1765-1784.

Stephens, C., 1992, 'Training Urban Traditional Birth Attendants: Balancing International Policy and Local Reality', *Social Science and Medicine*, 35(6): 811-817.

Straten, G.F.M., Friele, R.D., & Groenewegen, P.P., 2002, 'Public Trust in Dutch Health Care', *Social Science and Medicine*, 55: 227-234.

Sundby, J., 1997, 'Infertility in the Gambia: Traditional and Modern Health Care', *Patient Education and Counselling*, 31: 29-37.

Symonds, P.V., 1991, *Cosmology and the Cycle of Life: Hmong Views of Birth, Death and Gender in a Mountain Village in Northern Thailand*, unpublished doctoral thesis, Brown University: Rhode Island.

Symonds, P.V., 1996, 'Journey to the Land of Light: Birth Among Hmong Women', in P. Liamputtong Rice and L. Manderson (eds.), *Maternity and reproductive health in Asian societies*, pp. 103-123. Harwood Academic Press: Amsterdam.

Szasz, T.S., & Hollenger, M.H., 1956, 'A Contribution to the Philosophy of Medicine: The Basic Models of the Doctor-Patient Relationship', *American Medical Association Archives of Internal Medicine*, 97: 585-592.

Than, A.A., 2003, *Cultural Beliefs of a Group of Bamar Women Regarding Maternal Care: An Ethnographic Study*, unpublished master thesis, School of Nursing and Midwifery, La Trobe University, Melbourne.

Thurtle, V., 2003, 'First Time Mothers' Perceptions of Motherhood and PND', *Community Practitioner*, 76(7): 261-265.

Tiwari, K.C., Majumder, R., & Bhattacharjee, S., 1982, 'Folklore Information from Assam for Family Planning and Birth Control', *International Journal of Crude Drug Research*, 20: 133-137.

Townsend, K., & Liamputtong Rice, P., 1996, 'A Baby is Born in Site 2 Camp: Pregnancy, Birth and Confinement Among Cambodian Refugee Women', in P. Liamputtong Rice and L. Manderson (eds.), *Maternity and Reproductive Health in Asian Societies*, pp. 125-143. Harwood Academic Publishers: Amsterdam.

Tsianakas, V., & Liamputtong, P., 2002a, 'What Women From Islamic Background in Australia Say About Care in Prenatal Testing and Antenatal Care', *Midwifery*, 18(1): 25-34.

Tsianakas, V., & Liamputtong, P., 2002b, 'Perceptions and Experiences of Prenatal Testing Among Muslim Women in Australia', *Journal of Reproductive and Infant Psychology*, 20(1): 7-24.

Turner, V., 1967, *The forest of Symbols*. Cornell University Press: Ithaca.

Turner, V., 1979, 'Betwixt and Between: The Liminal Period in Rites De Passage', in W. Lessa and E.Z. Vogt (eds.), *Reader in Comparative Religion*. Harper and Row: New York.

Van Gennep, A., 1966, *The Rites of Passage*, University of Chicago Press: Chicago

Walraven, G., & Weeks, A., 1999, 'The Role of Traditional Birth Attendants with Midwifery Skills in the Reduction of Maternal Mortality', *Tropical Medicine and International Health*, 4: 527-529.

Weaver, J.J., & Ussher, J.M., 1997, 'How Motherhood Changes Life-A Discourse Analytic Study With Mothers of Young Children', *Journal of Reproductive & Infant Psychology*, 15: 51-68.

Weniger, B., Haag-Berrurier, M., & Anton, R., 1982, "Plants of Haiti Used as Antifertility Agents', *Journal of Ethnopharmacology*, 6: 67-84.

Whiteford, L.M., & Gonzalez, L., 1995, 'Stigma: The Hidden Burden of Infertility', *Social Science and Medicine*, 40(1): 27-36.

Whittaker, A. (2000). *Intimate knowledge: women and their health in North-East Thailand.* Sydney: Allen & Unwin.

Whittaker, A., 2002a, 'Water Serpents and Staying by the Fire: Markers of Maturity in a Northeast Thai Village', In L. Manderson & P. Liamputtong (ed.), *Coming of age in South and Southeast Asia: Youth, courtship and sexuality*, pp. 17-41. Curzon Press: Surrey.

Whittaker, A., 2002b, 'The Demise of Birth Attendants in Northeast Thailand: Embodying Tradition in Modern Times', in S. Rozario & G. Samuel (eds.), *Daughters of Hariti: Childbirth and Female Healers in South and Southeast Asia*, pp. 211-233. Routledge: London.

Whittaker, A., 2004, *Abortion, Sin and the State in Thailand.* RoutledgeCurzon: London.

World Health Organization, 1978, *Alma-Ata 1978 Primary Health Care'*, World Health Organization/United Nations Children's Fund, 6-12 September: Alma-Ata.

Yang, D., 1992, 'The Hmong: Enduring Traditions', in J. Lewis (ed.), *Minority cultures of Laos: Kammu, Lua', Lahu, Hmong, and Iu-Mien*, pp. 249-326. Southeast Asia Community Resource Centre: Rancho Cordova, California.

Yelland, J., Small, R., Lumley, J., Liamputtong Rice, P., Cotronei, V., & Warren, R., 1998, 'Support, Sensitivity, Satisfaction: Vietnamese, Turkish and Filipino Women's Experience of the Postnatal Stay', *Midwifery*, 14(3): 144- 154.

Zadoroznyj, M., 1999, 'Social Class, Social Selves and Social Control in Childbirth', *Sociology of Health & Illness*, 21(3): 267-289.

In: Reproduction, Childbearing and Motherhood
Editor: Pranee Liamputtong, pp. 35-46

ISBN: 978-1-60021-606-0
© 2007 Nova Science Publishers, Inc.

Chapter 2

IMMIGRANT WOMEN AND FERTILITY: GENDER UNDER RE-CONSTRUCTION

Tatjana Alvadj

INTRODUCTION

What happens to a woman who conceptualizes her gender and her fertility in a certain way when she moves from one social, cultural and political environment to another, characterized by disparate social constructions of gender and fertility? What factors encourage her to keep the previously structured identity? What factors force her into a re-construction or acculturation of her gender role and, therefore, a different conception of her fertility? How docs she negotiate these double expectations? What support does she need in order to be successful in that process?

These questions, identified through my community work[1] were the focus of the research project "Immigrant Women and Fertility: Rights and Responsibilities". I conducted the research to complete the academic requirements for the Master of Arts degree at the Department of Anthropology at the University of Alberta, but also to fulfil the obligations to Planned Parenthood Edmonton, the organization that I am affiliated with and that adopted the project and obtained funding from the Status of Women Canada. In that light, the research project brought together all four pillars of the competent community-based research: identified community need, the professional principles of research conduct, the relevant, client oriented non-profit organization that stood behind the project, and the sufficient financial support.

---

[1] In the pilot project "Immigrant women and sexuality: What do we need to know?" that I have conducted in December, 2005, I interviewed the immigrant women working in the area of settlement, who have identified the issues related to fertility important for the process of integration of immigrant women

THEORETICAL STANDPOINT

In the past two decades, feminist anthropologists have taken a closer look into the issues of women's fertility and related issues including pregnancy, medicalization of pregnancy, pregnancy loss, use of reproductive technologies within different cultural settings - Western societies, black and other minority communities in the Western world, and developing countries (Rapp, 2001). Authors such as Ginsburg and Rapp (1991, 1995), Petchesky (1995), and Browner (2001) employed a Marxist approach and perceived biological reproduction as a complex social activity, separate and distinct from the activity of child rearing and central to the reproduction of social life.

> By using reproduction as an entry point to the study of social life, we can see how cultures are produced as people imagine and enable the creation of the next generation, most directly through the nurturance of children. But, it has been anthropology's longstanding contribution that social reproduction entails much more them literal procreation as children are born into complex social arrangements through which legacies of property, positions, rights, and values are negotiated over time. (Ginsburg and Rapp, 1995: 1-2).

Feminist anthropologists criticized the fact that the knowledge about fertility, and social policies emerging from that knowledge and created to affect fertility across the world, rest on research done by demographers and human biologists (Ginsburg and Rapp, 1995; Greenalgh, 1995). It has been argued that these disciplines have taken a narrow approach to the issue of fertility by ignoring the complexity of relations and factors involved in reproductive decisions. From the mid 1980s, feminist anthropological thought has been focused on "politics of reproductive processes, and its implications for gender and cultural construction of the body, sexuality and procreation" (Greenalgh, 1995: 4). Collins (1990), Martin (1992), Ginsburg and Rapp (1995), Lock and Kaufert (1998), Petchesky and Judd (1998) and many other authors have taken a holistic approach to the issue of fertility by asking questions such as: how is agency constituted and how does it influence reproductive dynamics?; how is a female personhood constituted in regard to fertility?; how is gender shaped and re-shaped through reproduction and its control?; finally, how is the power and resistance played out in the context of agency. Inspired by these general questions, this particular research was designed to develop a broader understanding of complexity of reproduction in the context of cultural, political and economical transition from one society to the other.

Although upon their arrival to a host Western country, immigrant women are more likely to have less education and less work experience than their male counterparts (Boyd, 2001), they are more likely to obtain work in the new country before their partners, because the demand for unskilled low paid labour force is still high in the Western world (Buijs, 1993; Kibria, 2000). Pre-migration gender-role patterns and ideologies do not simply disappear; they continue to affect the lives of immigrant women by adding new challenges of racial and social oppression. Feminist scholars state that immigration often leads to losses as well as gains for women, and that patriarchal practices often continue to have an impact on women's lives (Kibria, 2000; Espiritu, 2001; Foner, 2001). The experiences of fertility and the body mirror the turbulences of social change. Strong social pressures coming from outside of the ethno-cultural communities are tied with women's involvement in a public arena (school, work). Consequently, immigrant women are forced to challenge their gender, and their reproductive behaviours.

THE RESEARCH FOCUS

In the research, I focused on the women born abroad, in the countries with significantly high birth rates, who arrived to Canada between three and ten years ago. The participants of the research were African, Haitian and Kurdish women, the visible minority women who as newcomers, despite belonging to different social classes and/or having a different level of education in their home countries, share similar experiences including a "triple burden: gender inequalities [are] compound by discrimination on the basis of class and race/ ethnicity" (Foner, 2001:1) upon immigration. Therefore, the term 'immigrant women' in the context of this research carries the notion not just of ethno-cultural background profoundly different from the Canadian one, but also the connotations of the specific social, economic and political status imposed on women coming from these specific backgrounds.

The participants (21) in the study were self-selected individuals who showed the interest in, and shared concerns about the status of immigrant women. They volunteered to participate in the study after the goals of the research were discussed with them. The majority of participants arrived to Canada between 1998 and 2001. Their age ranged from 25 to 48, with the majority in their thirties. They were all, except one, currently married. One woman did not have children at the time of the research, and one was pregnant with her first child. Other women had between one and eight children, with the majority having three or fewer children.

Being an immigrant woman (from Bosnia) myself, living and working in Edmonton, Canada, where I conducted the study, I did not need to leave my ordinary everyday life and step into the land unknown. Staying in my own and familiar environment, I carved the 'fieldwork' out of my existing reality. As some urban anthropologists have already reported (Martin, 1992; Spitzer, 1998), such fieldwork does not allow one to distance oneself physically or emotionally, to take a break or simply to go home to one's real life. In such circumstances, it is difficult to define when fieldwork has started and when it has finished. My professional experience in working with immigrant women began long before the formal beginning of the research. It continued after the data collection was completed. The opportunity to discuss the gender and fertility in the process of transition gave the necessary stimulation to some of the groups and individuals I have met that led to the individual action and community mobilization. These actions forced me to stay engaged in the process that we initiated together. With some of the women, I continued to meet regularly, assisting with the resources mostly related to family planning. In a way, the fieldwork has never stopped despite of formally completed data collection.

Having said that, it came natural to choose the method of data collection that will preserve the authenticity of the circumstances under which the study was conducted. Therefore, I followed the format of group gathering that some women previously have already established as a way of mutual support and turned it into a group discussion. This method enabled me a delicate transition from the informal gatherings that women were used to towards the formal dialogue that allowed me to collect the data. Individual interviews were used as the additional tool. They served the purpose of more personal interaction and a chance for exploring some of the issues that I sensed during the group discussions as important but not suitable for the group setting. Finally, with some of the women I spent time either meeting them at different community events, visiting them at home, accompanying them to the Birth Control Clinic, or talking on the phone with them. That gave me the opportunity to observe other aspects of their lives, and learn about their family circumstances.

In analyzing the data, my focus was on what the women said, how they related to their stories, and sometimes what they avoided to say. I paid attention to their emotions: frustrations, sorrow, irony, and humour. I searched for the signs of their power and strengths and the areas of struggle and vulnerability. I was aware and respectful of the differences among them: educated women, illiterate women, young women, mature women, black women, veiled women, political immigrants, refugees. Individually, the women were so different, and by coming closer to any of them, the construction of the whole "story" tended to take a different shape and direction. However, I was searching for the common ground I defined as a transition. The transition is not a clean, linear and uniform "progress" of a programmed integration and change. It is a messy, dynamic, contested and conflicting time of living and understanding, rejecting and accepting the change of identity, gender, body and mind. The challenge for the researcher is communicate the dynamics of conflicting forces that makes the experience of womanhood, immigration and fertility a complex social, political and cultural process. In doing so, I am aware that I had to insist on commonalities among women, on harmonizing and focusing their voices into a few precisely formulated "policy recommendations". So, my challenge was to be a "composer" who can create intelligible music that will communicate the important message about immigration, women, fertility and change, but also a listener of individual voices that carry their own life and their own story.

INVISIBLE WOMEN

The majority of respondents in the study defined qualities such as respectful, hard working, obedient, fertile, devoted to the husband, family and community as the characterizing features of their gender in the countries of origin When thinking back about their lives before migration, the women reported that being a "good wife" was not limited to an individual woman and her relationship with her marital partner, but included other responsibilities to the broader collective. Women simultaneously functioned on different levels of community involvement combining a private and public domain of life. The individual roles as wives and mothers were defined by their social involvement as active participants in the family and community life as well as by their social and economic contribution that includes producing a desirable number of children and, often, financial contribution through the paid work or dowry.

All the respondents reported that being the mother was the central point of the realization of gender role in the country of origin. Having children was often used as an instrument to fulfil social, economical, and political aspirations of the different factors involved within the broader collective. These factors may include god, ethnic group and its political and economic agenda, the local community, the extended family with the mother-in-law as a leading character, the husband and, finally, the woman herself and her own aspirations and biological abilities to reproduce. They seem to be placed around an individual woman in spiral circles, not necessarily all of them, or in the same particular order. They are connected by complex social, political, economic, cultural and spiritual links and "are as likely to be antagonistic as mutually supportive" (Browner, 2001: 774). In such circumstances where female fertility functions as an economic, political and social mechanism, the number of children is rarely limited.

> When you had a lot of children it was a wealth. …. Having a big number of children was a wealth and also a pride for the family… (Gaby)
> So, a good wife must have lots of children. Yes, because we are caring a new generation, we have to have more children. (Lisa)
> And it was also blessing to have kids. It was nobody's decision It was just natural thing to do…I don't think somebody had to tell [a woman] to get pregnant or not… (Linda)

The women's lives change after the migration, affected by different social circumstances and cultural expectations. Various priorities (need to learn the language and improve the standard of living, family obligations, childbearing and childrearing) compete with each other in a furious pace. The new social environment influences a new hierarchy of power: the distant, bureaucratic mainstream institutions take the place of the familiar patriarchal collective left behind in the countries of origin. These new establishments of power set the rules and policies that control the lives and oversee the integration process of immigrant women. At the same time, the diminished power of the collective in the country of origin contributes to development of new gender roles within the family where the woman, a newly established "individual", acquires significantly different authority in decision making process. This new situation simultaneously works to a woman's advantage and disadvantage. Acquired social freedoms are paid in social isolation and enforced choices. In many views, the new social order of power reflects the one left behind in perverted, up-side-down fashion.

As a result of migration and change of social and cultural context, the interdependence of women, fertility and collective social wellbeing has been distorted. The environment, where the whole community celebrates the role of a mother and wife, has disappeared after immigration. The female fertile body has been moved from the center to the periphery of the social universe. The physical, emotional and social experience of pregnancy and childbirth suddenly become characterized by pain, fear, and solitude. Lola claimed that "some women are afraid to have a baby here"; Linda recalled that "you are in so much pain and there is no support for you." Ruth added:

> When I gave birth [back home], everybody worried about me. Everybody had attention for the baby and me. I didn't need to think about the baby that much. Here, when I came from the hospital, I just opened the door and no one was at home. I was crying, oh my God…And the next day, my husband had to go to work, and I was alone all day. Nobody asked me if I had something to eat or drink… It is hard here.

The absence of the family and community turns childbearing and childrearing as a collective endeavor into often a sole responsibility of the woman. While husband is at work, she is the one who is left to deal with problems of loneliness, depression, financial problems and confusion over priorities. The time spent at home with her babies Linda describes as at first "*shocking*", and then "*a very, very lonesome time*". Angie says that by having children without help of the extended family "*you are killing yourself*". The absence of "the big family", as one participant described the community back home, deprives the women from the collective support, sense of belonging and emotional and social shelter. The new social world around the fertile female body changes its shape and function. Consequently, female fertility is getting a different meaning. Being a mother is still very important, but is now a lonely business that gives fewer benefits and many pressures. The prosperity of the family as a whole is based on fewer, not more children.

> I am on birth control. I am not going to have more…it is no way for me to bring more children. I need to upgrade my skills, I need to learn English and I need to go and have a job otherwise my children will not have a good life. (Selma)

The change in participants' tone when comparing the past and the present life, from cheerful enthusiasm about the number and role of the children in the family to rational recognition of the reality counted in dollars and personal sacrifices, is a result of not so much internally changed values as they are the consequences of the imposed reality that does not leave lots of choices. Handwerker (1990: 31) explains that the change in perspective and behaviour happens when access to resources is improved or optimized by that change. This study shows how fertility in the Canadian context starts to prevent immigrant women from achieving a better living standard, accessing education and obtaining work. Consequently, the role of fertility and women's reproductive behaviour is forced to change and find a new a meaning.

The same circumstances that initiate the feelings of loss and grief over the lost world of community support helped to establish new power relations within the family that promotes women to make individual decisions. The change in family dynamic is visible in different aspects of women's lives. The power of absent extended family and their influence on women's fertility is minimized. Many women in the study, encouraged by safe, physical distance from the rest of the family, reported firm confrontations with the family members, especially the dreaded mother-in-law, who before migration held the absolute power over their lives.

> Even now my mother-in-law says 'only two, only two' [children]. I say to her that two is enough. She is far away, so I can tell her that, but if I was there, it will be more difficult because there is more pressure from everywhere. By phone it is not a big problem (laughs), you don't see them or you can say 'wrong number, wrong number!' (All women laugh) (Lola)

However, the humorous interludes and jokes about in-laws do not hide the serious issues of personal transformation. The reproductive views and choices are the result of the search for an appropriate balance between the respect for the culture of origin and acceptance of Canadian reality. It involves confronting the building elements of one's own self, one's own past and presence, and complicated re-construction of identity. In that course of self-realization, women feel as winner and loser at the same time.

> It is a challenge sometimes. It is a conflict between our culture and Canadian culture. Family back home, they don't understand why you want only one kid. They don't understand how it is expensive. But, at the end of the day, you have to deal with that. You have that choice. (Lilly)

> Some are good changes for the women, in terms of giving them more independence. Bad changes are that we cannot have more children. (Moyo)

Husbands, often frustrated with the loss of social surrounding dominated by patriarchal kinship system that enhanced their individual power, discouraged by degradation of their professional status, physically squeezed in tiny apartments with their families, and, equally to their wives, isolated from the rest of the society, have also changed their role. The "boss", as Zoe defined her husband's role back home, has been transformed to more of an equal, intimate partner. In analyzing the change in the behaviour, the participants easily pointed out the influence of the new cultural and social surrounding.

> The husbands now stay more at home, spend more time with the kids and are more involved with children schooling. This is another thing that changed. (Marie)

Changes in the relationship with the husband are a result of the change of the social and political factors influencing and defining the relationship. Browner (2001: 774) describing the "conjugal dynamic", argues that in "any society, each individual women has her own particular political relationship with her male partner". I find this concept similar to Kandiyoti's (1988: 275) idea of "the patriarchal bargain" that even more precisely illustrates the new situation for immigrant women: the women are using "their heightened resources to cope more effectively with male authority" (Kibria, 2000: 188) within a still existing patriarchal order. In other words,

> [The traditional values] are still the same, but they modified to suit the life style here. That change is that we see more women working outside and more men staying home. That had change. Men don't get as much job as women here. Here, you still have to obey your husband, but here in the decision-making you have to be part of it if he disagrees on same thing he has to give a very good reason for that. (Ruth)

In such circumstances, the sense of self as an individual with individual power consequently rises, establishing, among other new realizations, the practice of using contraceptives not only as a way to limit the size of the family and maintain the optimum standard of living, but also to achieve desired personal goals in terms of education and work. Instead of a god given virtue and a natural circle of events, as they described childbearing back home, fertility becomes an ability that can be controlled and regulated by individual human actions. Lola, whose husband would like to have more than two children, explained:

> He understands because this is what I want. I hold the baby…yeah! We don't fight for that! He wants more, I want less…but, we don't fight for that. He knows that, if I don't want, we will not have because of me. I know how to control myself. It depends on me. He does not force me for that.

Although the majority of respondents reported having more decision making power over their reproductive choices, they state also that *"many women in the community are afraid of their husbands"* who do not allow them to use birth control. As one respondent points out, many women believe that by *"having fewer babies, you will not keep the husband"*. In addition, some respondents reported that they chose birth control out of fear and confusion.

Often, the choice of birth control conflicted with their personal beliefs about fertility, body and bodily integrity. Angie, in her emotional monologue, explains:

> I think that God gave me my body to keep as it is. I think God gave me my body and I want to return one day to him with my body. So, what happened after my last child? I had to take a bitter decision to have my tubes tied. I didn't want to have more because it is too much for me. For me, this option was more secure, because I didn't want to live with the stress of being pregnant again. So, I did it even though I didn't like it. I did it because of the society I am living in it and about the future I have to plan. It is not easy.

In the Western societies, choice stands for "autonomy, independence, and freedom of will, signifying women's sense of themselves as having an influence on the process in which they are engaged" (Becker, 2000: 243). Handwerker (1990: 25) correctly argues, "genuine 'freedom of choice' exists only when you can choose among selectively neutral alternatives". Women in this study often do not perceive the existence of 'neutral alternatives' as a part of their reality. This complex reality has been lost somewhere in the chaos of societal pressures, perplexity over the individual priorities, grief over lost identities and celebration of new empowerments. The real political challenge for immigrant women is how to communicate that reality to the mainstream institutions that shape the programs and policies for them based on completely opposite premises of organized rationality and undisputable existence of a clear choice.

The program of integration and adaptation to Canadian society provides immigrant women with language and work training, but does not incorporate any cross- cultural reference to female fertility. The mainstream institutions that control and regulate immigrant women's lives are shaped by the fundamental Western belief that the boundaries between biological, psychological and social aspects of a person are arranged in separate compartments and should be taken autonomously. The ideology of individualism and rationality, the obsession with separation of private and public life, accompanied with the notion of 'freedom of choice', do not allow these institutions to acknowledge the obvious disparity between the reality of immigrant women's lives and programs and services offered to assist them in their integration.. The programs and services are created on the basis of what Craib (1994: 91) calls 'functional rationality' of modern societies, a direct or indirect intervention of the institutions of power into the lives of the individuals and their relationships "through policies of economic welfare and social services" Under such circumstances, female fertility is perceived as a private matter, and women are forced by the system to choose between the private (family, pregnancy, childbirth) and public matters (education, work).

> For a woman, you cannot miss school, even when your child is sick or you are pregnant, or you have a baby. No! You cannot even be allowed to go to the washroom, because for the teacher you are disturbing the class. When I was eight months pregnant, the teacher told me to quit school, because I was asking frequently to go to the washroom. (Lisa)
>
> School…doesn't treat us as human beings. Some women even preferred to quit school instead of being abused by the system. (Moyo)
>
> Me, I didn't tell them that I was pregnant, I had to hide and during my practicum some time I couldn't do all the work but, I didn't have the choice. I couldn't have sick leave; otherwise I could lose my funding. (Mary)

The simple solution offered by a participant that those African women who want children should still have the chance *"to learn the language and be part of this society"* does not resonate in the rules and policies imposed on immigrant women. Pushed into the space where the individual, as Bhabha (1994: 47) describes, "speaks, and is seen, from where is *not",* immigrant women are unimportant and invisible in their true identities, in their full experience, and left in reality of representations, images, or, plainly, prejudices.

ACTION

The women who participated in the study have demonstrated noticeable areas of strengths: the strong dedication to successful integration, enhanced individual power in decision making-process within the family and community and openness for new knowledge and change. In addition, they spoke about the areas of present struggles: the social isolation, the challenge to integrate the fertile body into the newly established context of societal expectations, social discrimination and insufficient knowledge of and access to contraceptives. Their experiences helped to distinguish the foci of the future community actions and create the action plan that was developed to influence the upcoming efforts towards empowerment of immigrant women and improvement of their social status through the additional research as well as enhanced community work.

The issues of fertility of immigrant women cannot be isolated from the realm of domesticity and privacy. To leave it there means to deny its obvious social and political connotation and create the room for growing injustice and biases. To bring it out into the broad daylight of social attention requires the action of empowerment, enhancing the "ability to control our own lives" (Ristock & Pennell, 1996:1) on various levels: individual, communal, organizational and political.

The project's efforts stimulated the discussion about fertility among the participants and transferred the problem from the periphery to the center of interest. The individual experiences of coping with fertility in a process of integration have been validated and recognized as important in immigrant women's life. As a result, some participants have been encouraged to get involved in the attempts to "do something about it" and actively participate in the planning of the further actions. The others were motivated to consult on birth control options and asked for the support in the decision making process. In either way, there was an element of individual empowerment expressed in terms of stirring participation and enhanced access to the resources.

On the community level, the participants suggested further expansion of discussions, and creation of a stronger female network of support. Such a network would simulate the kind of support that they have had in their home countries and stimulate information sharing and mutual help in a form of regular meetings but also drop-in centres for immigrant women.

However, the community effort alone is not sufficient without the serious change in policies that regulate the programs for immigrant women. As a necessary step towards that objective, the organization of a broader political body, the mobilization of agencies serving immigrant women in a form of coalition that will facilitate the process of organizational and political change is necessary. These organization should come together to build a political front with an objective of presenting the issue of fertility as the critical question for immigrant women in the process of integration and settlement and advocating for chages that include:

- in-site and outreach, culturally appropriate counselling on reproductive health for women and their partners;
- culturally appropriate representation of reproductive health issues as a component of English as a Second Language courses and academic up-grading curriculum;
- educational and recreational immigrant women's drop-in centres;
- mandatory day care facilities;
- optional home-based English as a Second Language education for women with newborns;

CONCLUSION AND IMPLICATIONS FOR WOMEN'S HEALTH CARE

The focus of the research project "Immigrant women and fertility: Rights and Responsibilities" was on immigrant women's experience of integration into Canadian society through the lenses of fertility and reproductive decisions that they have chosen or they have been forced to choose. The participants emphasized both the social isolation and lack of support as a result of disappearance of the family and community and a new experience of the modern state that demands integration through programs and services characterized by ignorance and discrimination. As a result, childbearing becomes a barrier in the process of integration and, as such, creates the uncertainty over priorities and, often, the need for contraceptives as the instrument enabling them to limit the size of the family and create necessary opportunities. In the decision making process, immigrant women, although pressured by the society to make 'rational' choices, find some room for individual agency. Partly liberated from patriarchal dominance of the husband and extended family, they negotiate their new position within the society, considering the responsibilities to the weakened collective, but also the newly established individual rights that enable them to re-direct the course of their actions towards the goals that could eventually benefit their individual wellbeing.

This study was conducted not only to identify the issues related to immigrant women and fertility, but to put together the basis for further actions towards the policy change in the domain of immigrant settlement. These further actions include building the stronger voice of immigrant women through the collaboration of agencies serving immigrant women, focusing on creating a common political platform to address the need for gender appropriate programs and services, and advocating effective and immediate change of existing settlement practices. These changes are directed to the implementation of in-site and outreach, culturally appropriate counselling for women, mandatory daycare in all immigrant serving facilities, outreach, home based English As a Second Language education as well as recreational and educational drop-in centers for immigrant women. The work that is required to achieve these goals will give the extended life to this project that enters its second phase.

REFERENCES

Becker, G., 2000, *The Elusive Embryo: How Women and Men Approach New Reproductive Technologies,* University of California Press: Barkley Los Angeles London.

Bhabha, H., 1994, *The Location of Culture,* Routledge:London and New York.

Boyd, M., 2001, 'Gender, Refugee Status, and Permanent Status', in R. J. Simon (ed.), *Immigrant women,* pp.103-24. Transaction Publisher: New Brunswick (USA) London (UK).

Browner, C.H., 2001, 'Situating Women's Reproductive Activities', *American Anthropologis,* 102(4): 773 - 88.

Buijs, G., 1993, *Migrant Women: Crossing Boundaries and Changing Identities,* Berg: Oxford Providence.

Collins, P.H., 1990, *Black Feminist Thought: Knowledge, Consciousness, and the Politics of Empowerment,* Routledge: New York London.

Craib, I., 1994, *Importance of Disappointment,* Routledge: London and New York.

Espiritu, Y.L., 2001, '"We Don't Sleep Around Like White Girls Do": Family, Culture, and Gender in Filipina American Lives', *Signs: Journal of women in Culture and Society,* 26(2): 415 - 40.

Foner, N., 2001, 'Benefits and Burdens: Immigrant women and Work in New York City', in R. J. Simon (ed.), *Immigrant women,* pp.103-24. Transaction Publisher: New Brunswick (USA) and London (UK).

Ginsburg, F.D. & Rapp, R., 1991, 'The Politics of Reproduction', *Annual Review of Anthropology,* 20: 311 - 41.

Ginsburg, F.D. & Rapp, R., 1995, *Conceiving the New World Order: The Global Politics of Reproduction,* University of California Press: Berkeley, CA.

Greenhalgh, S., 1995, *Situating Fertility: Anthropology and Demographic Iinquiry,* University Press: Cambridge.

Handwerker, P. W., 1990, *Births and Power: Social Change and the Politics of Reproduction,* Westview Press: Boulder, San Francisco & London.

Kandiyoti, D., 1988, 'Bargaining with Patriarchy', *Gender and Society,* 2 (3): 274 - 90.

Kibria, N., 2000, 'Power, Patriarchy, and Gender Conflict in Vietnamese Immigrant Community', in K. Willis and B. Yeoh (eds.), *Gender and Migration,* pp. 177- 92. An Elgar Reference Collection: Cheltenham, UK and Northampton, MA, USA.

Lock, M. and Kaufert, P., 1998, *Pragmatic Women and Body Politics,* University Press: Cambridge.

Martin, E., 1992, *The Woman in the Body: A Cultural Analysis of Reproduction,* Beacon Press: Boston.

Petchesky, R.P., 1995, 'The Body as Property: A Feminist Re-vision', in F.D. Ginsburg and R. Rapp, (eds.), *Conceiving the New World Order: The Global Politics of Reproduction,* pp. 387-406. University of California Press: Berkeley, CA.

Petchesky, R.P. and Judd, K., 1998, *Negotiating Reproductive Rights,* Zed Books: London and New York.

Rapp, R., 2001, 'Gender, Body, Biomedicine: How Some Feminist Concerns Dragged Reproduction to the Center of Social Theory', *Medical Anthropology Quarterly,* 15(4): 466-77.

Ristock, J.L. and Pennell, J., 1996, *Community Research as Empowerment,* Oxford University Press: Toronto New York Oxford.

Spitzer, D.L., 1998, *Migration and Menopause: Women's Experience of Maturation in Three Immigrant Communities*, unpubblished doctorial thesis, University of Alberta, Canada.

In: Reproduction, Childbearing and Motherhood
Editor: Pranee Liamputtong, pp. 47-62

ISBN: 978-1-60021-606-0
© 2007 Nova Science Publishers, Inc.

Chapter 3

BURMESE WOMEN AND UNWANTED PREGNANCY: 'I THOUGHT MY BLOOD WAS STUCK INSIDE ME'

Suzanne Belton

INTRODUCTION

Pregnancy is not always welcomed or for that matter acknowledged. And while for most women who desire a baby, the first signs and feelings associated with pregnancy are joyful this is not the case for many women who live in the borderlands of Thailand and Burma. In 2002, I was asked by local Thai and Burmese doctors[1] in Tak Province, Thailand to study their patients who presented with pain, bleeding and infected miscarriages. Many Burmese women live in resource-poor settings, disadvantaged by political conflict and chronic poverty, and an unwanted pregnancy sets up a chain of difficult questions and circumstances to navigate. This situation is further complicated in that many Burmese women live in Thailand, often as undocumented migrant workers, stateless and in fear of deportation back to Burma. Without their immediate families for support and usual networks, they find resourceful ways to regulate their fertility which include traditional and cosmopolitan methods. The methods employed are reasonably effective but in the process of regaining a normal menstrual cycle, serious illness, shame, expense and worry are often endured. In some cases death is the result. This chapter will describe the cultural issues in unwanted pregnancy and fertility regulation by Burmese women who live in Thailand.

BACKGROUND

Unsafe abortion is a considerable cause of maternal mortality and morbidity (Nongluck Boonthai and Warakamin Suwanna, 2000; Ahman and Shah, 2002). It is most often found

---

[1] I would like to thank doctors Cynthia Maung, Coordinator of the Mae Tao Clinic and Dr Lek Nopdonrattakoon, Chief of the Department of Obstetrics and Gynaecology Mae Sot Public Hospital for their kind assistance with this study and their ongoing care of Burmese women.

where elective, legal abortion is not possible and those most affected are disadvantaged women (Ankomah et al., 1997; Bankole et al., 1998). Wealthy, educated women from resource-rich countries rarely die from botched abortions. Like many other causes of maternal mortality, unsafe abortion is entirely preventable with sexual health education, accessible contraception, communities who value women, trained health professionals to provide comprehensive reproductive care and a legal system which diminishes the likelihood of harm from unregulated abortion. The right to choose the number and timing of pregnancies is enshrined in the Convention on the Elimination of Discrimination Against Women (CEDAW), an international convention signed by 180 nations or over ninety percent of the members of the United Nations. Both Thailand and Burma are signatories to CEDAW yet women continue to suffer and die from reproductive related causes (Royal Thai Government, 1997; Union of Myanmar, 1999).

Burma is a rogue state, characterised by political conflict, widespread poverty and human rights abuses (Rotberg, 1998). Many Burmese are forced to migrate to Thailand to escape these events and find work. The deteriorating economic conditions in rural and urban areas in Burma are cited by men and women as strong reasons to leave the country. Burma's failing economy and food scarcity are well documented and contribute to poor health, malnutrition and people using trafficking practices to enter Thailand for paid work (Asian Migrant Centre & Migrant Forum in Asia, 2003; Federation of Trade Unions-Burma, 2002; World Bank, 1995 to 2002).[2]

There is an estimated one to one-and-a-half million migrant workers in Thailand, the vast majority from Burma (Royal Thai Government, 2001; Asian Migrant Centre & Migrant Forum in Asia, 2002). However, the figures are probably an underestimate (Wong and Singh, 1999). The number of work permits issued by the Employment Department never concurs with NGO estimates of the numbers of migrant workers in Thailand (Federation of Trade Unions-Burma 2002). Once in Thailand, women are often employed illegally in menial jobs such as petrol pump assistants, household servants, waitresses, unskilled factory workers, labourers or farm-hands. Their employment contracts, working conditions and wages are below those expected by Thai citizens (Darunee Paisanpanichkul, 2001; Pim Koetsawang, 2001; Chuthatip Maneepong, 2003). There is no maternity leave offered to illegal workers and they can be sacked at the employer's whim. If women hold a work permit it can be cancelled if they are found to be pregnant. Thailand offers an insecure sanctuary to convention refugees and migrant workers from Burma.

METHOD

With the help of local male and female research assistants, I interviewed Thai and Burmese health workers (20), traditional birth attendants (lay midwives) (20), women who were recovering after any type of abortion (43), and men (10). I conducted a retrospective medical record review of 232 cases of suspected abortion admitted to either the informal

---

[2] Human smuggling or trafficking is common and most people need the assistance of an employment broker to cross the border and locate a job. Thai and Burmese work as traffickers and Thai police are frequently implicated in organising illegal employment. The fee to engage a human smuggler is between 2,500 Baht to 6,000 Baht (Caouette et al., 2000; Federation of Trade Unions-Burma, 2002).

Burmese Mae Tao Clinic or the Thai Mae Sot General Hospital. I lived in Mae Sot town in Tak Province, Thailand for ten months during the research and took part in clinical and social occasions with Thai and Burmese people. This also gave me the opportunity to interview and discuss the situation with community leaders, women's groups and non-government organisations working in health and welfare. The results were fed back to local groups and key informants for further clarification and analysis and a report was co-authored with Dr Cynthia Maung and results presented in a doctoral thesis (Maung and Belton, 2004; Belton, 2005).

THEORETICAL STANDPOINT

As a feminist researcher I have privileged women's voices and considered women's right to decide the number and timing of her offspring according to international human rights theory and law. So I came to the research without notions of blame and some empathy to the plight of women. I am firstly trained in bio-medicine and my nursing and midwifery skills and knowledge were indispensable in understanding physical symptoms, interpreting medical records and talking with health workers. Western bio-medicine may appear theory-free but it is not. While many of bio-medicine's theories are proven we still cannot answer questions about the beginning of life in its embryonic form or why some pregnancies end, and in the developed world, women often tussled with these dilemmas. As a medical anthropologist I was tasked to listen and represent other forms of knowledge. Eastern forms of medicine also have long traditions and ways of comprehending the body and its functions in health and illness. I was interested in the nexus between the two and how women navigated their reproductive lives.

SOCIAL AND CULTURAL CONTEXT : WORKING WIVES

All the women interviewed were married and two thirds were already mothers. Women defined their own ethnic identity, some stating they had parents from different Burmese ethnic groups[3]. Ethnicity, therefore, is not necessarily a discrete category. Burmese was the most common language spoken and understood by informants, followed by Sgaw Karen. About a quarter of the women interviewed could not read basic Burmese or Karen languages and the rest only had three to four years of school. The vast majority of women interviewed were Buddhists but most religious beliefs were represented. The majority of women were long-term residents with three years of more in Thailand. Most of the women were in paid employment and contributed to the family income. Only nine out of thirty-five women in paid employment had valid work permits. Six women disclosed domestic violence in their relationship.

An abortion is defined biomedically as any loss of pregnancy before foetal viability. Foetal viability, the ability to live independently from mother, the uterus and placenta is

---

[3] The Burman state (Union of Myanmar) has over one hundred ethnic minority groups, some of whom continue a political or armed resistance to the dominant Burman majority. The Karen people form a large minority group some of whom are Buddhist, Christian or animist and who reject Burman state control of their affairs.

frequently defined by law (Rahman et al., 1998). Bio-medical foetal viability hovers around 24 weeks (or 500g) in environments where the best technological expertise and facilities are available (Petchesky, 1987; Llewellyn-Jones, 1999). In order for a very premature baby to survive, it needs piped oxygen, incubators, medicine and specialised nursing and medical care. The health facilities in the town were not able to provide intensive neonatal nursing, even in the Thai public hospital. The Thai obstetrician reported that neonates born prematurely at 28 weeks (7 months) have a poor survival chance in his neonatal intensive care unit. Therefore in this area, the pragmatic access to resources found more weight in defining a foetus' or infant's chance of survival than the law. In Western medicine abortions are defined as spontaneous or intentional (elective) and furthermore law defines them as illegal or legal.

In Tak province, it is difficult to identify women who are miscarrying (aborting) or at what stage in the process of abortion they are in, due to cultural understandings, the socio-political environment and the limited access to medical technology. Other research on abortion in similar environments does not mention the difficulties inherent in selecting research subjects other than stating that secrecy and illegality are barriers (Ankomah et al., 1997; Baretto et al., 1992; Chalida Gespradit, 2002; Huntington et al., 1993; Pongsatha et al., 2002). However, Tamang's (1996) hospital based survey in Nepal of 1,241 women does admit to incorrectly classifying 22 women during the research process as well as interviewing 103 women with a threatened abortion[4]. Tamang notes that women have the final option in defining the pregnancy loss rather than the clinician. Tamang found that 20% of the women interviewed in hospital had induced their abortion, which is a somewhat lower rate than for either Thai or Burmese women. An earlier article from 1992 in the same area also used a graduated taxonomy of abortion 'induced', 'possibly induced' and 'spontaneous' and found a rate of 10.5% non-spontaneous abortions in women admitted to hospital with abortion related complications (Thapa et al. 1992).

BLOCKED MENSTRUATION AND MORAL IMPERATIVES: RESULTS AND DISCUSSION

In Tak province, there is no common understanding of what an abortion is, either by health workers or women. Abortion is ambiguous in sites of low-technology. I argue that definitions and categories have cultural explanations which make sense, and the viability of the embryo, foetus or even neonate, is dependant on the perceptions of the woman and health care provider. Local understandings of foetal anatomy and physiology need to be included when analysing pregnancy loss, not just legal or bio-medical categories.

Women and lay midwives have their own cultural definitions of viability and abortion just as cosmopolitan medicine and national law does. Access to modern health knowledge and technology influences local understanding of fertility, pregnancy and abortion but may not replace cultural understandings. During interviews women, talked about their menstruation being 'blocked' for several months and taking herbal medicines to 'unblock' it. It would seem that they were indeed pregnant and had aborted themselves, but this was not always defined

---

[4] A threatened abortion is a transient episode, some small bleed that may or may not terminate the pregnancy. Beischer & Mackay (1986) suggest that 25 to 30% of spontaneous abortions are threatened, and some continue to a 40 week complete pregnancy; others end.

by them as an abortion. A married Burman woman with a five year old child who experienced a miscarriage after four months of amenorrhoea said:

> I thought my blood was stuck inside me. I didn't think I was pregnant but when it was nearly four months I thought I should come and do the urine test. Then I started bleeding for one day just a little. I thought 'Oh here is my period', then it stopped for four days but then it started again heavier. I was worried so I came here.

A naïve 31-year-old childless woman who had only been married for six months was admitted to the Thai hospital also with the diagnosis of an incomplete abortion. She was also surprised to be pregnant:

> This is my first pregnancy. I wasn't sure if I was pregnant or not – I only knew that my period was ten days late. I took Kathy Pan [5] ('hot' herbal medicine), ten tablets per day for two days. I took four packets or twenty tablets in total. The next day I bled a little. There was no pain. I never used it when I was single. My periods are normally regular. They always come at the same time of the month. Nobody told me to take it I just bought some by myself. I didn't have problems like vomiting or no appetite, you know, signs of pregnancy so I thought I wasn't. I don't feel anything about this pregnancy. I don't want a baby now. I am old I don't want to deliver a baby. I also thought I was too old to get pregnant. If I knew that I was fertile I would have used htou: zei[6]. After I got married I didn't use anything you see...I feel ashamed of myself because now everyone thinks I aborted my baby.[7]

Her intention was to regulate her period with the emmenagogue (*Kathy Pan*), not to abort as she did not think she was pregnant. A young lay midwife in the rural area who offers injections but insists she is not an abortionist, told us how to 'see the blood'.

> If a woman is single and she hasn't seen her period for up to ten weeks I give her Duoton Forte TP to bring down her blood. It's ok in women who have never had a baby but not ok in women who have. It is *thwei: zei purzee* – medicine to see the blood.[8]

She does not question why 'single' women had not seen a period in ten weeks. Menstruation can be erratic and the absence of regular periods does not always indicate a pregnancy. Fertility is not assumed and authors writing on women living in conditions of poverty confirm that fertility must be proven as malnutrition, mal-development, anaemia, and

---

[5] *Kathy Pan* is a common Burmese medicine for 'menstrual ailments' produced by a Burman business in San Chuang Township in Rangoon (Myat Chan-Tha Medical Hall, 2003). It is widely available in pharmacies, herbal shops and local markets in both Burma and Thailand. Myat Chan-Than informs the purchaser that *Kathy Pan* is made of 'rare, costly herbs'. They make no secret about the ingredients: Indian redwood tree, black pepper, nutmeg, cloves, sandalwood, camphor, and in smaller quantities, rosy leadwort, red sanders, white sandalwood, fennel, garden cress, and dill. Nutmeg is probably the active ingredient. It is found on the tree *Myristica fragrans*. Nutmeg is psychotropic narcotic. It is toxic if taken in large quantities and produces vertigo, flushing, stupor, and psychological disturbance such as hallucinations and altered consciousness – and one recorded death. It is also recorded as an emmenagogue and abortifacient (Weil, 1966). The very specific instructions for women that are included in packets of *Kathy Pan*) relate directly to humoral health, to the balance of hot and cold in the body, and to restore and promote the flow of blood.

[6] A Burman word glossed as a Depot Medroxyprogesterone Acetate intra-muscular injection such as Depo Provera or Depo Ralovera. The chemical is similar to the hormone progesterone.

[7] *Thwei: zei* is the Burman word for any 'hot' herbal emmenagogue.

[8] Progesterone 50mg Oestradiaol Benzoate 3mg –ampoule.

chronic infections can thwart fertility (Sobo, 1996). The widespread use of blood purifiers or *thwei: zei* (hot medicine) in Burma is common (Population Council and Department of Health Union of Myanmar, 2001; Skidmore, 2002) and it is common for women who experience menstrual irregularity or who fear it, to use these methods (Hull and Hull, 2001).

Without access to modern technology it is remarkably difficult to ascertain if conception, implantation and embryonic growth have occurred and prospective field studies in harsh environments show a foetal loss of between 14 to 45% (DeLuca and Leslie, 1996). In the area of the Thai-Burma border, Burmese women's own judgement on the matter prevails until they visit a health service provider and even then the issue may remain unclear as there is often no access to pregnancy testing or ultrasound. Amenorrhea glossed as blocked menses is found widely in the literature from Polynesia, Mexico, Malaysia, Afghanistan and Jamaica (Nichter and Nichter, 1998) Indonesia (Hull and Hull, 2001) and Thailand (Whittaker, 2000). The obstructed blood can be assisted to flow with traditional medicines and notions of the healthy uterus mechanistically opening and closing to allow the passage of blood (and also sperm) occur (Nichter and Nichter, 1998). Jamaican women take washouts to clear their 'tubes' which may end a tenuous pregnancy (Sobo, 1996). Native Americans practice similar forms of fertility regulation controlled by women:

> Within traditional societies and languages, there is no word that equals abortion. The word itself is harsh and impersonal. When speaking to traditional elders knowledgeable about reproductive health matters, repeatedly they would refer to a woman knowing which herbs and methods to use 'to make her period come.' This was seen as a woman taking care of herself and doing what was necessary (Maguire, 2003: 189-90).

Similarly Burmese women talk about blocked menstruation and take some measures against it, without necessarily acknowledging a pregnancy and the associated stigma of abortion. There is a small cultural loophole through which women may try to 'see the blood' again. This is analogous to Bangladesh, where mechanical 'menstrual regulation' in the early weeks of an unconfirmed pregnancy is legally and socially condoned and not called abortion (Lee et al., 1998). Another example of culturally mediated sanctioning of abortion is among Hmong women for whom children are cherished and large families desired. But as women age and have many children, they are 'allowed' to use herbal medicine to induce abortion. Herbal medicine is not given to younger women with few children and they do not have access to this information (Pranee Liamputtong, 2003).

FOETAL ETHNO-PHYSIOLOGY AND JUMPING SHRIMPS

The cultural rules of abortion not only pertain to the ambiguity surrounding menstruation but also the perception of foetal growth. Lay midwives were able to describe the development of the baby, where for several months it is 'only a blood clot' and later, in the third or fourth month, becomes human-like when it moves and looks like a 'jumping shrimp'. A Christian Karen abortionist was clear about when she felt she could offer a massage abortion. She had worked as an aide in a hospital in Burma:

Suzanne: How did you learn about massage – probably not in the hospital, right?

Lay abortionist: I learnt about massage from when I felt normal babies – you can feel if they are alive or dead, if they are already human. I don't do it if they are human only if they are blood.

Suzanne: How many months is that?

Lay abortionist: Two to three months – if they move you can't do it.

Movement is a key concept. This idea is similar to Western cultures, where in the past women defined their own pregnancies at 'quickening', sometime around the 18 to 20 weeks (4 to 5 months) when the baby was first felt to move (McLaren, 1990). Whittaker's Thai informant Nong is able to describe in Lao language this movement and realisation of another entity apart from her own body. "It's self-aware (*huu tuu*), right. It knows already. Just when it wiggles and wriggles (*yik-yaek*) and bumps and thuds (*pok-paek*) around" (Whittaker, 2002: 9).

Medical technologies have enabled people to see the foetus with ultrasound equipment, hear the heartbeat with a doppler device or test urine when the menstrual period is only three days late, and thus people's awareness and the culture of defining a pregnancy and its viability has changed over time[9]. When I asked the Thai obstetrician when he felt the conceptus was a 'life force', he replied that it was at the time he saw the heartbeat in the six week old embryo during ultrasound examination. So even for the urbane obstetrician, the movement of the heart was a key moment, just as the shrimp-like movement was pivotal for the women and their midwives.

The majority of lay midwives interviewed said they did not do abortion. Some conceded that they knew how to do it but they did not practice their knowledge or they knew other midwives who did do it. One aged eccentric Karen lay midwife was repelled by my question of whether she ever saw women who did not want their babies. She told me while pulling a disgusted face, "I never see women who don't want babies. They do that in the factory!" Another Muslim midwife acknowledged the illegality:

This is how they do their business. These things cause trouble. This is what they do. I know them but I don't want to point them out to you. They may cause trouble for me. They won't talk with you anyway or they will only talk about giving birth.

After many months, I did meet an abortionist in town who said she was Buddhist:

Suzanne: Are there any times that you say no to a woman, that you cannot do it?

Lay abortionist: I understand that my job is not a good one. I understand that it is dangerous. I do refuse sometimes.

Suzanne: I heard from some people that it is an unskilful act in Buddhism– what do you think about this?

Lay abortionist: In the Buddhist religion if you kill then it is an unskilful act. Buddhists should help people. If it were possible I wouldn't do it. I do help women to stay here with me.

Suzanne: Some lay midwives said to me that the earlier the better as the unskilful act is less – what is your idea?

---

[9] See also Rosalind Petchesky's (1987) article *Fetal Images: The Power of Visual Culture in the Politics of Reproduction* for further discussion of technology and its impact on the American abortion debate.

> Lay abortionist: In my experience four to eight weeks is difficult and it just doesn't work. I
> found that it works best at four months. Technically speaking it is easier. I have no
> instruments. I just use my fingers and a stem so the womb needs to be a certain size.[10]

Her main focus then was on the technical aspect of abortion and not with her birth into
the next life; her own karma. One mature lay midwife from the rural area told the parable of
the birds' nest by way of explanation of the negative karma associated with abortion. Her
story was that there was a little boy who saw a birds' nest and he climbed the tree and
knocked the empty nest to the ground. Then there was a little girl who saw another bird nest
in the tree and when she climbed the tree she saw the nest held eggs. She took a stick and
knocked the nest to the ground. The little boy was naughty but the little girl was naughtier.
Her story is easy to understand, the nest held the potential for life but the eggs were a greater
potential, and so the little girl had committed a greater transgression.

Buddhist theology suggests that everything is linked and interdependent and there is no
absolute right or wrong. The major ethical ideas include wisdom, compassion, skilful actions
and making merit. In Buddhism, unskilful acts (*akuśala*) such as transgressions outlined in
the following sentence can undo merit previously gained and good and bad are relative
concepts. The five basic precepts in Buddhism are "to abstain from taking life; to abstain
from taking what is not given; to abstain from sensuous misconduct; to abstain from false
speech; to abstain from intoxicants as tending to cloud the mind' but none of these are
absolute rules" (Keown 1998: 13). Furthermore, while abortion is a serious and unskilful act
as it involves the intent to kill, it is moderated by the gestation and development of the
embryo/foetus: the earlier the gestation the less negative karma is incurred (Keown, 1998;
Maguire, 2003). Buddhist theology is not a completely cohesive set of beliefs and is
interpreted in the context of everyday life. Barnhart extends Keown's interpretation of 'life'
to question the value of a conceptus or even pre-sentient foetus as the same as that of a human
being:

> On this view, the point of the First Precept is to disqualify intentional killing where the clear
> purpose is to end an individual life. Such an action can never be compassionate in Buddhist
> eyes. However, questions as to the status and nature of the lives one weighs in such tricky
> situations where interests clash are obviously relevant. If we are talking about the lives and
> interests of mothers and fetuses, fetuses and families, or fetuses and communities (such as in
> times of famine), then we are directly faced with the issue of the relative moral standing of
> different sorts of life. What I have argued here is that because Buddhism allows a distinction
> between the biological basis of life and its higher cognitive as well as affective aspects and
> insists that an individual human life requires the conjunction of all such aspects, no Buddhist
> need equate a presentient fetus with a sentient human (Barnhart, 1998: 293).

Additionally he considers the reasons surrounding the unwanted pregnancy are pertinent
and consistent with a compassionate Buddhist viewpoint.

Many of the women were keenly aware of the rules, social mores and religious views of
inducing an abortion. Women believed that there was less spiritual risk if the abortion
occurred in early pregnancy while it was still 'blood', the baby did not move or was already

---

[10] Leaf stems or sticks are used by lay midwives to induce abortion. Kapok trees or tobacco leaves are commonly
used in this area. They cause cramping, fresh blood loss and eventually infection, with fever and malodorous
vaginal discharge. The risk of perforation of the uterus, bladder or bowel is high.

dead. Hnin Hnin Pyne (Sen and Snow, 1994: 24) tells us more about the position of women from the Buddhist perspective. By "being a responsible daughter, supportive wife, and, most of all, a nurturing mother", a woman can improve her inferior spiritual status. Women who abort are not considered nurturing and disrupt the Buddhist worldview. Women said, "I worry that my other friends will know what I did. As I am Buddhist I made a very big mistake and I understand about the law which is why I did it secretly". Women spoke of it being a 'bad thing' in religion and in law and they believed that their behaviour contravened some social and theological rules. Another woman said:

> I mean, why not just give birth and give the baby for adoption? The religion says this is bad, you will have five hundred more lives and the unskillful act will stay with you. Karen people don't do this but Islamic Burmese women do it.

But a Karen woman who did induce her abortion with a lay midwife called _ahpwa: gji_ (old woman) warned her while laughing. "_Ahpwa: gji_ told me, 'Don't tell anyone that I did abortion for you or they will come and arrest me. I feel sorry for you so that's why I am helping you". Some women felt that there was an acceptable window of time for an abortion in the early stages of the pregnancy. A married Burman woman with two children cried as she told the story of her induced abortion. "I didn't feel anything for this baby because it was just blood. If it was four or five months I wouldn't have done it because already it would be like a person". One 19 year old Karen woman was surprised to see the maturity of her foetus after the abortion:

> If I knew I was five months I would not have tried to end it. I think I am lucky. I am scared and I won't do it again. I won't go back to that old woman. I feel so sorry for my baby when I saw it I realised he was older. I did it because I thought I was only two months and my husband had left me.

Women's friends confirmed the belief that if a foetus is small it is acceptable. 'I don't know what the problem is to do abortion. I am not educated. My friends said, "The baby is so small, go ahead do it - don't worry".

Five women I interviewed reported following Islam. The Koran elaborates foetal development and describes the creation of a human being originating from clay and semen which is then forced into a 'blood-like clot' which turns into flesh, then bones and develops (Maguire, 2003: 120). This theological recipe is not dissimilar to how the Buddhist women viewed their growing foetuses, simply clots of blood and later flesh. Some women believed that the lay midwife was able to tell whether the foetus was alive or not before the abortion. This Karen woman had a history of five recurrent miscarriages and had consulted her lay midwife:

> I was really ill the first time I miscarried at home. There was no hospital or clinic to go to so I had to look after myself. A _wan:zwe_ (lay midwife - Burmese) looked after me in my house. But I don't know how she knew things. She had a lot of experience with women giving birth. She can tell by just looking at the blood if the baby is dead or alive.

Foetal Autonomy and Baby Death

Some women imbued their aborted foetuses with autonomy as though they were able to control their destiny. As already discussed, it is difficult to know in this environment whether a pregnancy ends spontaneously or with intent. One Karen woman who had a complex obstetric history with ten pregnancies, four neonatal deaths, two living children, one intra-uterine death at seven months and three abortions described her feelings: "Anytime I bleed I feel scared and worried. I go to the clinic straight away but they can't do much. I wonder if the babies will stay with me or go". Her history would certainly make her wonder about her babies and she is probably referring to them pre- and post-birth in this statement. Other women had fewer complications. A Karen woman in her second marriage with three living children wanted to be sterilised and disclosed domestic violence, and probably induced her abortion. She said, "I feel sorry for the baby but it didn't want to stay with me". A Burman woman with three living children, who ended her interview abruptly after appearing uncomfortable with the questions explained:

> I thought that maybe I was pregnant but the baby did not want to stay with me. I went to stay with my friend and I told her to give me a massage because I had pelvic and back pain. My friend did the massage and a week later I bled a lot. My baby came out in my house on the 26th and the next day I came to the clinic.

The way she tells the abortion story is as though the foetus has already decided to leave her prior to her massage. The decision is not hers but the foetus'.

Some husbands referred to the foetus in a similar way. One husband, a father of two children and whose wife became pregnant while using an intra-uterine contraceptive device said, "I want to keep this baby but our situation is bad so my child cannot stay with me. If the baby lived it would have a poor situation and it wouldn't have a good life". A 40-year-old Burman woman, with four living children, who had only been in Thailand ten days after an arduous journey from Rangoon, spontaneously aborted her pregnancy at four months. She said, "I was sad to lose this baby. My husband said that the baby is not strong enough to live with us". These men and women talked about the foetus as though it could independently decide its own future.

The idea of foetal autonomy became apparent in one very tense moment during the fieldwork where my distressed research assistant inadvertently witnessed a stillbirth in a lay midwife's hut. The mother of the baby had been discharged in early labour from the Mae Tao Clinic, she was underweight and her baby was small for dates. It was not clear why the young woman was sent away from the Mae Tao Clinic; perhaps the health workers thought her birth was hours away. In any case, she went to one of the lay midwives in town who took her in, commenced an oxytocic drip and delivered a dead baby a few hours later. I decided to continue to talk with the lay midwife about her practice for several reasons. This story had already filtered back to the Mae Tao Clinic and some people were asking me to tell them which lay midwife had 'killed' the baby. It appeared to me that there had been a chain of unfortunate decisions by several people. Ethically, I could not disclose the identity of the lay midwife who had agreed to be interviewed, but nor could I sit back without investigating the circumstances. The research assistant and I rode to her house on our bicycles and sat down in her shanty hut for a heated discussion which involved challenging the lay midwife's practice.

After some conversational cut and thrust, the midwife became irritated with me and my aspersions. In frustration she blurted out:

> Well my ideas are not the same as your ideas! I tried to help her and to save the baby. I wanted to take her to the Mae Tao Clinic but she said no. One woman was in labour for five days and the baby lived. If the baby wants to live, it will live!

And so the small baby who died that day wanted to die and it was no-one's fault, not the mother's, nor the health workers' at Mae Tao Clinic, nor the lay midwife.

Abortion and infant mortality in this area are common. Baby autonomy seems to me akin to Scheper-Hughes' examination of the self-preserving distant mother-love given to infants on the alto of Bom Jesus in Brazil where infant mortality was allegedly extremely high. She talks of Alto women's "willingness to attribute to their own offspring an 'aversion' to life that made their deaths seem wholly natural, indeed all but expected" in the chronic poverty of the shanty town (Scheper-Hughes, 1992: 270). Abortion and infant mortality are common occurrences in Tak province and some Burmese women felt that their unborn babies had an aversion to life. In this area where there are high rates of spontaneous abortion, women may not emotionally engage with a tenuous pregnancy. Some of these women felt they were mere vessels in which the foetus could choose to stay or not, and often only in the later stages of pregnancy when women saw the foetus as formed, and not only blood, did some emotion emerge. Burmese women in this area do not generally test their urine just days after a missed period, nor would they receive routine ultrasonography; in fact most do not have any antenatal care, and so the idea of pregnancy unfolds slowly even for women who desire children.

Similar ideas of foetal autonomy pertain elsewhere. In the everyday speech of the people in Tanzania they say when "a stillbirth occurs or an incomplete baby is terminated by midwives, the situation is described as the 'the baby returned to where it came from" or "it was unable to go to the delivery room" (Wembah-Rashid, 1996: 87). Allotey and Reidpath (2001) note the large percentage of infant mortality with an unknown cause in Ghana and suggest the cultural belief in 'spirit' children accounts for many deaths. Mothers or other relatives kill newborn infants for a variety of traditionally held beliefs, often if the child displays unusual signs or behaviour, in order to protect the living members of the community. Likewise, Sobo (1996) notes that the category of monster or witchcraft babies could be invoked by Jamaican women when pregnancy was not desired. Mexican foetuses' unsatiated desires for particular foods cause their own demise as they become 'unsettled' and begin 'to move around too much' and can trigger contractions which end the pregnancy (Castaneda et al., 2003: 79). In these cases, the foetus and not the woman or her partner, is central in its own downfall. In some cases Burmese families also perceive unborn children to be unlucky and better dead.

AMBIGUOUS ABORTION AND
CROSS-CULTURAL CONFUSION: CONCLUSION

To summarise, there is diversity in the meaning of abortion from various perspectives in this area of Thailand. Abortion is not a consistently understood phenomenon. For researchers and policy-makers, this makes comparative analysis of results across regions or cultures questionable. For clinicians, it can mean miscommunication with their patients and poor quality post-abortion care. I argue that some definitions and categories do not 'fit' local understandings. The medical categories used by the health workers taken from cosmopolitan medicine, where elective abortion is decriminalised and safe, are quite different from the convoluted and ambiguous nature of attempted induced abortion as it presents on the Thai-Burma border and this leads to clinical confusion. The variations in gestation show the arbitrary nature of decisions concerning viability, while stemming in part from moral theological paradigms, more practically are related to technological issues. The access to technology, or the ability to pay the hospital bill for a premature infant that most likely will not survive or who may be disabled, is a greater arbiter of viability.

Women's nebulous understanding of menstruation and pregnancy provide an ambiguous space of several months for action in which they may decide if their menstruation is delayed due to 'blockage' and rectified with traditional emmenagogues. Undoubtedly, many 'blockages' are pregnancies, but in areas where there is no access to legal or safe abortion, it makes sense not to know or to be vague. There is no value in confirming a pregnancy when there are no legal or safe abortion services, antenatal care or maternity leave. Early pregnancy is a fragile liminal state. Burmese women end their pregnancies through various means and in specifically cultural ways. Women and lay midwives attempt to end the pregnancy in the early stages, when the foetus is motionless. If intention is important in Buddhism, then the intention to regulate menstruation rather than abort a potential human is clearly a wise spiritual decision that avoids demerit.

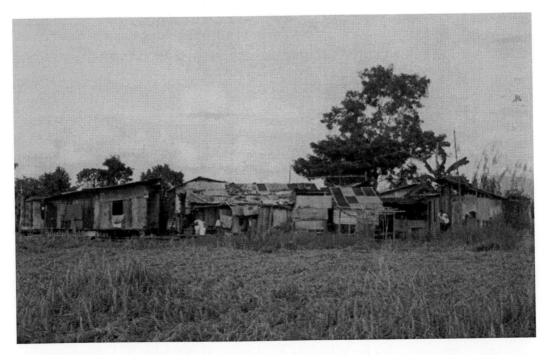

Plate 1. A typical shanty community for the Burmese community in Mae Sot (2001). Photograph by Suzanne Belton.

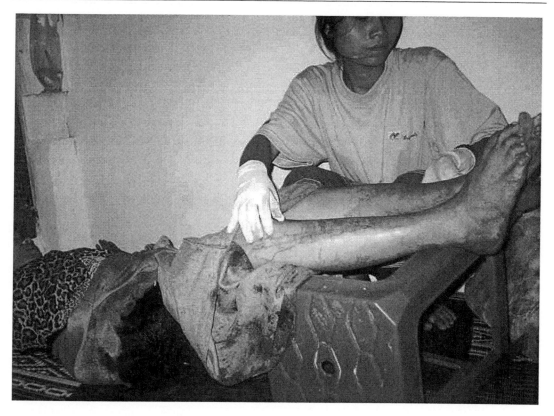

Plate 2. Emergency admission due to excessive blood loss and post-abortion care to Mae Tao Clinic, Mae Sot, Tak Province (2003) Photograph by Inge Sterk.

REFERENCES

Ahman, E., & Shah, I., 2002, 'Unsafe Abortion: Worldwide Estimates for 2000', *Reproductive Health Matters* , 10(19): 13-17.

Allotey, P., & Reidpath, D., 2001, 'Establishing the Causes of Childhood Mortality in Ghana: The 'Spirit Child'', *Social Science & Medicine*, 52: 1007-1012.

Ankomah, A., Aloo-Ounga, C., Chu, M., & Manlagnit A., 1997, 'Unsafe Abortions: Methods Used and Characteristics of Patients Attending Hospitals in Nairobi, Lima and Manila', *Health Care for Women International*, 18: 43-53.

Asian Migrant Centre & Migrant Forum in Asia, 2002, *Asian Migrant Yearbook 2001*, Asian Migrant Centre & Migrant Forum Asia: Hong Kong.

Bankole, A., Singh, S., & Haas, T., 1998, 'Reasons Why Women Have Induced Abortions: Evidence from 27 Countries', *International Family Planning Perspectives*, 24(3): 117-127 &152.

Barnhart, M. G., 1998, 'Buddhism and the Morality of Abortion', *Journal of Buddhist Ethics*, 5: 276-297.

Baretto, T., Campbell, O.M.R., Davies, L.J., Fauveau, V., Fillipi, V.G.A., Graham,WJ, Mamdani, M., Rooney, CIF., & Toubia, N.F., 1992, 'Investigating Induced Abortion in

Developing Countries: Methods and Problems', *Studies in Family Planning*, 23(3): 159-170.

Belton, S., 2005, *Borders of Fertility: Unwanted Pregnancy and Fertility Management by Burmese Women in Thailand*, unpublished doctoral thesis, Key Centre for Women's Health in Society, University of Melbourne, Melbourne.

Beischer, N. A., & Mackay, E.V., 1986, *Obstetrics and the Newborn: An Illustrated Textbook*, W B Saunders Company: Sydney.

Boonthai, N., & Suwanna, W., 2000, Induced Abortion: Nationwide Survey in Thailand, Department of Health, Ministry of Public Health: Bangkok.

Caouette, T., Archanvanitkul, K., & Pyne, H.H., 2000, *Sexuality, Reproductive Health and Violence: Experiences of Migrants from Burma in Thailand*, Institute for Population and Social Research, Mahidol University: Salaya.

Castaneda, X., Billings, D.L., & Blanco, J., 2003, 'Abortion Beliefs and Practices Among Midwives (*Parteras*) in a Rural Mexican Township', *Women & Health*, 37(2): 73-87.

DeLuca, M. A., & Leslie, P.W., 1996, 'Variation in Risk of Pregnancy Loss', in R. Cecil (ed.), *The Anthropology of Pregnancy Loss: Comparative Studies in Miscarriage, Stillbirth and Neonatal Death*, pp. 113-130. Berg: Oxford.

Federation of Trade Unions-Burma, 2002, *Migrant Workers from Burma*. http://www.tradeunions-burma.org/ftub/Migrant/Migrant_Workers%20_2000.htm#policy.

Gespradit, C., 2002, 'Abortion Approach', *Journal of Population and Social Studies*, 10(2). http://www.ipsr.mahidol.ac.th/content/Publication/Volunm_Journal/journal [Access date 16 August 2006].

Maneepong, C., 2003, *Dynamics of Industrial Development in Border Towns: Case Studies in Thailand* (Volume One Unpublished thesis), Faculty of the Built Environment, University of New South Wales, Sydney.

Hull, T. H., & Hull, V.J., 2001, *Means, Motives, and Menses: Use of Herbal Emmenagogues in Indonesia*', in T. H. Hull and V.J. Hull (eds.), *Regulating Menstruation: Beliefs, Practices, Interpretations*, pp. 202-219. University of Chicago Press: Chicago & London.

Huntington, D., Mensch, B., & Toubia, N., 1993, 'A New Approach to Eliciting Information about Induced Abortion', *Studies in Family Planning*, 24(2): 120-124.

Keown, D., 1998, *Buddhism and Abortion*, Macmillan: Houndmills Basingstoke.

Koetsawang, P., 2001, *In Search of Sunlight: Burmese Migrant Workers in Thailand*, Orchid Press: Bangkok.

Lee, K., Lush, L., Walt, G., & Cleland, J., 1998, 'Family Planning Policies and Programmes in Eight Low-Income Countries: A Comparative Policy Analysis', *Social Science & Medicine*, 47(7): 949-959.

Liamputtong, P., 2003, 'Abortion - It Is for Some Women Only! Hmong Women's Perceptions of Abortion', *Health Care for Women International*, 24: 230-241.

Llewellyn-Jones, D., 1999, *Fundamentals of Obstetrics and Gynaecology, 7th* edition, Mosby: Philadelphia.

Maguire, D. C., 2003, *Sacred Rights: The Case for Contraception and Abortion in World Religions*, Oxford University Press: New York.

Maung, C., & Belton, S., 2004, *Working Our Way Back Home: Fertility and Pregnancy Loss on the Border of Thailand*, Mae Tao Clinic (Report): Mae Sot.

McLaren, A., 1990, *A History of Contraception from Antiquity to the Present Day*. Basil Blackwell: Oxford.

Nichter, M., & Nichter, M., 1998, 'Cultural Notions of Fertility in South Asia and their Impact on Sri Lankan Family Planning Practices', in S. van der Geest and A. Rienks (eds.), *The Art of Medical Anthropology Readings*, pp. 268-281. Het Spinhuis: Amsterdam.

Paisanpanichkul, D., 2001, 'Burmese Migrant Workers in Thailand: Policy and Protection', *Legal Issues on Burma Journal*, 10(December): 39-50.

Petchesky, R. P., 1987, 'Fetal Images The Power of Visual Culture in the Politics of Reproduction', *Feminist Studies*, 13(2): 263-292.

Pongsatha, S., N. Morakot, & Tongsong,T., 2002, 'Demographic Characteristics of Women With Self Use of Misoprostol for Pregnancy Interruption Attending Maharaj Nakorn Chiang Mai Hospital', *Journal of the Medical Association of Thailand*, 85(10): 1074-80.

Population Council and Department of Health Union of Myanmar, 2001, *Perceptions of Reproductive Morbidity Among Women, Men and Service Providers in Pyay and Kalaw Townships in Myanmar*, Population Council & Department of Health Union of Myanmar (Report): Bangkok.

Thapa, P. J., Thapa, S., & Shrestha, N., 1992, 'A Hospital-Based Study of Abortion in Nepal', *Studies in Family Planning*, 23(5): 311-318.

Rahman, A., Katzive, L., & Henshaw, S.K., 1998, 'A Global Review of Laws on Induced Abortion, 1985-1997', *International Family Planning Perspectives*, 24(2): 56-64.

Rotberg, R. I., 1998, *Burma Prospects for a Democratic Future*, the World Peace Foundation and Harvard Institute for International Development and Brokking Institution Press: Cambridge, Massachusetts.

Royal Thai Government, 1997, *Second and Third Periodic Reports of State Parties Thailand TA 2-3*, CEDAW Committee United Nations: Geneva.

Royal Thai Government, 2001, *Improvement of Health Conditions of Migrants in Three Priority Provinces of Thailand*, Royal Thai Government: Bangkok.

Scheper-Hughes, N., 1992, *Death Without Weeping The Violence of Everyday Life in Brazil*, University of California Press: Berkley.

Sen, G., & Snow, R.C., 1994, *Power and Decision: The Social Control of Reproduction*, Harvard University Press: Boston.

Skidmore, M., 2002, 'Menstrual Madness: Women's Health and Well-Being in Urban Burma', *Women & Health*, 35(4): 81-99.

Sobo, E. J., 1996, 'Abortion Traditions in Rural Jamaica', *Social Science & Medicine*, 42(4): 495-508.

Tamang, A., 1996, 'Induced Abortions and Subsequent Reproductive Behaviour Among Women in Urban Areas of Nepal', *Social Change*, 26(3&4): 271-285.

Union of Myanmar, 1999, *Initial Report of State Parties Myanmar C/MMR/1*, CEDAW Committee United Nations: Geneva.

Weil, A. T., 1966, *The Use of Nutmeg as a Psychotropic Agent*, Retrieved October, 2004, from ww.erowid.org/plants/nutmeg_journal1.shtml

Wembah-Rashid, J.A.R., 1996, 'Explaining Pregnancy Loss in Matrilineal Southeast Tanzania', in R. Cecil (ed.), *The Anthropology of Pregnancy Loss: Comparative Studies in Miscarriage, Stillbirth and Neonatal Death*, pp. 75-94. Berg: Oxford.

Whittaker, A., 2000, *Intimate Knowledge: Women and their health in North-East Thailand*, Allen and Unwin: St Leonards, Sydney.

Wong, T-C., & Singh, M., 1999, *Development and Challenge: Southeast Asia in the New Millennium*, Times Academic Press: Singapore.

World Bank, 1995 to 2002, *Data by Country – Myanmar*, Retrieved 30 June, 2004, from http://www.worldbank.org/data/countrydata/countrydata.html

In: Reproduction, Childbearing and Motherhood
Editor: Pranee Liamputtong, pp. 63-77

ISBN: 978-1-60021-606-0
© 2007 Nova Science Publishers, Inc.

Chapter 4

REASONS FOR ABORTION AMONG MARRIED WOMEN IN INDIA

Lakshmi Ramachandar and Pertti J. Pelto

INTRODUCTION

In this chapter, we examine the complex of economic, cultural and other reasons underlying the choices for pregnancy termination (MTP) among rural Indian women. Our aim is to explore the complexities of motivation that lie beneath the (often) superficial explanations reported in the literature. The extensive abortion research literature in India is quite unanimous in noting that married women are the overwhelming majority of abortion seekers, and that "the majority of women opt for abortion because of "already many children" (Chhabra and Nuna, 1994: 39). Chhabra and Nuna cited a study by Khan and associates (1990: 39) which "...observed that 67 percent of the MTP acceptors had achieved their desired family size". More recently, Ganatra (2000: 197) summarized the abortion research in much the same language, saying that "the majority desire to limit family size and to space the next pregnancy--a telling indicator of the unmet need for contraception. She went on to mention some other reasons, including the observation that "in some cases, the woman may be considered 'too old' to have children". The same general picture emerged in a recent study in Rajasthan, which found that 65 percent of the abortion seekers did not desire any more children, and 21 percent said they desired spacing after the previous childbirth (Iyengar and Iyengar, 2002). All the recent summaries about abortion in India also mention sex-selection and "preference for male child" as another motive.

The picture emerging from the past 25 years of abortion research in India is that rural married women are, for the most part, resorting to abortion for "ordinary birth control". The recent Abortion Assessment Project - India has greatly increased our overall understanding of abortion practices, particularly with relation to married women (Barge et al., 2003; Barnes, 2003; Mallik, 2003; Hirve, 2004). The numbers and situations of abortions among adolescent girls and other unmarried women, on the other hand, are extremely difficult to study, due to the severe stigmatization attached to such cases. Very little research has focused on abortions among unmarried women (Ganatra and Hirve, 2002). Unanswered questions about the abortion situation in rural communities also include the vexing issue, "why don't the women adopt and use contraceptives?" We will take up that question in the later part of this chapter.

In our research, we have found that the superficial explanations usually given concerning abortion are a gloss for very complex systems of cultural concepts, economic factors, and social structural features which deserve careful attention. The phrase, "to limit family size" begs for much deeper probing about the thought processes, cultural expectations, and life situations of Indian rural women. Of course most of the data about "reasons for abortion" come from surveys, in which there is space and time only for short answers. We feel that deeper exploration of women's explanations about abortion, and about their intense suspicions concerning contraceptive technology, reveal a rich inner world of meanings and expectations. These cultural and social constructions help us to understand the ways in which individual experiential worlds interface with economic forces and the broad currents of cultural information carried in television and other media. Our aim in this study has been to explore in more depth the different layers of intentions and motives, taking the women's statements as much as possible in the language and style in which they spoke, and to bring out the wide range of variations and nuances in the "voices of the women".

Research on abortion in India is facilitated by the relatively liberal abortion laws, in existence since the passage of the Medical Termination of Pregnancy Act (MTP Act) in 1971-72 (Government of India, 1973; Chandrasekhar, 1994). The liberalization of the law was intended to expand women's access to low-cost and safe abortion services, in order to reduce the very high rates of morbidity and mortality from 'back street' abortions by unqualified providers. The liberalization also seems to have embodied some ideas of "population control", according to some writers (Hirve, 2004). In the past 30 years there have been large increases in legally recognized abortions, although the majority of pregnancy terminations continue to be done outside the officially registered, government certified, sector of medical services.

RESEARCH POPULATION AND METHODOLOGY

The first author (LR) carried out research in a rural district (Dharmapuri) in Tamil Nadu for approximately 15 months in 2001-2002 (Ramachandar, 2003). Dharmapuri is considered a "less developed district", as the health and demographic indicators are relatively low compared to the more developed areas of Tamil Nadu. For example, at the time of the research the district had a contraceptive coverage rate of 47 % (mainly sterilization), compared to about 55% in the state as a whole. The infant mortality rate was 50 per 1000 live births, which was considerably higher than the rates for Tamil Nadu state. Female literacy in the district was about 45 % in 1999 (Gandhigram Institute 1999; Dharmapuri district 2000, 2001).

Communities served by four different primary health centres (PHCs) were chosen for study, in locations ranging from peri-urban to remote, isolated areas. In each PHC area, comprised of several dozen villages, we received help from the village health nurses (VHNs) for identifying and contacting women who had had abortions in the past six months in their service areas. With that strategy we were able to interview 97 women in depth about their abortion decisions, their family situations, the choices of providers, and other information.

The families in our sample were of wide-ranging socio-economic status, from a few wealthy landowning families, to poor, landless agricultural laborers. In approximately one-third of cases the family owned some agricultural lands. More than half the women were literate (53), and one fourth of them had higher secondary education of nine years or more.

"STOPPERS", "SPACERS", "SEX SELECTION" AND OTHER PATTERNS

In terms of the usual categorizes of "reasons," the great majority of the women (68 of the 97) said that they did not want to have any more children, so we can refer to them as "stoppers" as sometimes labeled in the reproductive health literature. Another 10 women gave "spacing" as the motive for the abortion. We categorized seven cases as overt or covert "sex selective abortion.Twelve cases gave complex motivations which we have grouped in the category "cultural/religious reasons". A few women described "contraceptive failure", "health reasons", and miscellaneous other explanations.

People's explanations about their motives for doing things are in some ways analogous to the layers of an onion. There is the usual, "cover explanation," which the person hopes is sufficient to satisfy the interviewer. Beneath that first layer is a second "text", which helps to justify and elaborate the initial explanation. Further discussions, often in the form of conversations about the attitudes of other family members, and the overall social situation of the woman, bring out additional features that give more texture and nuance to the previous discourse. Each woman has, in fact, several reasons, several motives, for which there are sub-texts of explanatory materials.

Theme One: Poverty and Economic Hardship

When the women were asked about their reasons for terminating a pregnancy, many of them talked immediately of economic hardship. An agricultural laborer, Shanti phrased it like this: "Nambha vasadhikku thgundhamadhir kuzndhai gal irrukanom" (We have limited income, so, limit the [number of] children). Kaveri, a 26 year old, illiterate mother of two children, works her own lands with her husband, as well as doing wage labor on neighboring farms. She phrased her explanation directly in terms of economics:

> We do not want to have more children. Namakku sothu bothu kamiya irrukku (We do not have large economic assets). We are very poor and our income depends on our coolie work.[1] That is; the money paid for our labor. If we do not go for work we do not get money. During sickness we lose our wage. We have no regular income. The thatched hut that you see is all our wealth. Why should we have more children?

A small number of women were, indeed "rock bottom poor", so that "one more mouth to feed" was simply out of the question. A poor cobbler family who managed barely to have enough food from one day to the next, partly through the generosity of neighbors, certainly could plead "poverty", without further elaboration. But poverty and economic hardship are

---

[1] 'Coolie', sometimes written as 'kuuli' is a common word among Tamilians, referring to all menial wage work

relative concepts. Most of the families had some economic flexibility; some small windows of choice-making beyond simply managing daily food and shelter.

When we probed further about their poverty, more complex explanations came forth. Three women went on to explain that they are very poor because the husband drinks up all the family money. Chelluvamma spoke of poverty as the reason for her abortion, but then added angrily:

> All that he knows is go and spend the hard earned money on liquor and have sex and produce children. I am the one to feed them take them to the school, and see that they perform well in the school. We are not rich to have children. Everything is expensive these days and therefore I got tired being a machine in this stupid house. I have no strength in my body and I have become weak.

Chelluvamma's brief statement is loaded with a bundle of complex motives and feelings, including a major, developing concern among most families--education.

Theme II: Education of the Children

"Education of the children" was the most frequently mentioned theme in all the interviews. The case of Lalitha illustrates how the general answer, 'poverty,' is transformed into a focus on the children's schooling:

> When I asked the reasons for her abortion, she first said, 'Vasadhi illai' (Inadequate income). Then she quickly added, 'School fee structure is very high [so there are] increasing education costs. If I had not gone for abortion and got sterilised, pirkalathil Kuzandhaigalluku badhikka padum (the children would have suffered a lot).' Lalitha expressed a common theme, concerning taking good care of one's existing children. If one has more children, then all the children will have less food, clothing and other necessities, including less support for education.

In various ways the women's economic worries focused attention on education as a key element. There are school uniforms to be paid for (new uniforms to be purchased every year as the children grow); and the costs of books and various "extras" connected with school programs. The pattern of hiring tutoring to improve childrens' examination performance is spreading rapidly to rural families. Some of the families in our sample are paying the extra cost of sending their children to private schooling. The following excerpts further illustrate some of the rapidly changing aspirations about education:

According to Kalyani, in a scheduled caste village, she and her husband want to have only two children and not more. She said:

> I do not want my children to be engaged in this rope making business". The couple are interested in their children's higher education and therefore they are saving their income for the children's future. She said, "I want my children to study as much as they can so that they could go for government jobs.

Her father-in-law, who was present at the time of this interview, supported the idea that his grandson should study well. He did not want him to become a "coolie" like [the boy's father]. The father-in-law continued:

Education is very important these days to get good jobs and to improve the quality of life. We are ready to make sacrifices and devote our time to get some wage, so that we could invest in education. For a male, minimum requirement is completing 10th standard. We do not have our own land, therefore our big hope is children's education. If he is successful completing 10th standard it might be possible to get some government job.... these youngsters should understand the value of education.

In some families their educational aspirations are quite high, including university education for both boys and girls:

Menaka, in a comparatively well-to-do family, is happy with two children (a boy and a girl). She is interested in giving university education to her children. For higher education they have to save a lot of money since education is getting expensive. She says, "what if they do not perform well; we have to provide them with private tuition.

Valli, too, spoke of the high costs of education, and now her oldest daughter is wanting to go on to the university.

L: Tell me something about your children. Your older daughter is 18 years and she studying, what are your future plans?
V: We are interested to give higher education to my daughters and son. In fact this morning my daughter was saying that she would like to continue her studies. Me and my husband decide concerning their education. My older daughter says, that she will not get married but go for higher education Sometimes my husband says, that she should stop her studies since it is becoming expensive. But my daughter insists that she should continue her studies. Now if she has to go for her second year we have to pay 1200 rupees for her admission. Even this morning she was discussing this with her father. My husband said that he would need ten days to get the money.

Throughout much of India there is a rapid growth of interest in providing adequate education for children (cf. Saavala, 2001: 50-57). Even families with better incomes seemed to feel that they could only afford good education for their children if they kept the family size small.

Theme III: Sexual Activity and Pregnancy are Inappropriate When the Couple is "Old"

An important cultural concept in Indian and south Asian communities is the expectation that sexual activity, pregnancy and childbearing should be sharply reduced or ended when one's children reach puberty and are nearing marriageable age. This set of cultural ideas goes back to the ancient scriptures of the *Manusmriti,* according to which a 'man's' life is ideally supposed to be composed of four *ashrams* (stages of life) (cf. Kakar, 1996). The first period is that of the 'student' (*brahmacharya*), during which celibacy should be observed. After 12 years of *brahmacharya* the youth should get married, and assume the second phase, *Grihastha*, the role of married man and householder. This is the active phase of a man's life cycle, during which he should develop the balanced practice of *dharma* (correct social-religious practice), *artha* (economic actions), and *kama* (sensual enjoyment). The role of adult married man is ideally thought to last until the birth of the man's first grandson. With the birth of a grandson (ideally), the man and his wife should give up the householder stage and devote their lives to spiritual actions (India Mystica, 1995-98; The Laws of Manu, cited in Kakar, 1996). Although the main features of this ideal life cycle are no longer salient, the residual concept has remained throughout India--that it is socially inappropriate for 'older people' to engage in sexual intercourse, and it is particularly shameful for an 'older woman' to get pregnant. In her study in rural Andhra Pradesh, Saavala (2001:129-130) found that "the most important form of abstinence for fertility levels is the abstinence of elder couples who have married children or children of marriageable age. Intercourse between a wife and a husband is supposed to end by the time their child, either a son or a daughter, marries".

Our informants expressed the idea that it is unacceptable for a woman to be pregnant if her daughter (or daughter-in-law) might be pregnant at about the same time. Some people said that it would be shameful "to have two cradles in the same family". Several of our informants gave that as the main reason for their abortion and sterilisation. The following two cases, each of them with four daughters and no sons, expressed these cultural ideas in approximately the same language:

Yeshoda and her husband explained how important it was that she has an abortion and becomes sterilized:

> My daughter is married and in our community when the son-in–law visits our place it is shameful if I am pregnant. This is not acceptable and would appear awkward, having such grown up children if I were to conceive. Marumagan veetil irrukum podhu kevalamai irrukum (When the son-in-law stays at our place it will be degrading if I am pregnant). I would feel terribly shy to face my married daughter and her husband. Therefore it was decided by both of us that after getting an abortion I would get sterilized.

She noted that even the neighbors would laugh and make fun of her. The husband added that the married daughter would be ridiculed in her in-laws house (romaba kevalama irrukuum).

Theme IV: Sex Selective Abortion and "Son Preference"

There is now a great deal of discussion in India about sex selective abortion, particularly in the northern states. Laws prohibiting the use of ultrasound and amniocentesis technology for identifying the sex of the foetus, and also prohibiting the abortion of a foetus for sex selection reasons, were passed in 1994 (Hirve, 2004). Despite the law, researchers have continued to note widespread evidence of sex selective abortions (Ganatra et al 2000; George and Dahiya 1998; Khan et al 1999) as governmental authorities are bringing very few cases against the medical facilities that do the sex selective scanning. For example, in the entire swath of northern states there were reportedly only 21 cases brought against violators in 1999 (Mallik, 2003).

Some of the discussions about "son preference" present a rather simplified picture, as if people in general simply prefer boys and dislike girls. One does not need to scratch much below the surface of things to find that the actual motives are much more complex. Yes, there is a "son preference" motive deeply imbedded in the cultural framework of Hinduism. Regardless of the current motivations and attitudes of specific parents, *the religious doctrines specify that only a son can officiate in one's funeral rites*, and light the cremation fire. That one religious factor was mentioned time and again by women as they explained that "there must be at least one son."One woman was apparently unaware of the illegality of sex selective abortion, as she was quite open in her explanation. Mallika Murugan said:

Me and my husband had been to the clinic in Dharmapuri, and vythil computer vechhi parthanga, adhil penn kuzandhai therindhadhu adhanal dhan kalichuten (They put a computer inside my stomach and examined the sex of the child, it was female therefore I went for abortion).

Several informants made it very clear that the major concern about having "excess girl children" is the high cost of dowry and marriage. Kasiamma said it bluntly:

The reason for small family norm [and abortion] is on account of dowry. She recalled the amount of dowry that her sister gave to celebrate her daughter's wedding. These days the boy's family demands cots, steel file cabinet, clothes, jewelry, wristwatch, gold ring, two wheeler, utensils, ceiling fans and all household items to start the new family life.

Murugamma described the heated arguments she had with her mother and father, who were horrified to learn that she had gotten an abortion. She told them:

In those days [when she herself got married], men were not all driving around with two-wheelers [motor scooters and motorcycles], so her husband was satisfied with the goats and sheep. But now , at the time of marriage negotiations the groom and his family are not interested in goats and sheep or in bags of paddy....in the present day they "are demanding materialistic things...."----file cabinet like that (pointing), Hero Honda, TV, ceiling fan....and in addition to all that, they may ask for land... Another thing they are demanding is an STD booth...or else a Tempo [three wheeled passenger vehicle] to run a business. Or to put up a roadside restaurant business. In these days, even the girls are getting smarter...they witness the marriage, and what people get in dowry...Even if the groom doesn't demand, the girls are demanding—"you give this." So there is a big change now, between her time and her daughters' time: "namba pillai galae kaekkarango" (our children are demanding). So there is a pressure both from outside and from inside the house. So for her daughter'smarriage she will have to spend 50,000 rupees [over US$1100; equivalent to more than a year of family income].

Her case was not clearly a sex selective abortion, because she did not get a scan to determine the sex of the child. Like four or five other women in our study, who said they had "enough children", fear of having another girl child was the underlying reason, driven by the extreme escalation in costs of getting a daughter married. They do not "hate girls". In fact, some women said they preferred girl children, as they were easier to take care of, and are very helpful in doing housework. The powerful economic forces arise from the traditional patrilineal, patrilocal family structure, along with the high costs of marriages (which traditionally are paid for by the bride's family) both in dowry and direct payments for the wedding arrangements.

Theme V: Concepts of Pollution and Ritual Actions

Very complex ideas about "pollution" and "ritual proprieties" can become reasons for abortion, although they are relatively infrequent. Among our 97 informants there were three cases in which concepts of "pollution" came into the picture. At first the informants gave stereotypic explanations for terminating their pregnancies, before divulging the more complex underlying themes. The most interesting case was that of Sripriya, a young woman with an 18 month old daughter. She explained that she had gotten an abortion because her daughter is still too young, so it appeared to be a clear example of "spacing". At the end of the interview the mother-in-law invited the researcher (LR) to attend her second son's marriage, which was scheduled to take place four weeks later. She mentioned that it was due to the forthcoming wedding that Sripriya had to go for an abortion. This came as a surprise, to hear mention of a totally different reason for the pregnancy termination.

> I had closed my notebook and I was confused. What had the son's marriage to do with the daughter-in-law's abortion? I continued the interview and the mother-in-law said that she had requested Sripriya to get her pregnancy terminated because she is the oldest daughter-in-law and therefore had a leading role in the second son's marriage [LR field notes].

The mother-in-law explained:

> Being a widow I cannot do some of the rituals, and the other choice was to request my brother-in-law's son and his wife to perform the marriage. But I did not want them to be the main persons because Sripriya is my daughter-in-law. It is just like having butter in the house and going and borrowing ghee from the neighbor's house. She has to receive the new bride, nelungu idonom [decorate the feet of the bride], she has to do the arathi [a ritual enactment] for the bride. Who else is more eligible than Sripriya? Pregnant women are not allowed to conduct marriage rituals because a fetus is growing and that is considered pollution. Therefore we senior women decided that she had to go for a termination.

This case of "reasons for abortion" encapsulates a complex series of 'cultural rules' in Hindu society. The 'problem' begins with the fact that the mother-in-law is a widow, and therefore culturally barred from participating in many ritual situations. In such cases the eldest son (Sripriya's husband) is the ritual head of household, and the wedding proceedings require a husband-wife combination. However, for participation in these sacred events, the wife must be 'pure' and non-polluting. The *theettu* (polluting condition) therefore had to be removed so Sripriya could enact the leading female role. Sripriya's additional statement underlines the central importance of *family honor*. If the leading roles in the wedding ceremony had been enacted by a peripheral relative, the *punya* (ritual merit) would have gone out of Sripriya's family, and thus diminished their *kudumba gauravam* ("family honor").

The concepts of *theettu*, and the reasons for Sripriya's abortion are universally understood among Tamilians. Nichter (1989) has described the same concept in the neighboring state of Karnataka, where 'pollution' is referred to as *mailige*. Two other women in our study reported that they terminated their pregnancies because they wanted to participate in rituals for which they would have been 'polluting' if they had been pregnant at that time. In one case the conception had occurred in *aadi* month, which is a particularly inauspicious time. During *aadi* (in July-August) there is much fasting, avoidance of undertakings, and weddings are not celebrated in that period. The woman and her family feared that the "inauspicious pregnancy" was particularly dangerous to the health and welfare of the husband, so they decided on abortion.

Theme VI: Family Honor (*Kudumba Gauravam*)) and Proper Behavior

Throughout the various cases, and the different themes emerging as reasons for abortion, there is an underlying concern about *family honor*. This theme was especially evident in relation to "Theme IV", in which women repeated spoke of the shame and *loss of family honor* if a woman were pregnant at the same time as her daughter, or if there were "two cradles in the house". Family honor is also very closely tied to the proper conduct and purity of daughters. If a daughter were to have an illicit love affair, especially if she became pregnant, it would be a very severe shock to the family honor. At the same time, having unmarried girls in the family, after the "normal age of marriage", is a cause for shame and arouses gossip among one's neighbors. No wonder that women think about the marriage prospects for a daughter *even before the birth of the female child!*

Arranging good marriages for daughters is a huge concern in every family, and a "good marriage" includes very costly arrangements--lavish amounts of food, hundreds of invited guests, plenty of gifts of saris, jewelry and other items, and other expenses. Families must begin saving money for their daughters' weddings from the moment of childbirth, if not before.

Of course "family honor" is a concept of some importance in every society. However, in south Asia, in India and neighboring countries, these concepts are raised to a level of importance that is not easily grasped by the average European or American.

Theme VII: "The Small Family Norm"

For some of the women we spoke with, the concept of the "small family norm" is a motivating force in itself. It appears that most women (and their families) in Tamil Nadu and neighboring areas in south India have absorbed the idea that two children is the ideal family size, provided they have at least one son (Ravindran and Mishra, 2000). This corresponds to the aims of the national family planning programme (Visaria, 2000; Saavala, 2001; Ramachandar and Pelto, 2002). Chitra Narasimhan explained her abortion as follows:

Alavvukku   meeri   irundhal   samallikka   mudiyadhu   (excess   children   are unmanageable).Varumanatthuku thangundha madhiri irrukonam. (the number of children depends on the income) According to the government rules we should have only two children.

In the past the government advertisements were propagating two child norm. "Irruvar kku irruvar" (two for two) but now it is irruvarkku oruvar (one for two).

As noted in Chitra's statement, some of the government family planning messages are saying that one child is enough. One informant in a village, when asked about ideal family size remarked that, *"if you ask in the town, people will say 'one child;' here in the village they say 'two children;' in more remote areas they will say 'three...'"*
There is now a wide-spread feeling that having many children is somehow "improper" and "backward". Sharada Dasappa commented:

> Why more children? Akka pakka jana namanna nodinagtharae (the right side and left side neighbors would laugh at us). These days nobody is having more than two children. Some couples are going for operation after one child. If we keep producing children my neighbours would laugh at us.

One of the most expressive key informants summed up the recent changes like this:

> Their thinking now is: 'if we have two children, we could give them good food, better education, provide good clothes.' Earlier the concept was like if we have four children., one can go for grazing the cow and the goats, another one will look after the house, one will go and milk the cow, another one would work in the field. Then they saw the disadvantages in the large family size. Nagarikam valara valara janangal arivu adhigama ayirukku ('Modernisation' has resulted in greater awareness.)

Theme VIII: "Concerns about Weakness" and Reasons Women do not Use Contraceptives

Throughout their discussions about abortion, the women made frequent mention of "weakness" *(shakti illai)*. Some women included "body weakness" as one of the major reasons for not wanting any more children. One of the women with a recent abortion told us:

> I had already suffered jaundice during my previous child birth. Still my body is very weak. Two children are more than sufficient. Now I have decided to go to [the clinic] and get sterilized.

The same worries about weakness were a central theme in relation to avoidance of contraception. For some of the women, even sterilization was seen as likely to lead to weakness and inability to do their daily work. Many of the women worked as wage laborers at least part of the time, in addition to engaging in heavy agricultural work at home. Fears of being unable to work and earn daily wages were uppermost for many. They expressed widespread fears that IUDs or oral contraceptive pills would cause damage to the body, bringing about "weakness", and endangering their wage-earning. Mallika commented:

> My body is highly sensitive and therefore contraceptives are no good. My body is getting weaker and weaker and now I cannot sit for more than five minutes on the floor. I get severe aches and pains in my knees and other joints. Eating those pills might aggravate my sickness.

Jayam said:

I do not like all those temporary methods....[and] I am scared of sterilization. As it is my body has become very weak and what if something goes wrong with my health after operation? Who will cook food, look after my husband and children? They are still young and studying and I have to support the family by earning some money therefore I am not going to get operated. I do not want to orphan my children.

A woman named Baby told the interviewer that her husband did not allow her to use any contraceptives because she is not a housewife, as she assists her husband in carpentry. Sometimes she is engaged in tough jobs especially while fixing roofing, therefore they felt that these contraceptives could cause additional damage to her body. The couple fears that contraceptives might hamper her routine work and deprive them of daily income. She said, "I have to work hard and therefore my husband is totally against these family planning methods".

Weakness is seen as resulting from a wide variety of causes, including child bearing, child rearing, lack of proper food, over-work, reproductive tract infections (RTIs), abortion, sterilisation, and many others (cf. Gittelsohn et al., 1994; Ross et al., 2002).In the Tamil language the expression commonly used for weakness is *shakti illai* (no strength). The corresponding word in Hindi, throughout western and northern India, is *kamjori*, while in parts of eastern India (Bengali and Oriya speaking areas) and Bangladesh it is *durbolata* (Ross et al., 2002). Interviews with rural women about 'common health problems' usually find 'weakness' to be near the top in their lists (Gittelsohn et al., 1994). Nichter (1989) has described pervasive concerns about weakness in a population in Karnataka.

Many women spoke of their fears about having a foreign object (IUD) lodged inside their bodies. In most cases the women reported the things they had heard from other women who had tried IUDs. A young woman, Shalini, described to me about the side effects that she had heard from neighbors and friends. According to her informants the IUD does not stay in one fixed location in the uterus. It keeps moving all over the body. Some women believed that the IUD could migrate into the lungs or other organs and cause death. One of the rope-maker informants said that the IUD had gone inside the heart of a woman, and she died. Another informant, Tanuja, explained her fear of the IUD as follows:

I have heard one lady was complaining about severe abdominal pain. The IUD had moved from her uterus to the stomach causing stomach ache. Then she could feel the movement all over her body.

Similar ideas about the movement of the IUD in the body are found in other parts of India, Sri Lanka, and elsewhere such as Botswana, Kenya, Mexico, Peru and Tunisia (Nichter and Nichter, 1989: 71).

The general suspicion about having a 'foreign object' in the body also included fears that the IUD would deteriorate and cause infection in the body. When Pushpa was asked her reasons for not adopting the IUD, she remarked:

If we use loop our body will be dried up (Kanjipogum). I heard loop (loopu) will get rusted (thuru) inside the body. Some of the women in this village have tried and discontinued IUD. Any rusted item sitting in the body is going to cause infection and pus formation. Nobody wants to go for such contraceptives. Many of my neighbor women who used this loop have reported this matter to me.

The list of health problems mentioned by women in Dharmapuri is quite similar to the complaints and fears reported from other parts of south and Southeast Asia. Gammeltoft (1999) surveyed a sample of rural women in Vietnam and tabulated the following major complaints concerning IUDs: backache (55 percent), weakness (50 percent), menstrual disturbances (42 percent), abdominal pain (29 percent), vaginal discharge (29 percent), weight loss, headache, bleeding, and others. She also encountered the concept of the IUD moving about in the body, and 'rusting' and other deterioration as causes of problems (Gammeltoft, 1999: 97). In rural northeastern Thailand, Whittaker (2000, 2002) found frequent mention of weakness, white discharge, menstrual irregularities, and back pain, and other complaints associated with IUDs and tubal ligation.

At a more abstract level, several women in Dharmapuri expressed the idea that IUDs and other contraceptive methods, including sterilisation, are "suitable" for the bodies of some women and not others. Sukanya, who is 29 years old and operates a small restaurant, said that she does not use an IUD because, "for some women's bodies it is not suitable" *(othukaradhilai)*. Similarly, Kaveri said, "Copper T fits and adjusts to some women's bodies, but it does a lot of harm for many [because] it is not suited to their bodies". Ramani linked suitability to her occupation. She said, "for the agricultural work that I am engaged in those methods are not suitable".

The concept of "suitability" is a widespread idea, in which women have different physiological features, including differing humoral (hot-cold) characteristics. Concerning her Vietnamese research, Gammeltoft (1999: 105) wrote that 'the women often emphasised that "the structure of each person's body is different'—different women also have different physiologies, different states of health, and different needs". Whittaker (2000: 113) found similar concepts in rural Thailand; "women speak of contraceptives as either *thuk* (correct) for their bodies or not".

CONCLUSIONS AND IMPLICATIONS FOR WOMEN'S HEALTH CARE

Our data show that the women in south India often have very complex reasons for terminating their pregnancies, even though their initial answer in interviews may be simple and direct, such as "already enough children", or "too poor to afford any more children". Acceptance of the "small family norm" is now general, even in more peripheral rural villages. But the *reasons* for widespread agreement about having only two or three children include a greatly increased concern about education for children (particularly the costs), the extremely high costs of marriage of one's daughters, and many other factors.

The concerns about children's education, too, are a response to economic forces impinging from a wider world. Very few villagers expect or want their children to make their living in localized subsistence agriculture, in the model of their parents and grandparents. Education for the children has come to be seen as *an economic necessity* that arises from the "inflation of expectations", diminished availability of agricultural lands, and the structural displacement of employment opportunities more and more to urban areas. For many younger people in the local region, "urban migration" may only mean taking up non-agricultural work in the nearby market town. But, even that small shift of aspirations requires literacy and abilities with numbers that come with education.

While many of the reasons and motives underlying women's abortion decisions are related to economics and social structural features, there is an important sector of explanation that is based on specific Hindu cultural ideas. The beliefs about the inappropriateness of sex and pregnancy when children are nearing puberty, concepts of pollution (pregnancy as *theettu* or polluting condition), and *kudumba gauravam* (family honor) include layers of meaning and nuance that cannot be glossed simply with our corresponding English language concepts. They are among the deeper "layers of the onion" that some people might infer are the "real reasons" for pregnancy termination. However, in most cases *all of the different levels of explanation* are part of the complex system of motivations. Peoples' motivations are seldom unitary and simple.

Understanding women's decisions to seek abortion must also take into account decisions made much earlier, in the form of *rejecting* contraceptive choices. In some cases the women had little choice, as the rejection of contraceptive options was made by the husband and/or senior generation family members. In most instances, however, the women concurred in those decisions, and their reasons included a complex array of beliefs, particularly fueled by a *fear of weakness*.

Our intentions in this study have been to present as much as possible of the "voices of the women"---including verbatim quotations and paraphrases of the ways they spoke about their abortions. However, examination of their spoken words, the motivations and ideas they expressed, and other evidence from the women must also be examined in the light of other data about Tamilian culture, aspects of general Hindu culture, and other aspects of daily life in that part of Tamil Nadu. The statements of the women always contain "things taken for granted", that must be interpreted in the light of other information, including the researcher's own first hand knowledge of Tamilian culture. The women did not have to "explain" or expand certain statements because those nuances are "common knowledge". Fortunately, the first author (Lakshmi) is Tamilian by birth, and is familiar with some of the "taken for granted" contextual understandings needed to "fill in the blanks" in the women's statements.

Rural women's multiple layers of motives and explanations for terminating pregnancies must be seen in relation to their specific family constellations, intertwined with centuries-old cultural practices and expectations, and pushed in new directions by powerful forces emanating from national and international social and economic processes. The women themselves are well aware that their reproductive choices take place in a field of action that is much influenced by forces and processes emanating from urban centers, the national capital, and distant foreign places.

REFERENCES

Barge, S., Khan, W.U., Narvekar, S, & Venkatachalam, Y., 2003 'Accessibility and Utiliation' *Seminar* (Special Issue on *Abortion: A symposium on the multiple facets of medical termination of pregnancy.*) 532: 36-40. (New Delhi) www.india-seminar.com

Barge, S., Bracken, H., Elul, B., Kumar, N., Khan, W., Verma, S., & Camlin, C., 2004, *Formal and Informal Abortion Services in Rajasthan, India: Results of a Situation Analysis*, Population Council: New Delhi.

Barnes, L., 2003, *Abortion Options for Rural Women: Case Studies from the Villages of Bokaro District, Jharkand*, Abortion Assessment Project-India, CEHAT:Mumbai.

Chhabra, R., & Nuna, S.C., 1994, *Abortion in India: An overview,* Ford Foundation, New Delhi.

Chandresekhar, S., 1994, *India's Abortion Experience*, Allen and Unwin: London.

Dharmapuri District, 2001, *Family Welfare Programme*, General Information Book.

Gammeltoft, T., 1999, *Women's Bodies, Women's Worries: Health and Family Planning in a Vietnamese Rural Community*, Curzon Press: Richmond Surrey.

Ganatra, B., 2000, 'Abortion Research in India: What We Know and What We Need to Know', in R. Ramasubban and S. Jejeebhoy (eds.), *Women's Reproductive Health in India*. pp. 186-235. Rawat Publications: New Delhi.

Ganatra, B., Hirve, S., Walawalkar, S., Garda, L., & Rao, V.N., 2000, '*Induced Abortions in a Rural Community in Western Maharasthra: Prevalence and Patterns'*, paper presented at Workshop on Reproductive Health in India: New Evidence and Issues, Pune, March 2000.

Ganatra, B., & Hirve, S., 2002, 'Induced Abortions Among Adolescent Women in Rural Maharashtra, India', *Reproductive Health Matters*, 10 (9): 76-85.

Gandhigram Institute of Rural Health and Family Welfar, 1999, *Rapid Household Survey: RCH Project, Dharmapuri*, Ministry of Health and Family Welfare: New Delhi.

George, S., & Dahiya, R., 1998, 'Female Foeticide in Rural Haryana', *Economic and Political Weekly*, 33(32): 2191-97.

Gittelsohn, J., Bentley, M.E., Pelto, P.J., Nag, M, Pachauri, S, Harrison, A.D, & Landman, I.T, (eds.), 1994, *Listening to Women Talking about Their Health*, Har-Anand Publication: New Delhi.

Government of India, 1973, T*he Medical Termination of Pregnancy Act No. 34 of 1971, Acts of Parliament,* Ministry of Law, Justice and Company Affairs: New Delhi.

Hirve, S., 2004, *Abortion Policy in India: Lacunae and future challenges*, Abortion Project-India. CEHAT: Mumbai.

India Mystica (CD-ROM), 1995-1998, *India Mystica: Encyclopedia of Indian Culture, Traditions and Beliefs*, Magic Software: New Delhi.

Iyengar, K., & Iyengar, S., 2002, 'Elective Abortion as a Primary Health Service in Rural India: Experience With Manual Vacuum Aspiration', *Reproductive Health Matters*, 10(19): 54-63.

Kakar, S., 1996, *The Indian Psyche,* Viking: New Delhi.

Khan, M.E., Barge, S., Kumar. N., & Almroth, S., 1999, 'Abortion in India: Current Situation and Future Challenges', in S. Pachauri (ed.), *Implementing a Reproductive Health Agenda in India: The beginning,* pp. 507-529. The Population Council: New Delhi.

Mallik, R., 2003, *Negative Choice: Sex determination and sex selective abortion in India,* Abortion Assessment Project-India, CEHAT: Mumbai.

Nichter, M., (ed.), 1989, *Anthropology and International Health: South Asian Case Studies*, Kluwer Publishers: Dondrecht.

Nichter, M., & Nichter, M., 1989, 'Modern Methods of Fertility Regulation: When and for Whom are They Appropriate?', in M. Nichter (ed.), *Anthropology and International Health. South Asian Case Studies*, pp 57-82. Kluwer Publishers: Dondrecht.

Ramachandar L., 2003, *Decision-Making and Women's Empowerment: Abortion in a South Indian Community,* unpublished doctoral thesis, University of Melbourne: Melbourne.

Ramachandar, L., & Pelto, P.J., 2002, 'The Role of Village Health Nurses in Mediating Abortions in Rural Tamil Nadu, India', *Reproductive Health Matters*, 10 (19): 54-75.

Ravindran, S., & Mishra, U.S., 2000, '*Unmet Need for Family Planning in India: A Women-Centered Perspective*', paper presented at workshop on Reproductive Health in India: New Evidence and Issues, Pune, March 2000.

Ross, J. L., Laston, S.L, Pelto, P.J., & Muna, L., 2002, 'Exploring Explanatory Models of Women's Reproductive Health in Bangladesh', *Culture, Health and Sexuality*, 4 (2): 173-190.

Saavala, M., 1997, *Child as Hope: Contextualizing Fertility Transition in Rural South India*, unpublished doctoral thesis, University of Amsterdam: Netherlands.

Saavala, M., 2001, *Fertility and Familial Power Relations: Procreation in South India*, Nordic Institute of Asian Studies Monograph No. 87: Richmond Surrey.

Visaria, L., 2000, 'From Contraceptive Targets to Informed Choice', in R. Ramasubban and S. Jejeebhoy (eds.), *Women's Reproductive Health in India*, pp. 331-382. Rawat Publication: New Delhi.

Whittaker, A, 2000, *Intimate Knowledge: Women and Their Health in North-east Thailand*, Allen and Unwin, St. Leonards: Sydney.

Whittaker, A., 2002, 'The Truth of Our Day by Day Lives: Abortion Decision-Making in Rural Thailand', *Culture, Health and Sexuality*, 3(4): 1-20.

In: Reproduction, Childbearing and Motherhood
Editor: Pranee Liamputtong, pp. 79-96

ISBN: 978-1-60021-606-0
© 2007 Nova Science Publishers, Inc.

Chapter 5

PRIVATE MATTER, PUBLIC CONCERN: LIVED EXPERIENCES OF ABORTION AMONG YOUNG WOMEN IN HO CHI MINH CITY, VIETNAM

Hoa Ngan Nguyen and Pranee Liamputtong

INTRODUCTION

Vietnam has a relatively large number of young people: 20.5 per cent of 79,832 million Vietnamese people are aged between 15-24 years old (Executive Board of the United Nations Development Program and of the United Nations Population Fund 2000). Among this group of people, abortion rates and the number of new cases of HIV/AIDS are increasing: about 20-30 per cent of abortions in Hanoi and Ho Chi Minh city were performed on young unmarried women; and more than half of newly reported cases of HIV infection involved people under 25 years of age (Gammeltoft, 2002a; Giesing, 2002). These issues suggest the urgency of researching young people's sexuality in relation to abortion.

Since 1986, under the effects of economic reform (*Đổi Mới*), many social changes have taken place in Vietnam: more freedom for people to make their own choice, and more contacts with western cultural influences. This reform has led to changes in family relations. In particular, parents seem to lose some of their control over their young children when these children become financially independent. More contacts with western culture are considered an important factor leading to changes in society and culture (Khuat Thu Hong, 1998). In terms of being exposed to foreign influences, Vietnamese young people are considered the most vulnerable group in society (Gammeltoft, 2002b). Under the effects of social and economic changes, premarital sexual relations have been increasing among young people (Khuat Thu Hong, 1998). But, premarital sex and abortion are considered as products of moral corruption, instigated by western culture. Many parents and politicians have widely expressed their condemnation for premarital sex and abortion. Nguyen Thanh Loi (quoted in Marr, 1996: 18) argues that the concept of female virginity must be emphasized, and premarital sex is proscribed by parents and others in society as a way to protect young people from the invasion of western consumerist and libertarian ideas. Khuat Thu Hong (1998: 37-

38), however, argues that premarital sex and premarital abortion are evidence of changes in sexual behavior and in the understanding of sexuality among young people. As we have shown in previous writing (Nguyen et al., 2006), premarital sex has become more acceptable among young people in Ho Chi Minh City but they lack knowledge about contraceptives. Equipped with poor knowledge of contraceptive and sexual issues, young people rely on abortion as a mean to control their reproductive life.

In this chapter, we examine the reasons for having an abortion among young female adults and their lived experiences of this event. We also attempt to identify some implications for sexual education to improve sexual health for youth in Vietnam.

PERCEPTIONS OF ABORTION IN VIETNAM

Historically, Vietnamese people (called Annamese at that time) attempted to prevent abortion by allowing the man to marry the girl with the lower bride price. They believed abortion was not a crime, but only immorally-wrong people had it, and these people were punished by going to the ninth hell (Devereux, 1960). It is believed that if people conduct bad deeds, after they die, their spirits will be kept in the ninth hell. In this place, their spirit will be tortured due to their bad conducts. In Buddhist creeds, which are practiced by 70-80 per cent of Vietnamese people today, there is no mention of induced abortion (Johansson et al 1998). But abortion was seen as a severe sin by the community in previous time in Vietnam (Le Thi Nham Tuyet et al., 1996). During this time, abortion was practiced secretly by traditional healers for unfortunate women. In pre-colonial times, pregnancy termination was not a crime against the state, but it became criminalized with the introduction of western abortion law during the French colonial time (Johansson et al., 1998).

In 1954, abortion was legalized, but still rare at the beginning of the 1980s. Since 1986, the abortion rate has increased rapidly, especially after the enforcement of one-or-two-child policy, and peaked in the early 1990s at about 100 per 1,000 married women of reproductive age (Johansson et al., 1998). There is no public debate about the ethics of abortion in Vietnam (Johansson et al., 1998; Gammeltoft, 2001). The scientific view in which pregnancy is perceived as a biological process, a young fetus is "nothing" and a "fully formed" fetus is a human being, dominates publicly and officially expressed views on abortion (Gammentoft, 2001: 323). Thus, a moral difference is justified between menstrual regulation when the fetus is a "blood clot" or "bean seed" and later abortion when the fetus is formed (Gammeltoft, 1999: 89-90). In addition, from the points of view of young people in Gammeltoft's study (2001: 328), to have an abortion "means not living up to your obligations as a human being to show care and compassion towards others". Abortion is therefore seen as a violation of "human morality", a disrespect for "human feeling", and something which is "inhuman" and "immoral".

From the medical point of view, induced abortions are performed through two procedures. Menstrual regulation (*hut thai* or to suck out the fetus) is used by a suction procedure within six weeks from the last menstrual period, whether or not a pregnancy is identified. The term abortion (*nao pha thai* or to destroy the fetus) refers to the procedure performed from six to twelve weeks from the last menstrual period. The procedure for terminating the second trimester pregnancy is a "modified Kovac" in which labor is induced by extra-amniotic saline infusion using a condom-covered catheter without prior ripening of the cervix (World Health Organization, 1999: 2). Menstrual regulation services are available at some community health centers. The services are regularly or periodically provided by mobile teams coming from the district level. Most of second trimester abortions are performed at provincial and central hospitals (World Health Organization, 1999).

With the enactment of the one-or-two-child policy in 1988, abortion services are available in both state and private medical facilities (Goodkind, 1994). These services are affordable and safe in large cities. Providers do not require official documentation to confirm personal information on the client records (Belanger and Khuat Thu Hong, 1999). Despite this, premarital abortion is still stigmatized in Vietnam. And this indeed makes it difficult for young unmarried women to express their views and the need to keep their abortion secret and suffer in silence.

METHODOLOGY

This chapter is based on our larger study on sexuality and abortion among young people in Vietnam. Based on the social construction of sexuality, we attempt to explain how social constraints and cultural values affect and shape sexual practices among young people in Ho Chi Minh city. We also attempt to understand why youth engage in unsafe sex. A feminist framework, which not only advocates the use of women's voices to express their experience but also introduces "women issues" into sociological research, is employed in this research (Liamputtong and Ezzy, 2005). Therefore, the concern is the subjective meaning and interpretation which young people, particularly young women, give to their experiences about their sexual practices. In Vietnamese society and culture, premarital sex and abortion are very sensitive topics because of social disapproval of these practices, and of the privacy of sexual experience. Qualitative methods, which focus on meanings and interpretations given by people to events and things, offer an insight into how people make sense of their experiences (Liamputtong and Ezzy, 2005). Therefore, a qualitative approach, using in-depth interviews as a method (Gubrium and Holstein, 2003), was deemed appropriate for researching this topic.

Purposive sampling technique (Liamputtong and Ezzy, 2005) was used to recruit the participants. Interviewees were selected through criteria such as age, abortion experience, and present place of interviewees' living. Unmarried women who had experienced abortion, aged between 15 to 24, and had lived in Ho Chi Minh city were suitable to participate in this research. We attempted to understand why youth engage in unsafe sex and consequently have an abortion. The criteria described above were used to recruit participants for the research.

The hospital where we recruited and conducted the study is one of the biggest obstetrical hospitals in Ho Chi Minh city. It is located in the city centre. There are two kinds of abortion services here: one operates in working hours, another in after-working hours. The fees charged for abortion services here are affordable with 30,000 dong (about A$ 3) charged for abortion in working hours and 50,000-60,000 dong (about A$ 5-6) for abortion after-working hours. Abortion services here are evaluated as safe and of good quality. Given its popularity among women seeking abortion services, this hospital was suitable for us to use in the conduct of the interviews because we had limited amount of time to recruit the participants due to the nature of the first author's postgraduate study requirements.

After the obtaining of ethics approval from La Trobe University, and authorizing approval from the Hospital had been granted, the first author traveled to Ho Chi Minh city, and made arrangements with hospital staff for conducting the interviews with women coming to the hospital for a follow-up examination after having had an abortion. Key informants, working at the abortion ward of this hospital, made the first contact with the women who met the criteria for inclusion in this research. After women agreed to participate in this research, the first author made interview arrangements with these women. All interviews with these unmarried women who had had abortion experiences were carried out by the first author at the advisory room of the Hospital from 2 to 24 January of 2003. Each interview took about an hour.

We believed that recruiting some young unmarried men to this research project was deemed necessary because data collected should be compared in order to distinguish any gender differences in, for example, attitudes to sexuality and sexual practices. Through the study of such differences, the effects of gender on sexual life can be better understood. Sampling young unmarried men was also purposive. It was based on the same criteria as the sampling of young unmarried women, except for the requirement of having had an abortion experience.

Men in this study were either female participants' boyfriends or any man who met the criteria of this research. One male interviewee was a female participant's boyfriend. The first author interviewed him at the advisory room in the hospital while he was waiting for his girlfriend, who was leaving for a follow-up examination. The other men she contacted through a male key informant, a colleague at the Institute of Social Sciences in Ho Chi Minh city. After these men agreed to participate in this research, a place at which the first author could do the interview with the men was arranged. The rest of male interviews were carried out at cafés near the interviewee's home, in the later half of February, 2003.

A total of sixteen interviews were conducted, involving twelve young unmarried women and four young unmarried men. The socio-demographic characteristics of the interviewees are presented in Table 1.

All recording tapes were transcribed, and then translated into English by the first author. The transcriptions of all recording tapes were organized into three columns with the text (raw data) in the middle column. We used thematic analysis to analyze the data; this method includes three main coding procedures: open coding, axial coding and selective coding (Liamputtong and Ezzy, 2005). The open coding which includes the themes was made in the left column of the transcriptions by the first author. These coding themes were then discussed with the second author. Then, the first author started the next step, axial coding in the right column of the transcriptions of all recording tapes. In this step, the themes were connected together in a new way. When this step finished, axial codes were discussed again between the two authors. Finally, the codebook was developed carefully with more detail including the first author's note-taking.

In the process of translating into English, many subtle nuances of language could not be easily translated in English due to differences in expression between English and Vietnamese. However, we attempted to translate all interviewees' answers so as to represent their feelings, their ideas, and their views as accurately as possible.

Table 1. Demographic characteristics of the participants

Demography	Female No	Male No
Age (years)		
15-18	2	0
19-20	3	1
21-24	7	3
Religion		
No religion	5	4
Buddhist	4	0
Christian	2	0
Protestant	1	0
Region of birth		
Ho chi Minh city	4	1
South regions	3	2
Central regions	4	0
North region	1	1
Educational level		
Primary	0	0
Secondary	4	0
High	4	1
College	2	0
University	2	3
Occupation		
Student	5	2
Worker	4	0
Trader	2	1
Employee in governmental sector	1	1
Types of accommodation		
Living with family	5	1
Living with relatives	1	0
Living in rent house	6	3
Living in dormitory	0	0
Length of stay in Ho Chi Minh City		
0-6 months	2	0
6 months to 1 year	1	1
1-5 year	2	0
5- 10 year	2	2
10+	5	1

FACING PREGNANCY

Young unmarried women in this study engaged in premarital sex (Nguyen and Liamputtong, 2007) and rarely used contraception (Nguyen et al., 2006). When they became pregnant, it was a stressful experience for them. In this section, we will discuss how young unmarried women dealt physically and emotionally with their unwanted pregnancies, and how their boyfriends and their parents reacted to their pregnancies.

Lived Experiences of Unwanted Pregnancies

Almost all the young women recognized physical signs of becoming pregnant, except for the two youngest women and an older one. The first physical sign of becoming pregnant mentioned by most women was that their period was overdue. Additional other physical signs, such as headache, backache, craving specific foods, and feelings of nausea were considered as certain signals for young women to find a next step to confirm their pregnancies.

> My period was ten days overdue. I vomited and felt very tired. I felt very worried. And then I went to this hospital and saw a doctor [Huong, a 23-age-old college student].

To confirm their pregnancies, seven women bought a tool kit for testing pregnancy, and two women saw a doctor for advice. The two youngest women did not recognize the signs of being pregnant. It was their mothers who noticed their unusual physical signs and took them for a check up at the hospital. One woman learnt about her pregnancy through a periodic health examination.

For most of these young women, their first reaction to their status of becoming pregnant was perplexity. They questioned why this should happen to them:

> I had sex only one time. I thought I could not get pregnant at all. When my mother got me to hospital for ultrasound, the doctor told her I got pregnant. I was puzzled and did not believe in what the doctor said (Oanh, a 18-age-old high school student).

This bewilderment was followed by feelings of sadness and anxiety. Some of these women said they cried for a month, or they could not sleep and eat for a week after they learnt they became pregnant:

> After I got a positive result from my test of pregnancy, I was very depressed. I cried in night time for all month. My mother asked me why I looked so sad. I had to make up the story that my boyfriend and I had problem about our plan for future (Dao, a 21-age-old trader).

For these young women, becoming pregnant meant a termination of their pregnancies. But some did not take this too lightly. Xuan, a 23-age-old tailor, mentioned her feelings of her pregnancy and abortion that:

> Generally, until that time I did not like a baby… But when my sister had a baby, I bought a skirt for her baby without any reason. I found that I liked a baby very much, and very often I thought of a baby. Then I learnt that I got pregnant, I wanted to have a baby very much. I wanted to keep my pregnancy, but my circumstances would not allow me to raise a baby. I thought I had to do that [having abortion], but I felt guilty.

Reactions of Significant Others

Most women in the study conceded they did not inform their parents about their pregnancies. The reason for doing so will be examined in more detail in the next section. Two youngest women, whose pregnancies were known by their parents, remarked on their parents reactions that:

> When my mother knew I got pregnant, she was so disappointed. She cried and scolded me. My father did not say any word to me. In my family, the atmosphere was so depressed and sad. I was very sad and regretted. Several days later, my mother advised me to have an abortion (Oanh, a 18-age-old high school student).

Of twelve women in the study, almost all women, except one, discussed their pregnancies with their boyfriends. It is interesting that half of the women said their boyfriends felt both happy and worried about their pregnancies. Lan, a 23-year-old tailor, explained her boyfriend's feeling:

> He was both happy and worried. [...]He was worried because we haven't had a wedding ceremony yet. People would think badly about us. He was happy because he was 29 year old, and he could be a father.

The other half remarked that their boyfriends' reactions ranged from fear, sadness, anxiety, and keeping silent:

> He and I both were afraid. He was even more afraid than me. So confiding with him made me more afraid (Xuan, 23-age-old tailor).
> When my boyfriend knew I got pregnant, as far as I could remember, he was sad but kept calm. But he was caring for me (Ngoc, 24-age-old employee).

In the discussions between the women and their boyfriends, they also had to work out the best possible solution for them. Several women said their boyfriend had to inform their parents about their girlfriends' pregnancies in order to obtain the approval for marriage. For some women, this approval was not accepted by their own parents due to the fears of losing family reputation within a morally-right society.

> He said he would tell his family about my pregnancy and we would have his family's approval for marriage. But my mother said I would not allow him to tell his family any thing related to my pregnancy. My mother did not want his family to disdain me and my parents (Oanh, a 18-age-old high school student).
> For some women, their love was already accepted by both their families and their boyfriends' families. Marriage in the situation with an unwanted pregnancy was still undesirable:

> We will marry in April, 2003. I could not keep my pregnancy. If I keep it until April, my pregnancy becomes bigger. So my family will be disappointed (Linh, a 22-age-old hairstylist).

For women who were not certain about their future marriage, the choice of abortion was unavoidable:

Hoa: Did you think that your love was strong enough to get married?
Huong: I did not know what he thought. Actually, how could I know his true thinking? But as a girl, when I loved some one, I loved with serious emotion. But men were different. Some guys thought like that, but others did not. [...] I did not know his true thinking. I thought he just thought of having sex with me. I knew that, so I made the decision to have an abortion myself (Huong, a 23-age-old college student).

It is noted that all women mentioned 'difficulties in getting married while pregnant' as reasons for their choice of abortion. But none of these women thought of having a baby without a proper marriage.

ABORTION

In this section, we examine why young women actively made the decision to have an abortion, and how their parents, their boyfriends and themselves felt about their abortion, as well as how they were cared for after having an abortion.

Abortion: Making the Decision

Fears of parents finding out about their pregnancies were expressed as a main reason for making the decision to have an abortion. Mai, a 24-age-old trader, said:

We have already proposed ritually, and we will have the wedding ceremony in February, 2003. I was afraid that my pregnancy would be bigger by that time. My parents would kill me. So I made the decision of having an abortion. Inside my heart, I did not want to do it, but...
(in tears)

The women's fear was explained by the fact that their family could lose their moral reputation because of their pregnancies. Two other women told us that their mothers always asked them to maintain their virginity until their wedding ceremony because this was seen as a female proper code of conduct. Therefore, their parents would not accept their pregnancies. The following excerpts exemplify their situations:

My mother always tells me that I am a girl and I have to keep my virginity (Minh, a 20-age-old university student)

If I kept my pregnancy, my family would never accept me. All of my sisters and my brothers never have sex before marriage. Only I had it (Mai, a 24-age-old trader)

These women had to consider not only their family's reputation but also their moral reputation. Lan, a 23-age-old tailor, said:

We (she and her boyfriend) were afraid of people's saying badly about my pregnancy before my marriage.

Linh, 22-age-old hairstylist, also expressed this concern:

As I said before my parents are very strict. So I couldn't keep my pregnancy. [How about your boyfriend's parents?] They were very strict, too. [Could you explain why they are very strict?] They did not like... For example they would reject me if they knew I had premarital sex.

The fear of being known by the family was so strong that these women could not accept their boyfriends' offer to arrange a wedding ceremony. Ha, a 19-age-old college student, insisted on having an abortion even though her boyfriend's family asked her to marry him and to keep her pregnancy:

My boyfriend wanted me to keep my pregnancy. His family knew that I got pregnant. But my mother didn't know any thing about it. My parents wanted me to go abroad and get married with a foreigner. They didn't want me to love him, so I didn't let them know. [...] My boyfriend's family said I should keep my pregnancy...I thought I wanted to have an abortion and did not want to raise my pregnancy because my mother did not agree to arrange the wedding ceremony for us.

It is also apparent that the women's social position impinged upon their decision to have an abortion. Besides the fear of being known by their family, two women reasoned that they had an abortion because of their economic circumstances:

Then I knew that I got pregnant. I wanted to have a baby very much. I wanted to raise my pregnancy but I was not in any good condition to raise a baby. I thought I had to do it [having abortion], but I felt guilty. I thought carefully of my decision. I couldn't keep my pregnancy. I had nothing (Xuan, a 23-age-old tailor).

The perceived irresponsibility on the part of their boyfriends also prompted some women to make their own decisions. One woman made the decision of having an abortion because her boyfriend did not accept her pregnancy and would not do any thing for her:

After I knew I had got pregnant, I didn't talk with my boyfriend... I thought even if I talked with him, he couldn't do any thing for me. [...] He was studying in the university. He did not want me to have a pregnancy. So I did not say any thing with him (Huong, a 23-age-old college student).

Two other women were still in high school. They did not recognize that they became pregnant. Their parents were suspicious of their pregnancies and brought them to the hospital for a check up. Oanh, a 18-age-old high school student, said:

My mother told me that I had to continue my study at high school and had to terminate my pregnancy. I was afraid of making my parents sad. I accepted my mother's decision. My mother also asked me to stop my relationship with my boyfriend after having the abortion. I thought I should follow her decision.

Both of these women had to follow their mothers' decision of having an abortion. Both were so confused that they did not know how to deal with this stressful event. Their mothers, hence, became their decision makers.

The men's perspectives on the decision to have an abortion revealed some interesting trends. In our interview with Nam, a 24-age-old trader, he confirmed that his girlfriend insisted on having an abortion because of her fear for her family's moral reputation. The following excerpt illustrates this situation:

[What did you think when you knew your girlfriend had got pregnant?] I was happy. I told her to keep her pregnancy. But she didn't want to do it. And family... Her family did not want it. My family liked me to have a baby.

Hung, a 24-age-old employee, reasoned that most unmarried women facing a pregnancy decided to have an abortion because they did not want to depend on their boyfriends' commitment to marriage. He said:

I saw many girls in this situation [having pregnancy] chose that solution [having abortion]. Very few of them asked their boyfriends to marry them. When unmarried girl got pregnant, there were only two ways for them. Having an abortion was the first way, and asking their boyfriends for marriage is the second one. But the second one depended on their boyfriends. Actually, the first way was the most popular option these girls choose. When they chose it, they forgot about its effects on their health.

Other men believed that abortion had a negative impact on the women. Son, a 24-age-old university student, explained that abortion was not good because of its effects on unmarried women's health and emotion, but it was the fastest solution to end an unmarried woman's problem. Dung, a 19-age-old university student, seemed to attach moral disapproval to abortion among unmarried girls. When asked if he had a female friend who was not married but had an abortion, how would he think of her, he responded that:

Firstly, I thought badly of this girl... I thought there are many reasons for what she did. But firstly I thought badly. Later if I knew her more, my thinking might change... But firstly I had no sympathy for her.

Who Makes the Decision?

Most women actively made the decision of having an abortion except two younger women who had an abortion due to their mothers' decision. Before making the decision, these women discussed with their boyfriend and received support from them:

Of course, I did not think of getting pregnant. So I was puzzled. My boy friend said it was up to me. If I wanted to keep my pregnancy, he would tell his family. If I did not want to keep it, he would bring me to hospital. I said we had nothing; we couldn't live on our families' support. So he said we went to hospital [...]. He [my boyfriend] said he accepted my decision. He was afraid that I would regret if I kept my pregnancy. He respected my decision (Vy, a 20-age-old electronic worker)

However, Huong, a 23-age-old college student, made the decision of to have an abortion without discussion with her boyfriend because she thought her boyfriend would not support her.

When making the decision to have an abortion, most women were more or less aware of potential risks of abortion on their health. Ngoc, a 24-year-old employee, told us that:

> I thought... It was possible that I would not have a baby later on. If the fetus became bigger, it would have affected me. It caused death. If blood came out too much, it would have been very serious on my health. So I should consult a doctor before making the decision.

Cuc, too, remarked that:

> I only knew that after having an abortion, I would be weak. I also heard that it was possible I would be childless in the future.

During the field work, we observed that doctors working in the abortion ward asked all women who wanted to have an abortion to sign a form of voluntary commitment for abortion. Potential risks during and after carrying out procedures for an abortion were clearly stated on this form. These women were also consulted about which kind of procedures would be performed and which kind of procedures they preferred to have. It was obvious that medical staff wanted their clients to be aware clearly of potential risks if they had an abortion. They were more likely to want their clients to take more time to think about their decision. However, unmarried women in the study insisted on their commitment to abortion because they were under pressure to protect their family's moral reputation, and for their own reputation as well as some other personal reasons such as their studies and their unstable economic condition.

Reactions to Abortion

While conducting our interviews, many times the women would cry. Many times we had to stop the conversation because they became so distressed when they thought of their abortions. Most of these women felt sad, afraid and guilty. This excerpt illustrates these women's feelings:

> [When you made the decision of having abortion, what did your boyfriend think?] What I felt at that time was that he was very sad but kept calm. [...] He always remembers that day. [Then the interviewee started crying for several minutes] (Ngoc, a 24-age-old employee)

However, two women in high school did not mention their feelings of abortion. They just mentioned their mothers' sad feelings caused by them, and said they would stop their relationship with their boyfriend after having an abortion:

> I though that after having an abortion I would stop my relationship with my boyfriend for the rest of my life. I do not want this event to happen again. I was afraid of making my mother sad. My mother did not want me to love him. (Cuc, a 18-age-old high school student)

For two women who had had more than one abortion, their sad feelings seemed to be not as strong as those expressed by the women with first abortion. While Ha, a 19-age-old college student, said she felt normal after having an abortion, Linh, a 22-age-old hairstylist, said she felt a little sad.

Some of these women made remarks about their boyfriends' reactions to their abortion. Mai, a 24-age-old trader, said her boyfriend cried when he knew her decision to have an abortion. Vy, a 20-age-old electronic worker, told us that her boyfriend could not sleep for several nights when he learnt about her decision to have an abortion, and felt guilty.

Fears of the consequences of an abortion were mentioned by the women. Some women remarked that after they experienced an abortion they did not dare to have sex again. They would only do it after their marriage and would give birth if they became pregnant. These excerpts exemplify this fear:

> I did not dare to do it. After having an abortion, even our love was so strong, I had to keep away from sex. In addition, my boyfriend loved me too much, so he would sympathize with me. Generally, he loved me so much, he would accept my opinion (Mai, 24-age-old trader).
>
> As I have said before, some times I and my boyfriend couldn't control our emotions... After this time, my boyfriend said we would give up having sex [smiling]. He feared for me (Minh, a 20-age-old university student).

Their fears were also related to the consequence of an abortion including being childless in the future or being punished due to the act of "sin". These fears stemmed from a traditional belief that by committing a bad deed, this will result in bad consequences.

> I was afraid of being childless (Linh, a 22-age-old hairstylist)
> People said that the fetus was only a clot of blood but it had spirit. If it was terminated, it would follow me later on. So it was difficult for me to become better off. I just heard that. I was afraid, but did not dare to say to any one. I just confided with my friends and did not do any thing to relieve my fear. Both he and I were afraid. He even was more afraid than me... He was very sad and thought abortion is sin. (Xuan, a 23-age-old tailor)

One woman said that she would not have an abortion if her fetus was one month old:

> [saying in tears]...If my fetus were one month old, I would be overbold to run away from my house to give birth. But it was only two weeks old, so I though the fetus would forgive me. I felt very sad (Mai, a 24-age-old trader).

These women felt guilty because of their abortions but they said they had no choice in the circumstances

> I cried for all week. Every time I thought I had abortion, I felt guilty. I couldn't give birth in the first time I got pregnant because of our condition. We thought carefully of our circumstance. My boyfriend had to study abroad for two year. I did not want to distract him. Moreover, I did not want my family to lose the reputation because of my premarital pregnancy (Dao, a 21-age-old trader).

Care during and after having an Abortion

Among the women in the study, the two youngest women received care from their mothers. The rest of the women kept their abortion secret from their families. They received some kind of support from their boyfriends or their boyfriends' friends when they were in the hospital. Only one woman had no care from either her family or her boyfriend or any friend in hospital. For this woman, the main reason for having an abortion was that she was not sure about her boyfriend's emotion. She went to hospital alone with so much confusion.

> I did not know there were the counselors in the hospital. It was the first time I went to the hospital. On that day, I really wanted to ask someone, but I didn't know who I could ask something, and what I should do. I just know the phone line 1080. But I didn't dare to ask them. I was afraid that they were not specialists of this issue (Huong, a 23-age-old college student)

She returned home quickly after the procedures were performed. At her home, she had to try to behave normally in order to conceal the event from her parents.

The care that the women received from their boyfriend, both during and after the abortion, included such actions as going with them to hospital, paying fees for services and for medicine, and consoling them. Eight women said their boyfriends went with them to the hospital and paid all, or some of the fees for the services and medicine. One woman went to the hospital with her boyfriend's friend because her boyfriend worked in another city. However, many women did not even take an hour rest at the hospital as the hospital advised. Some would go to work or to class as normal on the next day:

> My boyfriend took care of me. I returned my home. I had a rest at the hospital for 30 minutes. I worked as normal (Lan, a 23-age-old tailor)
> The last time, my boyfriend went with me. This time he also went there with me and I continued to go to my class as normal (Ha, a 19-age-old college student)

Lan, a 23-age-old tailor, said she had to carry on her usual work as normal because it was difficult to have a day out of work in her company. She almost run out of money due to her difficulties to turn up for work. Having to keep their abortion secret made the women work or live as normal. Moreover, social disapproval made it difficult for them to ask for and to follow proper instructions for care after having an abortion.

DISCUSSION

It is clear in this study that choice of abortion was not easy for unmarried women. The most common reason for seeking abortion was the pressure of protecting women's families' moral reputation and their own. Within the social atmosphere of disapproved premarital pregnancy, unmarried women had to put their families' reputation and their own reputation in the first place. In addition, the disadvantages due to their age, unstable economic circumstances, and unfinished study pushed them to choose abortion as a solution. In some cases, marriage offers or a marriage plan could not prevent unmarried women from having an abortion. Therefore, these women were the prime actors making the decision to have an abortion, when their boyfriends could not find a better solution for them (cf. Boggess and Bradner, 2000). Facing premarital unwanted pregnancy and subsequent abortion, these women suffered much physical and emotional pain.

In Vietnamese society, the maintenance of women's virginity until marriage is the dominant moral idea. When young unmarried women engage in premarital sex, they are considered as "stained" and "spoiled", and are devalued morally (Gammeltoft, 2001: 329). In the society like Vietnam, public shame is used to control people's morality (O'Harrow, 1995). In this context, young people's sexual life is affected heavily by the dominant moral idea. Gammeltoft (2002:119) examines the effects of dominant cultural ideas expressed through "public opinion" on Vietnamese young people's sexual life. According to Gammeltoft (2002:119), "public opinion" which includes the moral evaluation of neighbor, shopkeepers, family members, and friends, is the factor most feared by young people when they engage in premarital sex. That is why all young women in this study actively made the decision to have an abortion to hide their engagement in premarital sex. It also explains why all women in the study mentioned their fear of being known about their engagement in premarital sex as a main reason to seek abortion. And that is why most women in this study tried to keep their abortion secret and, silently suffer emotional and physical pain of their embodied abortion experience.

UNDERSTANDING ABORTION FROM A GENDER PERSPECTIVE

It is obvious that using gender norms provides a framework for many aspects of social regulation of young people's sexuality. Under the pressure of public opinion, of government policies and slogans, and of sexual education programs within Vietnamese society, young people's access to information and services is constrained. Within a gendered framework, young people have to inevitably face the conflict between their own sexual agency and social forces.

Facing premarital pregnancy was a stressful experience, particularly for young unmarried women. In the social context of Vietnam, having premarital pregnancy means that a young unmarried woman violates both her family's moral identities and her own. Therefore, not only are young women devalued morally by public opinion, but also their parents are stigmatized because of their daughters' conduct. In these circumstances, it is not surprising that many parents reacted negatively to this event by reprimanding their daughters, by being disappointed, and sad when they learned about their daughters' pregnancy. Young unmarried women were under the double pressure of moral devaluation for both their family's reputation and their own.

When young unmarried women engage in premarital sex, they expose themselves not only to the risk of spoiling their family's moral reputation and their own, but also to the risk of damaging their chances for getting married with a suitable partner (CARE International and Vietnamese Ministry of Health, 1997). If a young unmarried woman becomes pregnant, she has three choices: asking for a marriage approval from their boyfriends' families and their boyfriend, having a birth outside marriage, and having an abortion. Having a birth outside marriage in Vietnam, where premarital sex is stigmatized and condemned, is an undesirable option because it is shameful, and totally damages the potential of getting married in the future (Gammeltoft, 2002a, b). The possibility of being married depends on the attitude both of the woman's boyfriend and his family. Having a marriage under these circumstances, the young woman is still regarded as being tarnished, and hence, not totally respected by any parent-in-law. By having an abortion, young unmarried women can conceal their premarital sex and hence protect the potential of getting married in the future. Hence, as remarked by one male respondent, Son, a 23-year-old student, abortion is "the fast solution to end all problems" for young unmarried women. That is why all young unmarried women in this study actively made the decision to have an abortion.

When having an abortion, young unmarried women face the fear of abortion procedure, of negative health consequences in the future, and emotional pain. Most women in this study were aware of the health consequences of abortion when they committed to have one. However, the fear of social condemnation and moral judgment outweigh the worry about health consequences when a young woman makes the decision to have an abortion. They have to put their family's moral reputation and their own in the first place and suffer the fear of health consequences. In addition, most young women in this study experienced emotional pain after having an abortion. They could not confide with any-one in their family. They cried in silence. Some of them felt guilty because they thought the fetus, which they could not keep, had a spirit. Some of them were depressed because they had their first pregnancy but could not give birth. Most women in this study suffered these pains in silence, and yet they had to live and to work as if nothing had happened to them. The suffering of emotional pain in silence makes women's abortion experiences more distressful indeed.

It is obvious that abortion is an inevitable consequence of the social and cultural constraints which operate under gender norms. By highly valuing women's chastity through public opinion, through educational institutions, and through government policies and slogans, young unmarried women find it difficult to obtain accurate knowledge related to contraception and sexual issues, and to overcome the invisible obstacles in negotiating, as well as in making the decision of using contraceptives to practice safe sex (Gammeltoft, 1999, Nguyen et al., 2006). Consequently, women have to suffer physical and emotional pain through their embodied experience of abortion.

When abortion was legalized in Vietnam, it was expected that women would have control over their reproductive health. The woman is the person who should make the decision to have an abortion in accordance with what she thinks is best for her. However, the assumption, which underpins all Vietnamese social structures, is that sexual relations for women should be within marriage only and women's chastity is highly valued wards off this right for unmarried women (Gammeltoft, 2002a, b, Zhang and Locke 2002). When a young unmarried woman becomes pregnant, she may make her own decision to have an abortion. However, her decision is a consequence of many social constraints as mentioned earlier. Furthermore, her voluntary commitment to abortion is also made under the pressure of protecting her family's moral reputation, her own, and her potential for getting married in the future. In this circumstance, a voluntary commitment to abortion is turned into a subtly involuntary commitment (Gammeltoft, 2002a, b).

IMPLICATIONS FOR WOMEN'S HEALTH CARE

Abortion with its health consequences and emotional pain raises concerns for many researchers and health professionals interested in improving sexual health for young people. But, how can young people's sexual health be improved in the Vietnamese context?

According to the new public health debate, definition of health encompasses wide-ranging social, cultural, political and economic factors (Baum, 2002). This perspective on health is useful for new public health, which focuses on populations rather than individuals. The Ottawa Charter, the foundation of the new public health, specifies five key strategies in directing health promotion (Baum, 2002). These strategies include the development of healthy public policy, the creation of supportive environments, strengthening community action, the development of personal skills, and reorientation of health services. To apply these strategies in the improvement of sexual health for Vietnamese young people, the first thing is to develop a supportive climate, one in which sexual issues can be discussed openly. It is evident that there is an association between the openness and permissiveness of social attitudes toward sex, and teenagers' success in preventing unwanted pregnancies (Hadley, 1996).

Policy was considered as a powerful tool of public health (Baum, 2002). The importance of good health policy is recognized because it can close health gaps between social groups and between nations, it can broaden the choices of people, and it can ensure supportive social environments (Baum, 2002). In the Vietnamese context, the government policies related to the provision of family planning services need to reach every individual regardless of their marital status. It is here we argue that young people's specific needs regarding family planning services are to be included. This will inevitably help young women to avoid unwanted pregnancies and hence abortion rates can be reduced. In order to do so, research plays an important role. It may offer an insight into young people's sexual needs, suggest appropriate approach for interventions, and question the established social attitudes and practices so as to provide preconditions for improving policies and services for young people in Vietnam (Gammeltoft, 2002b).

Health promotion aims to develop personal skills through providing information, education about health and helping people to develop the skills to make healthy choices (Ashton and Seymour, 1990). In this sense, improving sexual education in Vietnam is essential. In Vietnam, those in powerful positions believe that sexual education may encourage sexual experimentation and risky behavior among young people, hence it should not advocated (Marr, 1996; Population Council, 1998). From the public health point of view, when young people engage in sex, they will do so more safely if they have received the benefits of sexual education (Schwartz and Rutter, 1998). There are also some positive experiences which can be learned from the Netherlands. Sexual education in this country does not involve the provision of lectures, but accepts teenagers' sexual experimentation as one of facts of life; and most young women simply equip themselves with the means to avoid pregnancy when they are ready for sex. The Netherlands also makes contraceptives easily available to young men and women. In this context, pregnancy rate among Dutch teenagers is the lowest in the world (Hadley, 1996). Sexual education programs in Vietnam could be improved by helping people feel comfortable with sexuality topics, and by promoting the attitude that sexuality is a normal part of being human. Skills in negotiating and practicing safe sex should be one of main parts of these programs. In addition, to improving sexual health for Vietnamese young people, family planning services should be reoriented to provide more access for young people. Practically, this work can only be done when health policies related to family planning have been developed in the first phase.

In sum, we have demonstrated in this chapter that young people's sexual life is shaped and constrained by gender norms through political interventions, sexual education institutions, and moral judgment. Under the pressure of these norms, young people have to face many difficulties in order to practice safe sex, and hence come to rely on abortion as a mean to control their sexual life. We have shown here that abortion is not only an inevitable consequence of social constraints, but is also a doubled stressful experience when young women suffer it in silence. The task of improving sexual lives of Vietnamese young people, particularly women, involves a long road to travel. We have at least, in this study, started this long journey. It is hoped that further research will be undertaken to fulfill this goal. Only then many sexually active young people in Vietnam no longer suffer in silence.

ACKNOWLEDGEMENTS

We thank all the Vietnamese young people who took part in this study and were willing to share their private experiences with the researcher. Without their insights, this study would not have been possible. The first author thanks the Ford Foundation for sponsoring her study at La Trobe University and field trip to undertake her field work in Vietnam.

REFERENCES

Ashton, J., & Seymour, H., 1990, *The New Public Health*, Open University Press: Milton Keyness.

Baum, F., 2002, *The New Public Health*, 2nd edition, Oxford University Press: Melbourne.

Belanger, D., & Khuat Thu Hong, 1999, 'Single Women's Experience of Sexual Relationship and Abortion in Ha Noi, Vietnam', *Reproductive Health Matters*, 7 (14): 71-82.

Boggess, S., & Bradner, C., 2000, 'Trend in Adolescent Male's Abortion Attitudes, 1985-1995: Difference by Race and Ethnicity', *Family Planning Perspective*, 32 (3): 118-123.

Bowling, A., 1997, *Research Methods in Health: Investigating Health and Health Services*, Open University Press: Buckingham.

CARE International and Vietnam Ministry of Health, 1997, *An Audience Analysis of Women, Men (aged 15-25) and Providers' Knowledge, Attitudes and Practices of Contraceptive Methods in Rural Vietnam*, Ethnical Culture Publishing House: Hanoi.

Devereux, G., 1960, *A Study of Abortion in Primitive Societies*, Thomas Yoseloff Ltd: London.

Executive Board of the United Nations Development Program and of the United Nations Population Fund, 2000, DF/FPA/VIE/6. http://www.unfa.org.regions/adp/countries/vietnam/3vie0105.doc

Gammeltoft, T., 1999, *Women's Bodies, Women's Worries*, Curzon Press: Surrey.

Gammeltoft, T., 2001, 'Between "Science" and "Superstition": Moral Perceptions of Induced Abortion Among Young Adults in Vietnam', *Culture, Medicine and Psychiatry*, 26: 313-338.

Gammeltoft, T., 2002, 'Seeking Trust and Transcendence: Sexual Risk Taking Among Vietnamese Youth', *Social Science & Medicine*, 55: 483-495.

Gammeltoft, T., 2002, 'The Irony of Sexual Agency: Premarital Sex in Urban Northern Vietnam', in J. Werner and D. Belanger (eds.), *Gender, Household, State: Doi moi In Vietnam*, pp. 111-128. Southeast Asia Program Publication: New York.

Giesing, P., 2002, HIV/AIDS communication among youths in Hanoi, Vietnam. MA thesis. http://www.media.ku.dk/HIV/AIDScomm/HIVAIDvietnamMA.pdf

Goodkind, D., 1994, 'Abortion in Vietnam: Measurements, Puzzles and Concern', *Studies in Family Planning*, 25 (6): 342-353.

Hadley, J., 1996, *Abortion: Between Freedom and Necessity*, Virago Book: London.

Johansson, A., Nguyen Thu Nga, Tran Quang Huy, Doan Du Dat, & Holmgren, K., 1998, 'Husbands' Involvement in Abortion in Vietnam', *Studies in Family Planning*, 29 (4): 400 (1). http:infotrac.galegroup.com/itw/infomark/104/364/14308175w7/purl=rc1_EIM_0_A539

Khuat Thu Hong, 1998, *Study on Sexuality in Vietnam: The Known and Unknown Issues*, Regional Working Paper, The Population Council: Hanoi.

Le Thi Nham Tuyet, Johansson, A., & Nguyen The Lap, 1996, 'Abortions on Two Rural Communes in Thai Binh Province, Vietnam', in K. Barry (ed.), *Vietnam's Women in Transition*, pp. 93-109. Macmillan Press Ltd: London.

Liamputtong, P., & Ezzy, D., 2005, *Qualitative Research Methods 2nd edition*, Oxford University Press: Melbourne.

Marr, D.G., 1996, Vietnamese Youth in the 1990s, working paper # 3, Macquarie University: Sydney.

Nguyen, H.N., & Liamputtong, P., 2007, 'Sex, love and gender norms: Sexual life and experience of a group of young people in Ho Chi Minh city, Viet Nam', *Sexual Health*, 4: 63-69.

Nguyen, H.N., Liamputtong, P., & Murphy, G., 2006, 'Knowledge of Contraceptives and Sexually-Transmitted Diseases and Contraceptive Practices Amongst Young People in Ho Chi Minh city, Vietnam', *Health Care for Women International*, 27: 399-417.

O'Harrow, S., 1995, 'Vietnamese Women and Confucianism: Creating Spaces from Patriarchy', in W.J. Karim (ed.), *'Male' and 'Female' in Developing Southeast Asia*, pp. 161-180. Berg Publishers: Oxford.

Population Council, 1998, *Vietnamese Youth Reproductive Health Needs in the Doi moi Era: Challenges and Opportunities*, Population Council: Hanoi.

Sachdev, P., 1993, *Sex, Abortion and Unmarried Women*, Greenwood Press: Westport, CT.

Schwartz, P., & Rutter, V., 1998, *The Gender of Sexuality*, Pine Forge Press: Thousand Oaks, CA.

United Nations Development Programme, 2000, VIE/96/029. http://www.undp.org.vn/undp/prog/prodocs/gov/vie96029.pdf

World Health Organization, 1999, Abortion in Vietnam: An Assessment of Policy, Programme and Research Issue. http://www.who.int/reproductive-health/publications/HRP_ITT_99_2

PART TWO: CHILDBIRTH IN DIFFERENT CULTURES

In: Reproduction, Childbearing and Motherhood   ISBN: 978-1-60021-606-0
Editor: Pranee Liamputtong, pp. 99-112   © 2007 Nova Science Publishers, Inc.

Chapter 6

CELEBRATING SAFE CHILDBIRTH

Elizabeth Hoban

INTRODUCTION

Two dominant and diverging paradigms inform the discourse on childbirth. The biomedical perspective treats pregnancy and childbirth as an illness, requiring technological management by skilled professionals in formal medical facilities. In contrast, in non-Western and Western societies, where the two approaches may co-exist, pregnancy, childbirth and the post-parturition period are seen as natural, biosocial and life-crisis events that is:

> everywhere a candidate for consensual shaping and social patterning. In most societies, birth and the immediate post-partum period are considered a time of vulnerability for mother and child-indeed, frequently a time of ritual danger for the entire family and community. In order to deal with this danger and the existential uncertainty associated with birth, people tend to produce a set of internally consistent and mutually dependent practices and beliefs that are designed to manage physiologically and socially problematic aspects of parturition in a way that makes sense in the particular cultural context (Jordan 1993: 3-4).

Since the late twentieth century, the dominant cultural paradigm for doing birth has been biomedical with a risk-averse, surveillance and technocratic focus (Arms, 1975; Arney, 1982; Davis-Floyd, 1993, 1994; Jordon, 1993; Murphy-Lawless, 1998; Walsh et al., 2004). This approach to birth has been characterized by decreasing rates of maternal and infant mortality, and increasing rates of caesarean section, instrumental delivery, and intra-partum interventions (El-Nemer et al., 2006). Childbirth in most countries has moved from the private arena into the public domain, albeit political, ostensibly for the (physical) safety of mother and infant. Even in countries where efforts have been made to humanise birth, recent evidence indicates that the technocratic model remains strongly entrenched (Downe et al., 2001; Hildingsson et al., 2003). This shift has occurred despite the fact that high rates of maternal and infant mortality no longer exist in most Western societies, particularly post-war rates in advanced Western societies (Lane, 1995). In contrast, the high rates of maternal and infant mortality that continue to exist in many developing countries provides a clear justification for the introduction of a way of birthing which is predicated on the grounds of physical safety (El-Nemer et al., 2006).

The biomedical model of childbirth has assigned risk to individuals rather than structural and social conditions (Lane, 1995). This model assumes that the body is always ready to fail, even if it appears to be a low-risk situation. Biomedicine views birth as a medical problem that can result in pathology, disability and death at any stage of the pregnancy, birth and postpartum period. The individualization of risk has legitimized the routine use of interventions such as the adoption of the lithotomy position in delivery or labour, the pharmacological induction of labour and drugs for pain relief and labour (Wagner, 1994). Appropriate management can prevent some complications during the pregnancy, labor and the postpartum period; other women can be identified as being at risk, such as women who had complications in a previous pregnancy. However, most complications are difficult to predict, in fact, complications can occur among low-risk women. Therefore, it is not easy to determine which woman will develop obstetric complications and at what stage of her pregnancy or confinement these might occur. According to the World Health Organization (WHO) fifteen percent of all pregnant women will require skilled obstetric care, and in their absence they will suffer serious and long term morbidities and disabilities (WHO, 1998).

Limited research exists that explores, within the physiological/biomedical framework, the cultural perceptions of safety and risk in maternities in Western and non-Western societies, and how it impacts on women's choice of type and place of birth, and their birth attendant. The perception of risk is a social process and the different social principles that guide behavior affect people's judgment of what dangers should be most feared, what risks are worth taking, and who should be allowed to take them (Douglas, 1992). In all societies women make rational and pragmatic choices when developing their safety-first strategy, based on their experiential and embodied knowledges of pregnancy and childbirth (Hoban, 2003; Pilley Edwards, 2005). In Cambodia, local discourses of risk are informed by past experiences of medical interventions and contacts with institutions, understanding of the medical dialogue, the status of women, women's ability to maintain their cultural practices and their loss of autonomy and control over their lives. Cambodian women do not have difficulty deciding where to give birth and who will be their birth attendant; they are well aware of the economic, cultural, physical and emotional costs before making their decision. Women have their own method of calculating the proximal and distal costs and risks associated with each option, and they weigh them up against the likely birth outcome (Hoban, 2003).

Indigenous pregnancy, birthing and postpartum practices in Western and non-Western societies, including in Cambodia, have undergone considerable change due to the imported medicalized and institutionalized Western system of obstetrics. Empirical research demonstrates that elements of indigenous birthing systems survive, either in part or in full. In Cambodia, for example, women do not forsake what they perceive to be safe, reliable, effective practices, such as postpartum food prescriptions and precautionary behaviours that are based on humoral medical theory; they modify and adjust them to modern ways of giving birth, depending on the resources, options and sense of agency women are afforded.

In this chapter, I describe how Cambodian women trust and rely on universal preventative strategies, such as *ang pleen* (mother roasting), which begins immediately after childbirth and is terminated 5-10 days post-partum to ensure their safety. Mother roasting forms part of a suite of postpartum practices that include drinking Khmer herbs, eating 'hot' foods, postpartum massage to ensure women's humoral balance is returned immediately post-birth thereby preventing life-threatening pre-conditions such as *chiem chok* (stuck blood), or morbidities such as a weak and aching body in old age. At the cessation of mother roasting when the woman leaves the roasting bed, her family hold a celebration called *tumleak cǝǝŋ krañcǝǝ* (dropping the stove), which marks the postpartum woman's safety and the end of her confinement. A *saen doon taa* (ritual to thank ancestral spirits for assisting the woman in childbirth) and the *yiey maap* (grandmother midwife) and her spirit teacher are publicly thanked their role in ensuring a safe birth outcome. During this ceremony traditional knowledges and practices are transmitted between generations in a culturally safe place. I argue that these practices are based on internally consistent logic and experiential evidence, spanning over generations. Within the existing economic parameters of families, dietary restrictions, food prescriptions and precautionary behaviors are part of a holistic approach to maintain the hot-cold balance in the puerperium and ensure long-term physical well-being.

THE RESEARCH SETTING

Cambodia is a Southeast Asian country that borders Thailand to the west, Laos and Thailand to the north, the gulf of Thailand to the south, and Vietnam to the east. Cambodia experienced more than twenty years of civil war and internal conflict from 1975 until the late 1990s. Following the 1993 United Nations brokered democratic elections Cambodia has experienced relative political stability. Cambodia has a population of 13.1 million people with a fertility rate of 3.3 in 2004 (United Nations Family Planning Association, 2005). Cambodia's Gross Domestic Product is an estimated US$260 per capita. An estimated 36 percent of the population live below the official poverty line. The poverty line in Cambodia is approximately US$14 per capita per month, based on the consumption of 2,100 calories per day. In rural areas, 40 percent of households have per capita consumption below US$14 per month and another 40% of households have per capita consumption between US$14 and US$30 per month. The maternal mortality rate is 437 per 100,000 live births, with 32 percent of births being attended by trained personnel, 66 percent of births are attended by grandmother midwives, 38 percent of women receive antenatal care by trained personnel and 55 percent of women are not seen by anyone in pregnancy, and 66 percent of pregnant women are anaemic (Cambodia, Ministry of Planning and Ministry of Health, 2001).

Socio-economic change in Cambodia has brought new opportunities and influences, such as technological advances, foreign investment, regional trade agreements, including membership of the Association of South East Asian Nations (ASEAN). In this modernizing environment, Cambodian society is struggling to regain a sense of national identity and to hold onto traditional values and ideals, including traditional ways of doing birth. Perceptions of gender identity, especially for females, are closely related to notions of 'culture' and 'tradition', and resistance to changes in gender relations is often strong. Women are the 'cultural bearers' par excellence, and this ideology is linked to the proper behavior of women. Cambodian society is hierarchically ordered, with notions of power and status conditioning all social relations. Women are considered lower status to men; however, the status of women is also determined by age, religious devotion, marriage, childbearing and a woman's ability to manage the household. Men occupy a superior social status than women according to the secular legal code and Theravada Buddhist ideology, although women possess a considerable degree of equality, voice and independence in village life.

This chapter is based on fifteen months ethnographic research conducted in 2000-2001 in Chūp Commune (hereafter referred to as Chūp) Preh Net Preah District northwest Cambodia. Twelve months of this time was spent living in Chūp in particular the four villages where I focused my research activities, Krasung, Prasath, Rol Chruk and Krasung Chas villages (pseudonyms). There are 280 households and a population of 1,575 people in the four villages. Ethnographic research in these villages included participant observation, thirty five semi-structured interviews with nine grandmother midwives and their female assistants, *kruu kmae* (traditional healer), government and non-government health staff and thirty formal life-history interviews with the nine grandmother midwives. I conducted unstructured interviews with pregnant and postpartum women, grandmother midwives, traditional healers, village elders, referral hospital, health centre and NGO personnel and local authorities. In addition, a household survey was conducted in each of the 280 households to obtain demographic and reproductive health data from the study population. Community mapping was conducted at the same time as the survey over a six week period. Eleven semi-structured observation and interactions were recorded using a proforma on an *ad hoc* basis in the Chūp Health Centre and referral hospital to identify and accurately describe meaningful human interactions and processes between women and their midwife. All research activities were conducted by me in the Khmer language or with a research assistant.

Chūp Commune is forty minutes drive from the Banteay Meanchey provincial town of Sisophon. The four study villages are located along a laterite sealed secondary road. The all-weather road provides villagers in Chūp and neighbouring communes with access to the district market and Route 6, which connects Banteay Meanchey and Siem Reap Provinces. The primary occupation of Chūp residents is rice farming but most residents engage in other small-scale subsistence agriculture, fishing and livestock, in addition to rice production. The average household owns 2 hectares of agricultural land and 60 percent households had no rice at the end of the season. Twenty two percent of households have no agricultural land. Ninety six percent of women had their last birth at home and they were attended by a grandmother midwife. Forty six percent of the population has no formal education. The demographic profile of Chūp villages reflects the profile of Cambodia more generally.

Claah To□nlee (Crossing the River)

Childbirth in Chūp is a marked life-crisis event, evidenced by the use of the metaphor *claaŋ to□nlee* (crossing the river). The Khmer have always been aware of the hydrological and economic significance of their river system. The Mekong and the Bassac Rivers and the great Tonle Sap Lake form the main drainage system of the country and are the backbone of the economy, providing livelihoods for 80 percent of the population. Approximately 60 percent of water in the wet season originates from the Mekong River, causing the Tonle Sap to increase in size from about 2,600 kilometers square to approximately 10,500 kilometers square and its depth from 2 meters to 4 meters at the height of the flooding (Gartrell, 1997). Historical accounts of the ancient waterways of Cambodia confirm their might after the rainy season (Chou, 1992 [1873]: 39).

If we consider the magnitude of this river system, against the simplicity of the small water vessels used by most people, it is not surprising that the Khmer fear crossing rivers, especially in times of flooding: "The river is very big and there is nothing to compare it with" (grandmother Yeun). The journey of childbirth draws on metaphors of the dangers associated with crossing the river in a small craft, which are real and known to birthing women and their families: "If you crossed the river you were safe, and if you didn't, you died", and, "When you are crossing the river, you don't know if your boat will sink and you will drown" (grandmother Sim). People commonly say that a labouring woman is "crossing the river" and after the birth, her family would say she had "*claan haey*" (crossed already), or use another metaphor *niv pleen* (warming on the fire), indicating that the woman had already given birth and that she was now roasting. Emily Martin (1987: 157) suggests that concrete metaphors like a river "stress a process that develops from within and the continuity of this process with the past and future".

Nowadays, the metaphor crossing the river is used less often, especially by young people. Grandmother midwives, who have been trained by the NGOs, say that this term is used less often nowadays "because the *peet* (biomedical health personnel) have arrived in the area and there are many kinds of injectable drugs and objects to open the womb and new types of medicines to help women with severe pain and for things to be expelled from the woman's body" (grandmother Lum). Grandmother midwives who have received training know the *peet* have instruments to assist women with obstetric complications, "nowadays, if you are crossing the river and your condition is bad, you can stay alive if you go to the *peet*. You can get serum and energy medicine from the *peet* and they can help take the baby out if the mother cannot push the baby out herself. Nowadays, we only cross the creek" (grandmother Yeun). However, untrained grandmother midwives who have limited contact with the health system and minimal knowledge of the emergency obstetric care provided by *peet*, rarely refer women with childbirth complications to health facilities.

Many Chūp villagers know there are health services in the commune and district centers because family members have sought treatment when they are ill. Nonetheless, parturient women rarely access the private or government *peet* when they have childbirth complications; they continue to rely on the skills and agency of grandmother midwives, as did their ancestors. It was the grandmother midwives on whom women and their families depended to 'help' solve the woman's problem. If the grandmother midwives could not, then the woman died: "I am the boat's owner and I am called to take the woman to the other bank. She will be well if she is taken to the other bank. If the boat sinks when we are near the bank of the river, she will die. All those in the sunken boat die" (grandmother Choum). Grandmother midwives' skills were paramount. Women trusted these women and relied on their ability to help them through childbirth, "before we had no *peet*, we only had the grandmother midwives. No *peet* and no injection of medicines. We had nothing. Women were alive because of these ten fingers and Khmer herbs. We only had our hands. If our hands could help them, then their body was not in danger. It was more difficult than it is today. Today, it is easy" (grandmother Choum). Brigitte Jordan (1993: 192) notes that midwives' period of apprenticeship often involves acquiring knowledge that is "in the hands".

Similar stories were told and retold by village women and grandmother midwives themselves. All grandmother midwives are adamant that no woman has died in her hands. It was evident that they still fear certain birth complications, depending on their empirical experiences, such as a 'stuck baby' (obstructed labour) and a 'stuck placenta' (retained placenta). The grandmother midwives spoke of their traditional methods of dealing with birth complications such as obstructed labour, a breech delivery, a transverse lie or a retained placenta, and there was little variation between the techniques they referred to, whether or not they had been trained by NGOs. Old women in villages tell stories of women dying in childbirth from a 'stuck baby', 'stuck placenta' and 'stuck blood'. The maternal deaths reported to me during the study occurred in the past thirty years, but the most recent maternal death was in a nearby village a month before my arrival; the woman died from a postpartum haemorrhage.

EXPLAINING HEALTH AND ILLNESS

In Cambodia, as in Thailand, Burma and Laos, humoral medicine is derived from the Āyurvedic tradition introduced with Sanskritization (Manderson, 1981), perhaps as early as the last millennium BC. Humoral medicine in Cambodia, with its intra-cultural variations and inconsistencies, is primarily based on the classification of the body and foods as hot and cold, and the elements of wind and air. The three elements that maintain internal order are phlegm, bile and blood. However, a 'simple' hot-cold dichotomy is the dominant feature of Khmer medical beliefs, and the ranking of hot and cold by degree and the parallel classical differentiation of wet and dry, have largely disappeared among the general population, a trend noted by Manderson for other Southeast Asian societies, with the exception of Malaysia (1981: 517-518). In Chūp villages, I found a weak system of ranking, with villagers generally unable to name hot or cold foods; however they were vigilant in their adherence to dietary restrictions for certain illnesses, in particular, postpartum dietary requirements and behaviours.

Good health requires a person to maintain his/her individual balance of the humors and their qualities. Humoral balance is maintained, not only within the body, but also with external forces such as social relations, environmental and climatic conditions and relationships with supernatural deities. Illness is the result of humoral imbalance and extremes in hot and cold. It is classified according to where the illness originates, in the external or internal environment, however, even if the origin is external, such as anger or grief, the disorder upsets the internal environment, leading to illness. Food is coded according to hot or cold properties, in relation to their effects on the body, as are medicines (Western and traditional). Generally, hot foods heat the body and cold foods cool the body; the properties of the food do not relate to its spiciness, temperature or its raw or cooked state. Disease may be due to an excess of hot or cold, which may be caused by temperature heat from the environment, constitutional heat and heat from food, and they all combine to produce hot disease. Conversely, environmental cold, constitutional cold and "cold" foods combine to produce cold diseases. However, people differ in their concepts of the hot-cold attributes of food, herbs and medicines (Manderson, 1987). To restore health a diagnosis is needed: is the illness caused by excess hot or cold properties? According to the diagnosis, treatment requires dietary adjustment, changes to the external environment or medicines, sometimes all are needed to restore the humoral balance. Marcucci (1986) notes that, Khmer indigenous perceptions and understanding of humoral concepts are not expressed as explanatory models of health, illness and healing at the local indigenous level (also noted by

Nichter, 1980, for South Kanara, India). Thus, for the Khmer and similarly for other Southeast Asian societies, attempts to draw general explanatory models of illness perceptions and practices based on formal humoral theory, albeit culturally syncretic, should be approached with due caution. Therefore, although Khmer medicine has traits of Chinese and Western medicine, it is the explanatory model perceived at the local level, the indigenous level that is most important for understanding medical decisions (Marcucci, 1986:168).

HOT AND COLD IN PREGNANCY AND THE PUERPERIUM

The *klu☐n* (human body) is perceived as a cavity supported by bones that are covered by skin. Under the skin are *saasay* (string-like structures including fibres, nerves, blood vessels and tendons), through which circulates the *chiem* (blood), *tik* (water) and *kyal* (wind). Wind moves blood and water through the *saasay. Taa* (grandfather) Mok, a traditional healer, once told me, "the body is like a motor and the *saasay* are the pipes. The *saasay* need to be continually cleared otherwise they get blocked". When there is disequilibrium of wind, the humors of bile, phlegm and blood are correspondingly disturbed. Wind and its association with blood circulation affect the humoral condition that heats and cools the body (Marcucci, 1986). The humors are not seen as the cause of the illness, however; instead, they are the signs of physiological disequilibrium. Illnesses caused by wind can be due to a variety of factors: foods; emotional states such as anger, sadness, anxiety and grief; hard physical work; changes in the environment and climate; and alteration of body status such as pregnancy and childbirth.

Wind is by far the main physical concern for Khmers. According to grandfather Mok, "Wind is in the blood, and if the blood slows down because the body is cold, the wind will get stuck in the body and cause illness". Illnesses, with mild symptoms of wind, are called wind and they can result in headaches, dizziness, vomiting, diarrhoea and fatigue. The more serious conditions of wind, referred to as *kyal thom* (big wind), occur when the wind stops or freezes, thus affecting the circulation of blood throughout the body. This condition can be local, such as in the chest area around the *beh dooŋ* (heart), where blood flow slows down and causes *beh dooŋ ksaoy* (weak heart) or the extreme condition known as *steah beh dooŋ* (blocked heart), a life threatening condition that requires immediate treatment. *Chiem cok ŋaop* (death from stuck blood) is a serious condition feared by postpartum women and grandmother midwives. It occurs when wind is blocked, stopping the flow of blood at the site of the uterus. Mild to moderate symptoms of the illness include palpitations, dizziness, headache, body spasm and cramps, numbness in the limbs, inability to sleep, poor appetite and feeling 'internally cold'. This life-threatening condition needs immediate treatment by the traditional healer, utilizing Khmer herbs and cupping, pinching, coining and dermabrasion to release the wind and blood. The more severe form of stuck blood is said to resemble a trance-like state when the woman's body is rigid and she plucks at the walls and straw mat where she lies and speaks nonsense language. John Marcucci (1986), in his study with Khmer refugees in Dallas, United States, describes the illness *kyal cok* (frozen wind), which I also found to be a concern of Chŭp villagers. This serious illness occurs because the movement of wind is stopped or frozen, thus affecting the circulation of blood. This life threatening condition must be treated with acupressure within thirty minutes from the time of onset, otherwise the person will die. *Kyal cok* (stuck wind), as noted by Marcucci (1986) is similar to stuck blood; however, in Chūp, the latter relates specifically to the postpartum illness.

Khmer women regard pregnancy as a hot state. Unlike women in some other Southeast Asian societies, Khmer women generally do not pay special attention to dietary precautions during pregnancy to ensure hot-cold balance; instead they eat food that gives them energy. Pregnancy is not considered a very vulnerable time, as compared to childbirth and the puerperium, and dietary restrictions are frequently ignored, although, as Mark Nichter (1987: 377) writes for Sri Lanka, "attempts are made to ensure that an excess of hot or cold does not dominate any meal (or series of meals) except when warranted to counterbalance existing states of excess", and I believe it also applies in Chūp. Pregnant women know it is desirable to maintain the hot-cold balance in the body and the best way of doing this is by drinking Khmer herbs. However, women are poor and are not in a position to choose between hot and cold foods; they eat what is available and affordable.

Childbirth is a time of natural and supernatural danger, when a woman's physiological state is altered, causing humoral imbalance and disharmony. Childbirth depletes the woman of heat, blood and wind, placing her in a vulnerable state and subjecting her to illness due to cold, wind, magic and disease (Manderson, 1981, Manderson and Mathews, 1981; Pillsbury, 1982; Whittaker, 2000). Wind is particularly important during childbirth, because it can enter the woman's joints and ligaments at a time when they are the most permeable. During childbirth, the woman's *saasay* become *kcey* (unripe) due to a loss of heat, blood and wind, "*saasay kcey* women only have blood, because the wind has been lost" (grandfather Mok). The birthing process also puts the *saasay* under considerable stress. It is only when the body's humoral balance is restored, by eating hot foods and drinking hot medicines and mother roasting, that the *saasay* become *cah* (almost ripe) and wind returns to the blood. As childbirth is a marked life-crisis event, it requires strict adherence to dietary and behavioural practices in order to restore humoral balance, otherwise the woman will develop illnesses such as stuck blood.

Toah is a general classifier for illnesses that result from a relapse that occurs when postpartum woman loose body heat that results in disequilibrium of humors, namely wind. The symptoms of relapse *toah* are similar to "wind illness" described by Muecke (1979) for Thailand. Relapse can be short term (three to six months) or long term (years) and many women have *toah ram ray* (chronic relapse), often into their old age, due to a chronic disequilibrium of humors. There are five main types of relapse and they include: *toah mhoop* relapse due to eating "cold" food; *toah saasay* relapse due to performing heavy work; *toah damneek* relapse from coitus; *toah kum* relapse that occurs after experiencing emotional distress and fear; and *toah sansa□m* relapse from touching dew or moisture.

Postpartum women know it is in the best interest of their health, in the immediate and long-term, to conform to these precautions for as long as possible. Well-off women are able to do so; and so they are envied. However, the majority of postpartum women in Chūp have little choice but to recommence hard work as soon as they leave the roasting bed, between the fifth and seventh day postpartum. Old women know from personal experience that commencing physical work and being exposed to the environment and climatic conditions when they are *saasay kcey* will result in a relapse in the immediate term, and aching bones and joints in later life. They advise young women to adhere to the traditional practices, but often their advice is ignored. Poor women in Chūp know that if they adhere well to the minimum precautions, such as mother roasting, drink several liters of Khmer herbs, and eat three bowls of hot *babaa* (rice soup), salt and pepper each day, for the first three to five days postpartum, they will restore their body heat and maximise their chance of maintaining optimal health in the short and long term.

CELEBRATING A SAFE BIRTH:
TUMLEAK CƆƆƞ KRAÑCƏƏ (DROPPING THE STOVE)

Merit is right action and it is manifested through conforming to standards of appropriate behaviour. In merit-making festivals and ceremonies, such as *tumleak cƏƏƞ krañcƏƏ*, right-actions involve ritual offerings and other gifts to the monks, spirits and celebrants such as the grandmother midwife and her spirit teacher. Rituals performed during the *tumleak cƏƏƞ krañcƏƏ* provide a path to the supernatural deities. Life-cycle events and their associated ceremonies often combine offerings to spirits and monks, and appeals are made to both Buddha and animist spirits in times of trouble, for example childbirth.

Tumleak cƏƏƞ krañcƏƏ is a folk ceremony that marks the end of women's postpartum confinement to the roasting bed and her release from the physical and spiritual dangers that surround her childbirth. All the *tumleak cƏƏƞ krañcƏƏ* ceremonies I observed were made up of two discrete components: firstly, *saen doon taa* (Plate 1), which is dedicated to the couple's ancestral spirits who were called upon to help the woman during labour; secondly, the *tumleak cƏƏƞ krañcƏƏ* which marks the end of a postpartum woman's vulnerability. During the *tumleak cƏƏƞ krañcƏƏ* the woman and her husband thank the grandmother midwife and her spirit teacher by offering them gifts for taking the woman safely through childbirth, and they apologise to the midwife for having contact with the maternal blood during and after the birth. Grandmother midwives are responsible for the woman's obstetric care and the *tumleak cƏƏƞ krañcƏƏ* marks the end of her contract as the birth attendant. The ceremony is remarkably universal, with slight variations only in the prayers offered by the celebrants to the ancestral spirits. A local traditional healer is responsible for the *saen doon taa*. Food, water, wine and incense are commonly offered to the spirits, whether they are benign or malevolent. The female elders are responsible for the domestic arrangements such as making the *cƆƆm buen* and preparing the food, usually Khmer noodles, to share with family and friends after the ceremony. *CƆƆm buen* consists of sixteen areca leaves, with four leaves placed in each corner of the plate, together with four cigarettes, four slices of betel nut, and four candles and *tray pram* (five flowers and five incense sticks rolled up individually in five banana leaves) placed on top of the *cƆƆm buen* (see Plate 2).

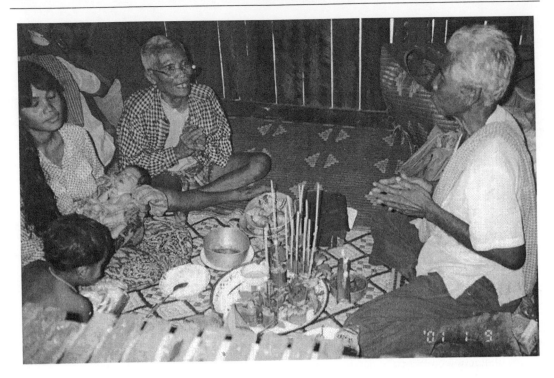

Plate 1. *Saen doon taa* ceremony.

The *tumleak cɔɔŋ krañcɔ̄ɔ̄* ceremony takes place when the postpartum woman is ready to leave the roasting bed, but not on Saturday, the unlucky day of the week. The day is set after consulting villagers who are knowledgeable about Buddhist and supernatural cosmologies, and in Chūp villages this is either the traditional healer, the most important ritual specialist. Postpartum women usually roast for a minimum of five days before the *tumleak cɔ̄ɔ̄ŋ krañcɔ̄ɔ̄* ceremony takes place. Thereafter, they may roast at night, sometimes for several months, depending on the wood supply, climate and a husband's willingness or ability to care for the fire. *Tumleak cɔ̄ɔ̄ŋ krañcɔ̄ɔ̄* are family celebrations, with the inclusion of village elders. Depending on household economics, the event can range from an elaborate gathering with an abundance of cooked food to offer the spirits and the guests, and generous gifts for the grandmother midwife, to simple rituals attended by close kin. Very poor families may not hold a *tumleak cɔ̄ɔ̄ŋ krañcɔ̄ɔ̄*, because they cannot afford the *saen doon taa*, the *cɔɔm buen* and material gifts for the grandmother midwife.

There are two *cɔɔm* associated with childbirth. The first is usually money, between 20 and 100 Baht, and it is given to the grandmother midwife immediately after the delivery and before she leaves the birthing place; it is payment for her midwifery services. The second is called *cɔɔm buen*, the gift given to the grandmother midwife by the postpartum woman and her husband during the *tumleak cɔ̄ɔ̄ŋ krañcɔ̄ɔ̄* ceremony. The amount of money received with the first and second *cɔɔm* is not significant.

When *yiey* assists women in childbirth, the mother has to do something in return to thank her, to do a good deed for her in return. This is why they give *yiey cɔɔm*. They give *yiey* these gifts and beg her pardon. The *yiey* who assists women in childbirth receives merit. *Yiey maap* is the driver of the boat and she has guided the woman across the river and she has made the other side safely. The *cɔɔm* is the gift for guiding her across the river to safety" (traditional healer in Chūp).

Golomb (1985: 78) notes that in Thailand and Malaysia, when practitioners request the assistance of ancestral spirits during consultations, they have to propitiate the spirits of former gurus at least once a year by holding feasts in their honour. The clients must present token donations to the ancestral spirits each time they request their assistance. These donations are separate to the fee they pay the practitioner. The situation noted by Golomb (1985) parallels that of Cambodia. All grandmother midwives have spirit teachers, "if you don't have your spirit teacher with you, you can not be *yiey maap*" (grandmother midwife Lum). In times of trouble it is the spirit teacher who guides grandmother midwives through the birth process.

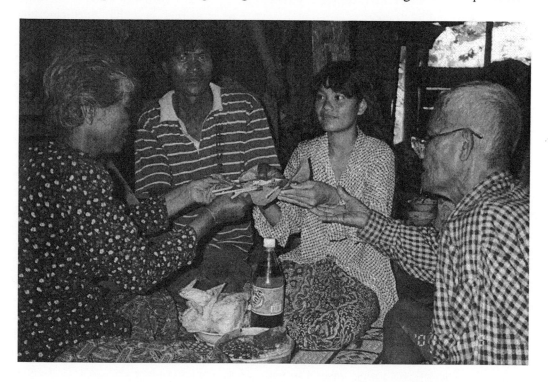

Plate 2. Wei presents grandmother midwife Yeun with *cɔɔm buen* during *the tumleak cɔ̄ɔ̄ŋ krañcɔ̄ɔ̄* ceremony.

OLD TRADITIONS AND NEW WAYS: A CONCLUSION

The health care system in Cambodia is modernizing, and government health providers, including those who work privately, are encouraging women to attend antenatal care during pregnancy and give birth with trained health personnel either at home or in health facilities (Hoban, 2003). The emphasis on biomedical obstetrics in Cambodia brings with it technologies such as lithotomy position for labour and delivery, the pharmacological induction of labour with drugs such as Syntocinon, the near-universal use of intravenous therapy for all deliveries, and the widespread use of drugs such as Ergometrine immediately post-birth. Government health staff are trained in biomedicine and the majority of midwives have turned away from traditional therapies such as mother roasting, Khmer herbs and postpartum massage by grandmother midwives in favour of Western medicines and treatments. It has been a difficult transition for many midwives who privately maintain and respect the philosophical standpoint and practical value of humoral medicine; this is particularly true in rural areas. However, for trained midwives' business to flourish (in both public and private sectors), they have to accommodate many traditional practices, for example postpartum practices that maintain women's humoral balance, especially those considered benign such as postpartum dietary precautions.

Conversely, women do not reject outright the utilization of modern medicine. They know that many Western drugs used during childbirth and in the postpartum period have similar actions to Khmer herbs, such as Vitamin C, which is classified as a 'hot' medicine, and Ergometrine which assists women expel blood from the uterus and therefore prevents 'stuck blood'. It is not uncommon to see young and well-off women roast for two or three days, and utilize adjunct therapies such as 'hot' injections, like calcium, vitamin B complex, vitamin C, and take antibiotics such as ampicillin that are quick acting and efficacious. Poor women have limited choices and their only option is to follow the traditional dietary and behaviour practices. Despite poor women in Chūp knowing the efficacy of Western medicine, it is outside their means.

Pregnant women have limited contact with government health facilities; it is an alien medical system. Women attend antenatal care because they are told to by trained grandmother midwives, or because they want drugs such as ferrous sulphate, only when they are not well. Women do not attend antenatal care for preventative services, such as tetanus toxoid immunization. Pregnant and postpartum women seek out trained midwives or doctors only when they have an obstetric complication. Women's primary choice is to give birth at home and in the care of a grandmother midwife. When they give birth in hospital they have to forsake their traditional practices and move into a vulnerable and unknown space, one that promotes expensive Western treatments over affordable traditional therapies. Women are forbidden to mother roast and drink Khmer herbs while in hospital; instead they place hot rocks, wrapped in cloth on their abdomen, dress in many layers of clothing and wrap a cotton scarf around their head to avoid excess heat loss. Hospital authorities have banned mother roasting because the maternity ward fills with smoke which causes discomfort for other inpatients, and it is a potential fire hazard. In addition, mother roasting is considered to be an ancient Khmer tradition that has no scientific proof of its efficacy. If women want to maintain their humoral balance in the postpartum period health personnel can provide them with 'hot' injections, for a fee. It is only well-off women who have 'hot' injections in hospital; poor women receive tablets such as vitamins C and B complex, which they consider are second-best and have minimal effect on their humoral balance. Khmer herbs, on the other hand, are considered to have questionable efficacy and may exacerbate fluid retention, especially for women with pre-existing conditions such as hypertension and oedema. Hot rice soup is condoned.

Women rarely stay in the hospital for more than 24 hours after a normal birth, and when they return home they immediately commence mother roasting, Khmer herbs, eat hot rice soup and the grandmother midwife begins the postpartum massage. Women who birth in hospital also have a *tumleak cə̃ŋ krañcə̃ō* ceremony when they leave the roasting bed; the same guiding principles apply for all postpartum women. If the grandmother midwife plays any role in the woman's care during childbirth or in the postpartum period she is included in the *tumleak cə̃ŋ krañcə̃ō* ceremony. However, if a woman's birth and immediate postpartum period is medicalized, either at home or in a health facility, the contract is between the government midwife and the postpartum woman. The contract ceases once the fee is paid for the service; the government midwife is not included in the *tumleak cə̃ŋ krañcə̃ō* ceremony. However, the majority of birthing women in Chūp, especially poor women, take proactive steps to stay outside the tentacles of the expensive and untested government health system for fear that their engagement with modern medicine may result in life-threatening illnesses such as 'stuck blood' or a relapse; a situation that could have been prevented, if they were able to exercise control of the birthing process and environment. Women, who choose to birth in their home environment, are supported by their family and assisted in birth by their preferred birth attendants. Women are able to execute safety-first strategies, such as up hold dictary restrictions, food prescriptions and precautionary behaviours to maintain the hot-cold balance in the puerperium, avoid financial debt due to hospitalization, and accrue merit by appeasing ancestral spirits and thanking the grandmother midwife and her spirit teacher during the *tumleak cə̃ŋ krañcə̃ō* ceremony for the role she played as a safety agent during childbirth.

REFERENCES

Arms, S., 1975, *Immaculate Deception: A New Look at Women and Childbirth*, Bantam Books: New York.

Cambodia, Ministry of Planning and Ministry of Health, 2001, *Cambodia Demographic and Health Survey 2000*, Ministry of Planning, National Institute of Statistics/ Ministry of Health, Directorate General for Health: Phnom Penh.

Chou, Ta-Kuan, 1992, *Customs of Cambodia*. Siam Society: Bangkok.

Davis-Floyd, R., 1993, *Birth as an American Rite of Passage*, University of California Press: Los Angeles.

Davis-Floyd, R., 1994, 'The Technocratic Body: American Childbirth as Cultural Expression', *Social Science and Medicine*, 38: 1125–1140.

Downe, S., McCormick, C., & Beech, B., 2001, 'Labour Interventions Associated With Normal Birth', *British Journal of Midwifery*, 9(10): 602–606.

Douglas, M., 1992, *Risk and Blame: Essays in Cultural Theory*, Routledge: London.

El-Nemer, A., Downe, S., & Small, N., 2006, 'She Would Help Me From the Heart': An Ethnography of Egyptian Women in Labour. *Social Sciences and Medicine*, 62: 81-92.

Gartrell, A., 1997, *Resource Management in the Cambodia Mekong Basin, The Mekong Basin Series*, Murdoch University Asia Research Centre: Perth.

Golomb, L., 1985, *An Anthropology of Curing in Multiethnic Thailand*, University of Illinois Press: Urbana, Chicago.

Hildingsson, I., Waldenstrom, U., & Radestad, I., 2003. 'Swedish Women's Interest in Home Birth and In-Hospital Birth Center Care', *Birth,* 30(1): 11–22.

Hoban, E., 2003. *'We're Safe and Happy Already': Traditional Birth Attendants and Safe Motherhood in a Cambodian Rural Commune*, unpublished doctoral Thesis, The University of Melbourne: Melbourne.

Jordan, B., 1993, *Birth in Four Cultures: A Crosscultural Investigation of Childbirth in Yucatan, Holland, Sweden, and the United States*, Waveland Press: Illinois.

Lane, K., 1995, 'The Medical Model of the Body as a Site of Risk: A Case Study of Childbirth', in Gabe, J. (ed.), *Medicine, Health and Risk,* pp. 53-72. Blackwell Publishers: Oxford.

Manderson, L., 1981, 'Roasting, Smoking and Dieting in Response to Birth: Malay Confinement in Cross-Cultural Perspective', *Social Science and Medicine*, 15B: 509-520.

Manderson, L., 1987. 'Hot-Cold Food and Medical Theories: Overview and Introduction', *Social Science and Medicine*, 25(4): 329-330.

Manderson, L., & Mathews, M., 1981, 'Vietnamese Attitudes to Maternal and Infant Health', *Medical Journal of Australia*, 1: 69-72.

Marcucci, J.L., 1986, *Khmer Refugees in Dallas: Medical Decisions in the Context of Pluralism*, unpublished doctoral Dissertation. Dallas, Southern Methodist University: Texas.

Martin, E., 1987, *The Women in the Body*, Beacon Press: Boston.

McClain, C., 1982, 'Toward a Comparative Framework for the Study of Childbirth: A Review of the Literature', in M.A Kay (ed.), *Anthropology of Human Birth,* pp. 25-60. F. A. Davis Company: Philadelphia.

Muecke, M., 1979, 'An Explication of "Wind Illness" in Northern Thailand', *Culture, Medicine and Psychiatry*, 3: 267-300.

Murphy-Lawless, J., 1998, *Reading Birth and Death. A History of Obstetric Thinking*, Cork University Press: Cork.

Nichter, M., 1980, 'The Layperson's Perception of Medicine as Perspective into the Utilization of Multiple Therapy Systems in the Indian Context', *Social Science and Medicine*, 14B: 225-233.

Nichter, M., 1987, 'Cultural Dimensions of Hot, Cold and Sema in Sinhalese Health Culture', *Social Science and Medicine*, 25(4): 377-387.

Pilley Edwards, N., 2005, *Birthing Autonomy. Women's Experiences of Planning Home Births*, Routledge: New York.

Pillsbury, B., 1982, '"Doing the Month": Confinement and Convalescence of Chinese Women After Childbirth', in M.A. Kay (ed.), *Anthropology of Human Birth,* pp. 119-146. F.A. Davis Company: Philadelphia.

Wagner, M., 1994, *Pursuing the Birth Machine: The Search for Appropriate Birth Technology*, ACE Graphics: Camperdown.

Whittaker, A., 2000, *Intimate Knowledge: Women and Their Health in North-East Thailand*, Allan & Unwin: St Leonards.

World Health Organization, 1998, 'Improve the Quality of Maternity Health Services. Safe motherhood. World Health Day'. http://www.who.int/whday/en/pages1998/whd98_ 08.html.

United Nations Population Fund, 2005, *Cambodia at a Glance. Population, Gender and Reproductive Health*, UNFPA: Phnom Penh.

World Bank, 2006, *Halving Poverty 2015? Cambodia Poverty Assessment 2005. Consultant Draft Report*, World Bank: Phnom Penh.

In: Reproduction, Childbearing and Motherhood
Editor: Pranee Liamputtong, pp. 113-125

ISBN: 978-1-60021-606-0
© 2007 Nova Science Publishers, Inc.

Chapter 7

BIRTH IN PAKISTAN

Margaret Chesney

INTRODUCTION

As a UK midwife, I have made nine field trips to work in a Red Crescent Maternity hospital in the interior of the Punjab, Pakistan. Following the first four field trips, an evaluation study was carried out (Chesney, 1994), thereafter research was undertaken on women's experience of birth in Pakistan (Chesney, 2004). During the first out of nine subsequent field trips to Pakistan, birth practice in the hospital was observed and provided the backdrop to the research. Babies were pushed, pulled and cut out, without even the basic necessities to resuscitate. During the first visit to the District General Hospital patients were found lying on charpoys (string beds) outside the buildings; they told us that they were unable to gain entry because they were too ill. There were no doctors available. Nursing staff were afraid to take responsibility for the patients in case they would be blamed for their demise. Inside the hospital the corridors were lined with patients on the floor. I remember specifically a ten year old boy with a gangrenous arm gained from touching a live wire and a fourteen year old girl who had full thickness burns to her lower abdomen and vulva. Both these accidents occurred due to 'load shedding'. This is when electricity is rationed because there is insufficient in the national grid for continuous use: so it is turned off for many hours, then back on unexpectedly. The boy was connecting a wire to the neighbours' electricity supply; the girl had been carrying boiling milk when the electricity went off and left her in darkness. These stories give the reader some idea of the health facilities in Pakistan. There is no National health or social support system and as a consequence many of the poor die before getting to a hospital, most because they cannot afford the transport or the cost of treatment.

METHODOLOGY AND THEORETICAL STANDPOINT

The aim of the research was to provide insight into women's experiences of birth in Pakistan. Swanson-Kauffman (1986) describes this as 'living inquiry', which is the parallel of living knowledge. According to Reason (1996:18), living inquiry is "passionate, committed, involved and personal". Research such as this is not just to gain knowledge to contribute to an existing body of knowledge, or development of theory; it is knowledge for the sake of relating to people in a different way, to improve understanding and impact positively on practice.

Guba (1990) and Lincoln (1998) judge there to be four philosophical paradigms of inquiry. These can be loosely mapped along the subjective, objective continuum.

Objective ◄───────────────────────► Subjective
Positivist   post positivist   critical theory   interpretivist / constructivist

Inquiry, whether from the positivist or interpretive paradigm, is based upon standards that relate to the answer to questions about ontology, epistemology and methodology (Guba and Lincoln 1994). For each research paradigms there are different ways of viewing the world (ontology) and distinctive beliefs of what is knowledge (epistemology). The methodology chosen was based upon my own ontology and what was considered authoritative knowledge of birth in other cultures (Jeffery Jeffery and Lyon, 1988; Jordan, 1993; Sizoo, 1997). The researcher's ontology may be anywhere on the objective, subjective continuum, with the positivist believing that truth can be objectively discovered using deduction from a hypothesis. The interpretivist/constructivist believes answers to research questions are relative to the context or mental framework and are interpreted or constructed. Thus, a persons' ontology describes how they view the world; some believe there is one reality that can be discovered (realism), others would argue that reality is socially constructed (relativism) (Guba 1990). Denzin and Lincoln (1994: 111-112) define the constructivists ontology as;

> ...relativist, in that the constructions are as alterable as the reality, the pistemology as subjective, whereby findings are literal and knowledge is created among the investigator and the respondents. The methodology of the constructivists is dialectic aimed as reconstruction of previously held constructions.

My philosophical position would, in Guba and Lincoln's (1994) and Denzin and Lincoln's (1994) terms, be described as that of a constructivist relativist, as the women's stories were constructed relative to the context of the individual experience, within the theoretical perspectives of the available knowledge. Ultimately, my ontological position has influenced both the theoretical underpinning empirical content (epistemology) and the methodology of the study on women's birth experiences in Pakistan.

The methodology of choice was interpretive ethnography (Denzin, 1997) with an anthropological bias. This was in keeping with the relationship between anthropology and midwifery. Reflection was an important element of the research methodology and a reflective diary was kept throughout the data collection period (Alvesson and Skoldberg, 2000).

THE SOCIAL AND CULTURAL CONTEXTS OF THE PARTICIPANTS AND THE FIELD SITE

The sample included two groups of women who were interviewed, one in Pakistan, Shah (n 6 + 1 Dr Q), and one a North of England town, UK (n10). The sample was one of convenience using a snow ball technique (Lee, 2000). Five of the ten women interviewed in the UK, self-selected following my attachment to an over-fifties luncheon club in the centre of the local Pakistani community . (Taz, Fari, Shab, Farn, Naz). The other five came though networking and community knowledge of the research (Ria, Bas, Ina, Ami, Dil).

Data has also been gathered through participant observation at the over fifties group in the UK and attachment to a women's hospital in Saiw Pakistan. A reflexive field note/diary was kept throughout the study period. All seven women interviewed in Pakistan were approached through a mediator, usually the interpreter (Kad). One participant (Aia) was the mother of a man we had become firm friends with. His second wife was also interviewed in the UK; another woman was interviewed on a bus journey from Lahore to Saiw (Shu). Three women were interviewed at the maternity hospital, the doctor, the dai and a woman who was accompanying her sister-in-law (Sha). The last woman was interviewed at our accommodation in Pakistan, where her husband was the gardener (Shad).

BIRTH PRACTICES IN A RED CRESCENT HOSPITAL IN PAKISTAN 1989

Officials in the hospital orchestrated the first visit to the Maternity Hospital. There was only one woman in the postnatal ward, she sat on top of a bed that had a mattress and sheets on. Whilst greeting the mother and admiring the baby, I lifted the baby's shirt to confirm my suspicions; the cord was off, this suggested the baby was 7 to10 days old. Both the mother and the baby had been brought in to the hospital especially for our visit. Later that same night, I called back unexpectedly and with the permission of the doctor stayed all night. All the beds were full, each had at least one woman and maybe a baby or small child lay on it, groups of women and children of all ages huddled around each bed. The women in the labour room lay flat, attached to drips and there were no mattresses or pillows, let alone linen on the beds. However, the temperature was above 40 degrees centigrade so the rubber covered mattress would have been more uncomfortable that the open spring base.

All the women had intravenous drips put in their arms; these were not held in place by strapping. The needle introducer was left in the cannulae and the women kept their arms still. The IV contained a drug to stimulate labour (even if they were in spontaneous labour). This IV was not calibrated, nor was the labour monitored in any systematic way. I was informed this was "modern western practice". I stayed with one woman who was so obviously in great pain. Her contractions were not intermittent as they should have been, this would have given both her and the unborn baby the vital rest needed to cope with the labour and birth. Instead her abdomen rose and stayed contracted stimulated excessively. I surreptitiously slowed down the drip. The 'staff nurse' conducted a vaginal examination putting on an un-sterile glove, the second vaginal examination in half an hour, following this she declared the woman 'ready'. The woman was then wheeled on a tin trolley to join other woman who was just giving birth in the delivery room. The relatives were not allowed to accompany us.

There followed a scene that was to haunt me forever. The labouring woman was put into lithotomy position, although there were no stirrups or leg supports, her large and second toes straddled the rusted upright lithotomy poles and her buttocks drawn to the edge of the bed. The woman's back lay directly on the metal (without any covering) bed. Two women pushed on the top of her abdomen and the doctor manually dilated her vulva, after putting on gloves that were draped over the sink. The baby was pushed and pulled into the world; there was no waiting restitution or rotation. My estimation of the baby's condition was Apgar of 4. She was placed on a hard chair at the side of the delivery bed, cord still attached. I asked if there was any oxygen to revive her and staff nurse wheeled in a large very old cylinder, someone offered a bowl of water into which a filthy catheter attached to the cylinder was placed. It did not bubble, and there was no oxygen. I looked round for some means to suck out this grey gasping baby. Before I gave mouth to mouth resuscitation, I was informed by a shrug of the shoulders that suction again was not available. As I leaned over to put my mouth over the baby's, someone placed my duppata (scarf) between the baby and me. Staff nurse returned with a syringe and proceeded to inject the still attached cord. The look on my face was answered with the name Decadron – a cardiac stimulant. As the placenta delivered the baby whimpered. Far from well she went home with the mother an hour later on the back of a motorbike.

On reflection, it was not the practice that shocked me as much as the staff behaviour towards the women. Staff treated the women and their relatives as if they were dirty. One woman whose membranes ruptured on the way to the toilet was shouted at for making a mess. Her relatives were called to retrieve her wet trousers from the floor. There was virtually no communication or dialogue between the women and the staff, orders were given to relatives only. I found out later that caesarean section births were carried out using Ether or Katamin as an anaesthetic. The woman doctor would undertake up to six abdominal tubal ligations twice a week. Her skill was obvious; the women would walk into and out of theatre. The number of births per year at this hospital was over 3,000.

All women admitted to this hospital had to supply medication, cotton wool, cord clamps, giving set, intravenous fluid, dettol, cord clamp and so on. This was bought by the relatives of the woman at the drug store in the bazaar on admission. The women who use this hospital are either the local poor, or those sent by the Dai (traditional birth attendant) from the suburbs or nearer rural villages. The births I witnessed in Pakistan may or may not be representative of birth practice in other Pakistan hospitals; however, they were the impetus behind me returning to work with the hospital staff to improve both the care and management of women in labour and to study women's experiences of birth in Pakistan.

THE DAI

The title, Dai, is often synonymous with traditional birth attendant (TBA) (Manglay-Maglacas, 1986; Maine, 1992; Minden, 1993; Fleming, 1994; Murray, 1996). Global confusion around terms and definitions of traditional birth attendants (TBA) led to a study by WHO (1992), which does little to clarify the issue. Literature from Pakistan (UNICEF, 1989) confuses, as it classifies 'trained' Dais and midwives collectively, with no mention of the TBA. Later research (Chawla, 2000) clearly recognised the untrained Dai as being 'with women' and defined her as an "indigenous birth attendant". Further differentiation comes through reference to the midwife as "being trained for 12 months", thereafter introducing yet another descriptor, "the auxiliary midwife" (Kamal, 2000). If the definition of midwife is taken literally, from the old English "wif (with) woman" (Collins 1994), then the Dai is indeed a "midwife" as she is "with woman". The statistics to uphold this are recorded by Fikree, Jafarey and Kureshy (1998), Chawla (2000), Kamal (2000) and Kasi (2002), each confirming that between seventy-five and ninety per cent of women who give birth in Pakistan are attended by the Dai. Further clarification of the definition that links to the role of traditional midwife describes her as being "a woman skilled in aiding the delivery of babies" (Kamal, 2000; Kasi, 2002).

The definition of Dai taken which applies to the responses from women interviewed, was that of Chawla's (2000: 41): "The Dai is seen as indigenous specialist in women's well being". This was because of the wider family links and health role and responsibilities (not covered here) the women referred to. Additional to this it is important to recognise that the characteristics of the Dai as told by the women included her being, untrained and uneducated (in a western sense), yet infinitely skilled and experienced. She was often older, may be blind, from the lowest social class (except the family Dai) without the support of a family.

However, the Dai was considered 'ignorant' (Naz) and was frequently blamed for "mishandling women" (Naz's granddaughter & Dr Q). Most of the women interviewed about their birth experiences in Pakistan agreed with Chawla's (2000) definition of being special. The Dai is the person they all called in labour, she was the specialist in birth. The women did not use the term "specialist"; more often the descriptor that was attached to the Dai was that of "family". It was evident in both the frequency of referral to the Dai and in the positive reverence, that the Dai was as important to the childbearing woman as the close female relative. The importance of the Dai being a relative, or part of the family, with or without blood or kinship links had clear emphasis within the women's words.

Thus, it was expected that some of the women would refer to the Dai when interviewed about their birth experiences. However, the frequency and extent to which the women referred to the Dai was not expected. All told stories of how the Dai were part of their birth experience, many referred to the Dai as part of the family.

THE DAI A FAMILY THING

It was evident from the women's narratives that Dais are trusted, special and influential members of the extended family and community. The role she undertakes was clearly understood by all the women interviewed; The focus of the role involved the Dai coming to the woman's home when she was in labour and performing duties that no one else was prepared to undertake. The mother-in-law or other female member of the family would have already made the diagnosis of labour.

Due to the social status of the Dai who cared for women outside her own family, there was incongruity in the Dai role. Taking on the role of Dai as work identifies the woman as unsupported.

Comments from the women interviewed on the Dai

The dai was my dad's auntie…she live in our street, only a few homes away…she is looking at me. Farn
My aunt (dad's sister) is also my mother-in-law…she is the dai. Naz
The dai was very kind, she delivered all my brothers, I got six and one sister. Fari
..Yeh… they (Dai) looked after her (grandmother)…the family system,…most of the family used to look after her when she was in labour" "The women in the family…because it was quite a big family they looked after her… Sam granddaughter of Taz
She, the Dai is in the same village, her mother was also… Bas
My sister became a Dai, it was the only way to get some money. Naz
My mother was a dai, but only for the family. Dil
The Dai was a family thing." Ami Riz's mother

According to Islam (Salahi, 1993: 78)

A woman is not required to work in order to earn her living. Her husband is responsible to ensure a decent standard of living…

A woman is not required to work in order to earn her living and if working affects the family, especially the children, then her husband has the right to prevent her from working.

As a working woman the signal to the rest of the community is that she does not have the support of a family. If the Dai was not of the extended family she would be from the same community as the women, sharing the same cultural values and social norms.

Although the women wanted and trusted their 'family Dai' some families would not support a family member becoming a Dai.

It is not something you would like your family to do…it is in the family, but not every family allows it…the families that do are on the poor side or may have no husband…being a doctor, now that's something else. Taz

Families who have access to education want a member of the family to be a doctor. Doctors did not generally want to work in the rural areas choosing to work in the more affluent towns with their amenities of water and electricity. Educated women can afford the services of a doctor and the cost of travel to a health facility in the large cities. However, it was interesting to note that nine of the women interviewed chose to give birth at home cared for by the family Dai. The social mix of the sample ranged from mathematics professor (wife of doctor) to cleaner (with 3 jobs). Calling the Dai and giving birth at home was seen to be the 'best' option, by virtue of the elder generations trust in the Dai and her practices. It was the mother-in-law who made the decision who to call or where to go for the birth. However, one woman's mother who was a Dai wanted the doctor to attend her daughter.

My mum used to take her cases to the doctor when there were problems; she did not take anything (money) from us (when she delivered her) …just for the medicines… Shad

Although the role of Dai from and within the family was a respected role it was still lowly. If the Dai was related to the family of the women giving birth, it may be necessary to call another Dai to undertake the 'defiling' role of cutting the cord and dealing with the placenta. As Sha says, "this is why the Dai is called – to deal with the cord and placenta". There was also a belief that the placenta and cord was capable of being sucked back in the woman's body with the potential to harm the mother.

> ...Of course we must call the Dai (for the birth), none of us can cut the cord. The cord is cut only after the placenta is delivered, otherwise it could go back inside, back into the tubes and the poison would spread and kill her. Ami.

Decision making during labour appeared to be grounded in a community of women, discussing what is to be done. Jordan (1993), in her text on birth in four cultures, confirmed that decisions about labour and birth are made jointly between the woman, her helpers and the midwife. Decisions such as, whether the woman should have something to eat, which position she should adopt, when she should push, whether she was pushing hard enough, what constituted reasonable effort, what is unsatisfactory progress and what should be done about it, were all taken by the women attending. The decision emerged as a negotiated consensus. The sas (mother-in-law) or aunt and the Dai may, as they did for Ria, make the ultimate decision to take over from the doctor. As it was Ria's first birth, and she was under the influence of a drug to stop her vomiting, she was aware, but not involved, in the decisions being made. However, with subsequent births she may be included or consulted. Similarly, Jeffery and colleagues (1988: 108) found that the birthing mother rarely features in the decision- making.

> Birth is a socially managed process, the labouring woman plays little part in the discussion about how her labour is progressing or any intervention...she might refuse a chosen treatment, whether hot sugar water or squatting on bricks, but management of the labour is not in her own hands. Usually the labouring woman's sas (or other senior attendant) calls the Dai only once she considers labour to be well established. Before that she (sas) may have examined the labouring woman's belly or tried to hasten the delivery through various domestic remedies.

It is noteworthy that the role of the mother-in-law (sas) and close relatives in Pakistan is much more important for birth in the home than the hospital. They will stay with the woman, cooking and caring for children. Relatives come with the woman to hospital and camp in the hospital grounds; they care for the woman's children and bring her food from the bazaar. The relatives will not be allowed to be with the woman in the labour room, let alone contribute or make decisions on care. Similarly, in a western managed labour, the woman herself may play little part in decision-making. Choosing the time to involve other health care professionals or when to send the woman to hospital is influenced by social cultural and religious beliefs.

EAST AND WEST TIME

Time may have very little meaning in a culture that believes that God sets the agenda. In Pakistan, the saying when arrangements are being made is "in shala", meaning, "with God's blessing" or "if God wills it". However, this statement has come to mean "only if God wants it to happen" and is used to frame the "maybe" with arrangements. There is a subtle different between God's blessing for all that may happen and God being responsible for it happening or not. Both are within the belief systems of Pakistani women, so these need to be understood by western carers.

When time is out of the control of the individual, it may cease to have the same meaning. No shame or loss of credibility occurs if appointments are not kept, as God has willed the 'other' to happen. Two stories which link this concept with the strong cultural norm towards hospitality are given here. A woman about to leave her house to attend her antenatal appointment, as she opens her door visitors arrive. The visitors take priority over the antenatal appointment and the woman will take her coat off and meet the needs of the visitors by feeding and entertaining them. This has implications for a hospital time controlled systems. The woman fully intended to keep the appointment; she was not missing it purposely. However, her priority lay with the social norm of community reputation based upon hospitality and God's will. A further second example of the responsibility for hospitality, even in the hospital, arose when Vez and Shab received a neighbour as a visitor just prior to the birth of their son. Neither of them could ask the neighbour to leave, even though she had changed the dynamics in the birthing room and Vez no longer seemed at ease.

Time was also found to be an important theme in Pairman's study (2000). She said it takes time to develop relationships and for trust to build. The Dai has developed relationships with the birthing woman and her family being of the family or of the community. The professional, employed midwife in the UK, even in the 'ideal' situation of one-to-one midwife and woman on a labour ward has many time constraints placed upon her by medicalisation that may come between herself and the labouring woman, such as shift changes, meetings and other responsibilities of being employed, as well as family life, childcare and running the home, all have the potential to detract from the time to build trust. The Dai also has multiple calls on her time, elderly relatives, grandchildren, housework; it could be argued that in an extended family network these responsibilities are more easily shared. However, geographical distance or death of in-laws and supportive relatives can create extra pressure upon a family, whether in Pakistan or the UK. It is usual for the men in Pakistan to travel for work. Most of the women in the research told of their husbands working away from home. It was more unusual for the women to be away from home, although Mrs. A lived with relatives whilst she studied. For the men folk to travel to seek work was seen to be an economic necessity, whilst the extended family supported those left at home. For women who had neither a supportive extended family nor a husband, the need to have some income was vital. There is no infrastructure of social or economic support in Pakistan. The paid work available and acceptable for the uneducated woman appeared to be limited to cleaning or becoming a Dai.

According to Kristeva (1982) female subjectivity appears to be linked to cyclical time (repetition) and monumental time (eternal). Both offer ways of conceptualising time from the perspective of motherhood and reproduction; cyclical from the menarche and through biological rhythm, menstruation to menopause and the monumental changes these bring. Further time differences could be linear, for example over history. The birth experiences for the women interviewed spanned three decades in history, from the 1950's to the 1990s. Three generations of women were involved in some interviews (Naz, Ina the midwife, Taz and Aia).

When birth takes place in the home in Pakistan, all those in the room are known to each other and share the same beliefs. Close female relatives are able to respond to the woman's needs; needs that do not need verbalisation. The woman's desires are known, the connection is spiritual, and there is engagement and trust. This contrasts strongly with birth in the hospital whereby women are cared for by strangers who they do not trust.

The midwives at the hospital were no good and they only complicated cases to get money Relatives are not allowed to be present during the birth

> They stayed outside for the births in hospital... I did say come inside... but the doctor said no there were already women there and them (relatives) being there would not make the pain go away. They stayed at the door saw me through the glass ...even if the pain was bad they wouldn't let anyone come in. Shad

BIRTH STORIES AND PARABLES

The research offered the opportunity to observe life and woman-to-woman interaction; to hear stories that symbolised what birth meant to women: Stories that had a message, demonstrated a point, had moral meaning, upheld a principle or parallel that could be applied to other situations. Within the stories there were powerful visual messages that stirred emotions and gave enlightenment that fed into my practice as a midwife and latterly as a teacher, in some way justifying the importance of undertaking the study. I would like to share three of the stories that constituted learning for practice.

Anaemia

This story is about a woman who visited her GP. She was severely anaemic and when the doctor asked her how many children she had given birth to, the woman replied 'two or three'. The doctor knew that the woman knew exactly how many children she had given birth to, however, she was purposely choosing to be vague. The doctor needed to know before giving treatment whether the woman had an anaemia brought on through recurrent pregnancy or not, so he subsequently questioned the woman's relatives, learning that the woman had nine healthy children. Giving birth had depleted the woman's already limited iron stores; the doctor could then treat this with simple iron. In seeking an explanation as to why the woman could not tell the doctor of the nine healthy children, it was revealed that if she spoke of her good fortune in having all the children alive and healthy that she would be tempting fate and this may affect the health of her children. This reminded me of my own belief system regarding cot death, when I gave birth to my eldest child in the early mid 1960's, which was connected to cot death when I was convinced if I 'prepared' myself by asking or even thinking about cot death that I would somehow make it happen.

The learning that emerged from this story was that women will go to great lengths; even endanger their own lives to protect their children from real or perceived risk.

Test with a Fly

The link between science and education has been considered indisputable. However, scientific thinking can exist without education, as we know it. This is evident following direct experience of asking a grandma why she was spoon-feeding the new-born baby what looked like dirty water from a spoon. When asked why she was not advising her daughter to give the mothers' milk the grandma replied:

We have tested the mothers' milk by putting a fly into it and it died, the milk is poisonous.

Although grandma had never attended a school for her education, life had taught her to question, to test and to problem solve using scientific principles. Her obvious lack of knowledge (to us) around drowning made me reflect upon the gaps in my own knowledge. The moral to this story is that embodied knowledge is authoritative, "what counts" (Jordan, 1993) is not certificates or degrees.

Like Mud

Dil told the story about mud coming from a woman who had been left to die by the doctors. This was when she was working as Family Welfare Worker in Pakistan:

One day I went to the village very far away and there was a girl, doctor said she would not live a month, she was very thin, I said how long has she been like this, they said two years, I said you put anything into her, I said all right don't blame me, I am not saying it is a fact…I will try that is all, to cure her. They said what will you do, I said I want some hot water, oil and I had some tablets, she had a temperature. First of all I tried oil; with my Dai we massaged all girl's (body). I said my God… it was like mud that came out of her, honestly when you were massaging it was coming like mud, that is the reason she was so ill…I threw away all the old bed sheets. I said give good food.

Major social implications awaited the poor dying woman:

I treated her like a child…it was like mud that came out of her… After a month she came back (got better), her mother-in-law was going to give her a divorce because she was ill. She wasn't doing the house job, not giving husband intercourse, so they said to me they would have to give divorce, her father was praying he was a very poor man. (Dil)

Poor sick women in Pakistan are about as low on the social scale as one can get. There is a well known saying in Pakistan that depicts how alone a sick woman can be: "Even a woman's shadow deserts her when she is sick". However, simple massage, good food, analgesics and cleanliness saved this woman's life. The meaning for me within this story was that basic tender loving care, healing hands and limited medication is a treatment regime that is relatively cheap, yet grossly undervalued. More lives could be saved.

CONCLUSION AND IMPLICATIONS FOR HEALTH AND SOCIAL CARE

The implications for health and social care are multiple. One main implication is increased knowledge and understanding of what birth means to women in Pakistan. Tandon

(1989:7) says how alternative research such as this contributes to knowledge production by answering certain questions like, what is life and birth like for women in Pakistan? He also opens out the purpose of research beyond seeking truth.

> The dominant system of knowledge describes its purpose and answer to the question, 'For what?' as the pursuit of truth. In contrast, alternative systems of knowledge production are involved in answering questions of daily survival and providing insights into the daily struggle for life and living, or ordinary people in a struggle...(Tandon 1989: 15)

The quality of the knowledge that has come through memorable stories and the narration of personal experiences could never have been imagined or predicted. Telling stories that have a meaning opens up thinking outside the normal. The women considered the Dai to be the defining person for labour and birth, however, she was also present to undertake defiling duties such as cutting the cord and dealing with the placenta. Having a Dai present at birth who may be 'of the family' but not necessarily, was judged to be essential. The professionals in the hospital blamed the dai for the poor condition of women on admission, using the pejorative 'dai handled', when it was so obvious the health of the women was compromised before childbirth by poverty and malnutrition. Undoubtedly recurrent childbirth exacerbated the woman's ill health.

Knowledge of the difference between East and West time has implications for the planners and providers of Health and Social Care. Appointment systems are not culturally sensitive or understanding of competing cultural norms such as hospitality. Punative treatment of women who miss appointments does little to encourage high risk women to attend for antenatal care. In Pakistan the saying when arrangements are being made is, 'in shala', meaning, 'with God's blessing'. However, there is a subtle different between God's blessing for all that may happen and God being responsible for it happening or not. Both are within the belief systems of Pakistani women so need to be understood by western health and social care providers.

Observing birth practice in one Red Crescent Maternity hospital unveiled what 'modern' western influence can have on mortality when there is a total lack of basic infrastructure which western hospitals take for granted. What was considered 'modern' western practice specifically the use of Oxytocin injections and or Syntocinon to excelerate labour was one of the major concerns that formed the seed to begin this research on birth in Pakistan. The influence the West has for the leading the way in 'modern practice' in developing countries is common knowledge. However, little action has been taken. It is interesting to note that drug companies do not advise that a hospital should have oxygen, suction or resuscitative equipment before drugs are used.

Women were treated with disdain by professionals in the hospital; without making excuses for the staff's behaviour I have pondered over how I would protect myself from the daily tragedy of working in a hospital like this, with women and babies suffering and dying so frequently. Distancing and blaming may be the only strategy that is effective. We in the West have so much to be grateful for, we have so much to learn I began by listening to the voices of women who have given birth in Pakistan.

REFERENCES

Chawla, J., 2000, *Crossing Boundaries and Listening Carefully Motherhood and Traditional Resources*, Information, Knowledge and Action, Final Report MATRIKA, Jan1997-March 2000 Pakistan.

Chesney, M., 1994, 'Midwifery in Pakistan', *British Journal of Midwifery*, 3(12): 661-664.

Chesney, M., 2004, *Birth for some Women in Pakistan, Defining and Defiling*, unpublished PhD Dissertation, Sheffield University: Sheffield, United Kingdom.

Denzin, N.K., 1997, *Interpretive Ethnography. Ethnographic Practices for the 21st Century*, Sage Publications: Thousand Oaks, California.

Denzin, N.K., and Lincoln, Y.S., 1994, *Handbook of Qualitative Research*, Sage Publications: Thousand Oaks, California.

Fikree, F., Jafarey, S.N., and Kureshy, N., 1998, 'A Community and Hospital Based Study to Examine the Magnitude of Induced Abortion and Associated Gynaecological Morbidity in Karachi Pakistan', *MotherCare*, Aga Khan University: Karachi, Pakistan.

Fleming, J., 1994, 'What in the World is being done about TBA's?; An Overview of International and National Attitudes to Traditional Birth Attendants', *Midwifery*, 10: 142-147.

Guba, E.G., 1990, 'The Alternative Paradigm Dialogue', in Guba G (ed.), *The Paradigm Dialogue*, pp. 17-30. Sage Publications, Newbery Park, California.

Guba, E.G., Lincoln, Y.S., 1994, 'Competing Paradigms in Qualitative Research', in N.K. Denzin and Y.S. Lincoln (eds.), *The Handbook of Qualitative Research*, pp. 9105-9107. Sage Publications: Thousand Oaks, California.

Jeffery, P., Jeffery, R., and Lyon, A., 1988, *Labour Pains and Labour Power*, Zed: London.

Jordan, B., 1993, *Birth in Four Cultures. 4th edition*, Waveland Press: Prospect Heights, Illinois.

Kamal, I., 2000, *Situation Analysis of Midwifery Training in Sindh*, UNICEF: Pakistan.

Kasi, A.M., 2002, 'Pakistan's Federal Health Minister's Address to the International Day of the Midwife', *National Committee for Maternal Health Newsletter*, August 2.

Kristeva, J., 1982, *Powers of Horror, an Essay on Abjection*, Trans.Roudiez L S, Columbia University Press: New York.

Lee, R.M., 2000, *Doing Research on Sensitive Topics*, Sage Publications: London.

Lincoln, Y. S., 1998, 'The Ethics of Teaching in Qualitative Research', *Qualitative Inquiry*, 4(3): 315-327.

Maine, D., 1992, *Safe Motherhood, Options and Issues*, New York Center for Population and Family Health. Columbus University: New York.

Manglay-Maglacas, A., 1986, *The Potential of the Traditional Birth Attendant*, World Health Organisation: Geneva.

Minden, M., 1993, 'TBA Training in Nepal', in *Proceedings of the International Confederation of Midwives 23rd Congress*, Vancouver.

Murray, S., 1996, *Midwives and Safer Motherhood*, Mosby: London.

Pairman, S., 1998, *The Midwifery Partnership. An exploration of the Midwife - Woman Relationship*, unpublished Master thesis, Victoria University of Wellington: New Zealand.

Reason, P., 1996, 'Reflections on the Purposes of Human Inquiry', *Qualitative Inquiry*, 1(2): 15-40.

Sizoo, E., 1997, *Women's Life Worlds, Women's Narratives on Shaping their Realities,* Routledge: London.

Swanson-Kauffman, K. M., 1986, 'A Combined Qualitative methodology for Nursing Research', *Advances in Nursing Science*, 8(3): 58-69.

UNICEF. 1989, *Statistical Profile of Women in the Punjab*, prepared by the Punjab Economic Institute, Shaheen Attiqurehma: Lahore.

Vincent Priya, J., 1992, *Birth Traditions Modern Pregnancy Care*, Element: Massachusetts.

In: Reproduction, Childbearing and Motherhood
Editor: Pranee Liamputtong, pp. 127-141

ISBN: 978-1-60021-606-0
© 2007 Nova Science Publishers, Inc.

Chapter 8

WOMEN, CHILDBIRTH AND CHANGE IN WEST NEW BRITAIN, PAPUA NEW GUINEA

Naomi M. McPherson

INTRODUCTION

In 1981, when I began ethnographic research in Bariai, West New Britain, Papua New Guinea, women and men elders well remembered their personal experiences under the German and Australian Administrations that colonized their minds and their bodies, the coming of the Catholic missions that colonized their belief system, and the Second World War that exploded on their beaches. They welcomed western medicines and clinics, but were ambivalent about the advent of independence and nationhood in 1975. They were (and are) disappointed by unfulfilled postcolonial promises of a better life in a modernized and globalized economy. Even though the Bariai were aware of being in the midst of these profound social and cultural changes, the effects of those changes on their individual and collective lives are only realized in retrospect some (often long) time after the fact. Over the past 115 years, these changes have affected the people of Bariai in both subtle and unsubtle ways (see for example, McPherson, 2001). In this chapter, I focus on changes in Bariai women's experiences of pregnancy, childbirth and childrearing and whether those changes have been beneficial to women (cf. Jordan, 1993). My presentation is roughly chronological, based on data collected during my ethnographic research in Bariai in the 1980s, 2003 and 2005 primarily through observation and participation in village and clinic birthing, and unstructured interviews and discussions with women and men, traditional birth attendants (TBAs), Health Clinic nurses, and various aid post attendants.[1] I have also gleaned data from census reports (incomplete as they are) created by the patrol officers who worked in the area during the mandate (1921-1975) of the Australian colonial administration.

---

[1] I am grateful to the Social Sciences and Humanities Research Council of Canada for financial support for this research during my 1981, 1982-83, 1985 and 1993 (in Australia) research in Bariai, and to the Grants-in-Aid of Research fund from Okanagan University College for financial support of my 2003 and 2005 research. As always, I am profoundly grateful to the people of Kokopo who make me welcome, share their lives and thoughts with me, and who continue to teach me about being Bariai.

The Bariai, whose population is about 1700 (census statistics are not always accurate or current), are located in ten coastal villages on the north coast of West New Britain province, Papua New Guinea (PNG). There are no airfields, roads, regular shipping, or amenities such as electricity and piped water in the area. The nearest hospital and only urban centre is approximately 200km east by sea at Kimbe, the provincial capital, and the local health clinic is about 50km west by sea (longer via the walking track). The Bariai are subsistence horticulturalists, depending primarily on taro, sweet potato, sago, cassava, coconut cream (for cooking) and bananas for the bulk of their diet which is augmented by a plentiful supply of fish, shellfish and other sea foods, pigs (raised as wealth and food), seasonal fruits and nuts, wild fowl and animals hunted in the bush. Hunger can be an issue during the rainy season when the gardens are not producing and the seas are too high to fish, or during periods of drought, which can be severe, when the monsoons fail to manifest.

The Bariai continue to live in houses made from bush materials harvested from the forest, although the historical changes mentioned above have had a huge impact on the structure of hamlets and villages, and thus, on gender relations. Colonialism and missionization in particular effected changes in the gendered use of space inside and outside the domestic (woman's) dwelling and the abandonment of residential sexual segregation has altered the constitution of the household (see McPherson, n.d.). Married men no longer sleep or socialize in the men's ceremonial houses (*lum*) but eat, sleep and socialize in women's houses (*luma*). Previously, the domain of a woman/wife and her children, the matrifocal household has shifted since 1981 to a focus on the cohabiting marital pair as the core of the patriarchal nuclear family.

Before getting into changes that have occurred in the Bariai system of reproduction since 1981, I present a very truncated version of the Bariai theory of conception and gestation, and birthing practices.

CONCEPTION, GESTATION AND BIRTH

Conception theories are never just about how babies are conceived; they are also about gendered bodies, gendered roles and a gendered ontology[2]. Bariai pre-Christian mythology tells how humans were created by the otiose Creator Being *Upuda* (B: 'our source', 'basis'). After creating the land, forests, and sea, Upuda took a branch of the *asi* tree, shaved off the bark (the shavings became the flora and fauna of the land and sea), and cut the stick in half. Upuda carved a male and a female from the two halves of the branch and breathed life into them. The first couple had fifty sons who married and became the ancestors of all the Bariai today.[3] While made of the "same stuff" and thus, a shared humanity, male and female bodies are different. Bariai use a garden metaphor to describe these sex differences: The female body is soft, cool and moist, an ideal environment for conception and gestation; the male body is hard, hot and dry, a hostile environment for planting and nurturing new growth. The female body also has a tube or "rope" that attaches the womb to the breasts. When a young girl's breasts get heavy and fall, the 'rope' has loosened and stretched thus indicating that the girl's

---

[2] See Jorgensen (1983) for theories of conception in Papua New Guinea.
[3] Where the wives for the fifty sons came from and where Upuda went when creation was complete is of no concern to the tellers or listeners of the myth.

body is mature and flexible enough to conceive, carry and deliver a child. Young men are considered mature enough to father a child with the appearance of facial and body hair and they have proven their ability in gardening, labour and exchange.

The mature female body naturally contains menstrual blood just as the mature male body contains semen;[4] conception occurs with the amalgamation of these two substances, which also contain the 'life force' or 'vital essences' (B: *sulu*). Adult men and women are considered innately fertile. Male sterility is impossible and inability to conceive is blamed on the woman who is believed to have interfered with conception through birth control, abortifacients, adultery, or sorcery. A woman's blood and internal organs must be 'strong' to envelope semen so it is not flushed away during her next menstrual cycle. A man's semen must be 'strong' to nourish the developing embryo. Conception requires multiple acts of sexual intercourse so that blood and semen form a coagulated mass called *avei ipata*, 'the shell of the tree.' At two months gestation, the foetus is *ital nakuie*, 'rat-like' with the beginnings of appendages and a tail. As the foetus grows the woman's body also undergoes changes, such as darkening nipples, from which others infer that she is pregnant. In many cultures, including our own, pregnant women crave and eat non-food substances, a condition called pica. Bariai women often crave a particular type of clay called *tano kaieau* (*tano*, earth, land; *eau* water), or clay from the Kai River.[5]

The couple continue to have sexual intercourse to "nourish the foetus" until the woman feels foetal movement (B: *gergeou iuad gau*, the child hits/kicks me) and her breasts are swollen with lactation. Given the anatomical "rope" that attaches womb and breasts, semen can also enter her breast milk. Semen is poisonous to the child. Therefore, at this point in the pregnancy, the couple cease sexual relations until the child is weaned from the breast (some 2-3 years) to safeguard the child from illness and possible death (cf. Counts and Counts 1983). Unfortunately, colostrum was also considered to be polluting seminal fluid and, until the mother's milk came down, another lactating kinswoman nursed the baby. When a child is born coated with vernix caseosa (B: *ikangkanga*), which women define with revulsion as coagulated semen, the mother is accused of liking sex too much to observe sexual abstinence during this latter stage of pregnancy. The vernix is polluting to women and is removed quickly by the attendants in order to avoid the contaminating effects (to mother and child) inherent in it. The configuration of the female body that attaches womb and breast, and the notion that semen can thus enter and contaminate breast milk is the basis of the postpartum taboo on sexual intercourse from the time of foetal movement to weaning. The taboo is observed primarily by the mother to protect her child's health. If the child becomes ill, the mother is considered at fault for not observing the taboo. The father's sexual relations with another woman, however, do not affect his nursing child and fathers were never as conscientious as mothers in observing the postpartum taboo. The postpartum taboo can be a time of great marital stress as women are concerned (with reason) that their husbands will seek other sexual partners.

---

[4] This is of course not the case in all Papua New Guinea cultures. See, for example, Gilbert Herdt's early (1981, 1987) contributions to this subject, where males are not born with semen but must acquire it from older men.

[5] Women periodically collect the clay from the river bank and prepare it by wrapping and hanging it in the house rafters over the hearth where it will dry to a chalk-like consistency. No other preparation is needed and the clay is eaten as desired. This clay is also used medicinally, as a curative for stomach ailments (indigestion, heartburn, reflux). Women's cravings (for the clay or other foodstuffs) are simply seen as peculiarities associated with pregnancy and are accepted as such. Women are quite clear, however, that it is they who crave not the foetus.

Prior to the advent of the local health clinic in 1982, women birthed in the village with the assistance of older women, primarily their mothers, elder sisters, grandmothers and other female kin. Knowledge and expertise in the reproductive system was the exclusive domain of women and no men were allowed to witness or participate in the process. Male exclusion from the birthing area and from women's knowledge mirrors women's exclusion from the men's ceremonial house (B: *lum*) and the secret-sacred knowledge that it signifies. Young women are also excluded from attending/witnessing a birth, primarily because the elders want to shield the young from being frightened of becoming pregnant themselves. Women maintained their daily schedule until well into second stage labour (or beyond) before sending for their mothers for the final stage. The labouring woman ate and drank to keep up her strength and walked her contractions until she was ready to deliver. Then she would assume a squatting position, balanced by holding on to a rope slung from the ceiling beams. Women surrounded her, front and back, soothing her with massage and quiet words; her mother or a village midwife crouched in front to monitor the dilation, presentation position, and to catch the baby as it emerged. Throughout labour and delivery women maintained their sense of modesty and never exposed their genitals keeping themselves discretely covered with a piece of cloth draped over the knees. At no time does a birthing woman cry out, moan, groan or thrash about. This is not the way of a "true" woman who, during labour, must be quiet, calmly efficient, and not express pain[6].

Although they do not define pregnancy and birthing as pathological conditions, Bariai women and men are aware of the potential risks associated with the reproductive process, but these risks are not necessarily related to the physiological process. Difficult births, retained placenta, malpresentation, haemorrhage, and maternal and infant deaths are caused by sorcery or the interference of ghosts and malevolent spirit beings. Women's lore and experienced village midwives are usually able to achieve a positive outcome through spells and the application of extensive acquired knowledge in dealing with birthing and its eventualities. Information contained in the colonial administration patrol reports suggests that TBAs were quite effective at preventing maternal mortalities.

BARIAI PATROL REPORTS

Patrol reports contain a record of the Australian Administration's presence in New Guinea. The reports were written by young male officers, known as *kiap*s who travelled throughout the Territory making contact with the people and the terrain. The reports contain census data, not only of people (mainly for purposes of labour recruitment), but also of palms, pigs, plantations, and crops. The census reports count people according to age, sex, marital status, and included information about births and deaths. The census data for Bariai is not complete—some archival material has been lost and patrol officers did not visit the area regularly—but what is there, is of some interest.

In 1950, Patrol Officer (PO) Leabeater notes only one maternal death of a young woman "whilst giving birth to a stillborn baby girl" and then follows up with the statement that

---

[6] Not all women achieve this degree of stoicism and comportment during the birthing process and those who don't become the subject of women's talk about her "strength" of character.

"deaths of females in child birth are agreeably small".[7] Patrol Officer Copley notes in 1952 that there is a hospital at the new Catholic Mission in Ongaia[8] and that the Catholic nursing sisters were planning a maternity ward when the mission itself was completed. But, it is not until 1968 that PO Batho notes, "Infant and Maternal welfare clinics [MCH] are conducted on a regular basis by the Sister-in-Charge and nurses from the Kilenge Catholic Mission Hospital". Regular visits might have been the goal. However, during my time in the village from 1981-1985, I witnessed two MCH patrols: one by a Catholic sister in 1981 and one by a nurse from the Health Clinic at Cape Gloucester in 1983. In 2005, the male aid post attendant at Gurisi travelled to Kokopo to conduct a Well-Baby clinic for 0-5 year olds (see Figure 5). He did not attend to pregnant women.

Patrol Officer T. Dwyer reports in 1954 that throughout the Bariai area, children in the age group 1-4 are at greatest risk of death from pneumonia after an attack of malaria, that most adults die of "senile decay", and that there are "very few females die in childbirth". PO Goodger reports the Bariai population in 1956 to be 582 "souls", dispersed among 9 villages, including 40 births (18 male and 22 female) and 22 deaths that year. He lists deaths by age group: 2 neonates, 2 under one year, 7 in the 1 to 5 year old, 3 in 5-8 year old, 2 in the 9-13 year old, and 6 over 13 years old (which includes adults of all ages). He notes there were no maternal deaths. In his 1959 patrol report, Haywood notes the Bariai population had reached 665 (an increase of 83 in 3 years) including 26 births (11 male and 15 female), 14 deaths (1 neonate; 2 under 1 year; 6 from 1-4 years; 1 from 5-8 years, and 4 from 13+ years), and 2 maternal deaths. Haywood (1959 #6) also reports an average of 2.2 children per family in 1959. Finally, Haywood remarks that the Bariai "suffer badly with malaria" due to the number of swampy areas in proximity to village sites.

Despite the incomplete census data for the Bariai, these few instances make clear that maternal mortality is very low and that primary cause of death for infants and children in the 0-5 year group is a consequence of the effects of malaria: low birth weight, low immune system, pneumonia, high fevers and convulsions, dehydration. In November of 1982, a maternity (delivery) house was built at the Health Clinic at Cape Gloucester, 50km by sea from the village. Women were encouraged to attend the clinic to give birth, which meant they had to present during the last 4-6 weeks of their term or "risk" (from the clinic perspective) delivering the baby on the footpath, in a canoe enroute, or in the village. Some women attended the clinic; most did not for reasons of convenience, lack of transport, the system's denigration of their womanhood and traditional knowledge. I have discussed this more fully in my previous work (see McPherson, 1994). Since the maternity clinic opened in November 1982 up to July 2005, there have been 251 pregnancies in the village of which only 42 (17%) have delivered at the Clinic and 209 (83%) delivered in the village. There was one maternal death (0.04% of deliveries)[9], one maternal and infant death enroute to the hospital in Kimbe from severe oedema[10], and 30 (12%) deaths in the 0-30 day age bracket, including 4 stillbirths and 9 miscarriages.

---

[7] Patrol reports pages tend not to be numbered; however, those wishing o pursue this information will find it in the census comments in the patrol reports cited by patrol officer's names.

[8] Ongaia is a Kilenge village with a Catholic Mission and Clinic and was the nearest source of medical care for the Bariai until the Health Clinic was built at Cape Gloucester in 1982.

[9] The young primipara died almost 4 weeks after birthing her daughter; the child died two months later as a consequence of low birth weight, malnourishment and dehydration.

[10] This was a third pregnancy and the woman and the twins she was carrying died shortly after arriving at the hospital in Kimbe.

The implementation of Maternal Child Heath care delivery system (MCH) in this rural area was targeted at women, who were misperceived to be dying in childbirth at a high rate as a consequence of their traditional system of birthing. Women's birthing knowledge and lore, indeed, women themselves were deemed inadequate to the task of delivering healthy babies and mothers (see McPherson, 1994). The provision of the maternity house and obstetric nurses trained in the western biomedical model of childbirth would thus prevent maternal and infant deaths. From the data gleaned from patrol reports and my own experience in the field, Bariai women rarely die in childbirth and neonatal death is not due to complications such as malpresentation, haemorrhage, or traditional practices that endanger the woman's health, but from complications of malaria. Bariai remains extremely malarial, yet no governmental or health offices seem to be supporting programs to reduce malaria.[11] I argued elsewhere (McPherson, 1986, 1994) that efforts would be better spent supporting and training village birth attendants (VBAs) to assist mother and child *in situ*, thus combining the best of both the biomedical and traditional systems. It seems someone read my article.

In 1995, AusAid, as part of its 5 year Kandrian Gloucester Integrated Project (KGIP) implemented a program to train Bariai village birth attendants.[12] Mary, one of the village women involved in the project, told me how she understood the project was to unfold. The trainers were a nurse and a doctor from Popendetta, Oro Province. They chose Mary to be a "Motivator", someone to learn VBA skills to assist at village births and then to be a trainer of other women VBAs. The plan was to train two women from each village, these two who would then train two more for a total of four VBAs per village. Mary attended training at the MCH facility at the Health Clinic at Cape Gloucester where she was taught to deal with all aspects of birth including breach and arm presentations, and to recognize potentialities for extreme blood loss and the necessity to transport to the Health Clinic. This assumed, of course, there was village transportation available, that is, gasoline for outboard motors to make the 50 km trip. In addition, she was taught how to perform episiotomies (which Clinic protocol maintains must be performed on all primiparae whether they need it or not) and to stitch tears. After this initial training, she was to attend at Popendetta for more training, but did not go because, she said, the aid money ran out and the VBA project ended.

Village birth attendants were to receive remuneration for their work from the 'government', probably the Department of Health, but payment never eventuated, so the trained women quit working as VBAs. As Mary put it: "I am not a fool" ['mi no fool']. Why should I do the same work for no pay as the nurses [at the Health Clinic] who receive a government wage". So, the women stopped formal assistance although, if asked/needed, they still "attend and assist at village births as there is no transport for the women to go to the health Clinic anyhow". Mary described one instance when she visited a village young woman

---

[11] In the 1980s the state sponsored antimalarial DDT spraying on a regular basis in all villages. The outcry about the use of DDT in developing countries eventually saw its use curtailed. To my knowledge, no other program has been initiated to rid villages of malaria carrying mosquitoes. There is little local knowledge about potential mosquito breeding grounds and how to clean them away (removing containers with stagnant water, filling swampy areas and so forth). Malaria attacks are frequent in the village population. People have no funds to purchase over-the-counter malarial prophylactics and resistant mosquito strains are increasingly unaffected by such medicines.

[12] The majority of the KGIP took place in the Kilenge area of Cape Gloucester and around to the south coast Kandrian area, it did not include the Bariai district except for a village birth attendant course, and the construction of a ferro-cement water catchment tank to provide potable water within the village. The tank project failed; when I arrived in 2003, it was a rubble of smashed cement. Ultimately the VBA project has also failed.

whom she knew was close to delivering her third child. She found the woman in labour and in agony as the baby was in a transverse lie with arm presentation. Mary pushed the arm back in and manipulated the baby to proper presentation; the baby was born dead. The mother was not transported to the Health Clinic and despite losing a great deal of blood, she did recover and the following year delivered a healthy child (again in the village).

Nowadays, women's expertise, knowledge and control over this aspect of their lives have been diminished. Midwifery has become paid employment and VBAs expect to receive money, like the nurses at the Health Clinic, as compensation for their work. Since money is scarce, village women prefer not to announce their labour but to birth by themselves or with only the assistance of their mothers, or even their husband. Mary related her experience with a young woman who was having a very hard time delivering her second child. When Mary tried to help, the woman's mother and husband refused her entry. Mary was angry: "Why would they close me out when she was having such a bad time?" Finally, Mary was permitted entrance and immediately recognized the young woman was in dire straits, very "swollen" (oedema?) and unable to deliver the child. Mary called for gasoline for an emergency transport to the MCH Clinic at Cape Gloucester. They arrived in the middle of the night and Mary let herself into the locked MCH maternity house. She put the woman on the delivery table, searched for instruments to perform an episiotomy and delivered the baby. The mother was badly torn during her labour and when the nurse came in the morning, she praised Mary for her expert work delivering the baby and repairing the tears. In this instance, the woman and her family had no choice but to compensate Mary for her work as a VBA.

Most women consider themselves capable of birthing unassisted after their second child. This was the case with Mili who, in 2005, was ready to deliver her sixth child. She laboured quietly most of the night and morning and birthed her child alone outside her house. She sent an older child to find the father to cut the umbilicus. On his way to fetch me to bring tea and sugar for his wife, he alerted Mili's mother and sister to help. Both mother and child were fine (see Figure 1). The presence of the husband as midwife violates the traditional system of male exclusion from the birthing process. I suggest that this is a consequence of the biomedical system that denigrates women's reproductive knowledge and experiences as backward, old-fashioned, full of superstition, and dangerous to mother and infant, and thus, making it feasible for husbands (who claim modernity and want their wives to deliver at the MCH Clinic) to participate in the birthing process. Mili's husband also prepared a sleeping platform on the ground near the house where she could rest and recuperate beside a warm fire until the postpartum fluids ceased. The fire would help to "dry" her "too damp" body and assist her internal organs to return to their pre-pregnancy shape.

When I asked Mili if she had put the child to the breast yet, she explained she was waiting until she felt less tired, perhaps later in the afternoon she said. Concerned that the infant would miss out on the colostrum Aunt Agata (see Figure 3) and I reminded her of the visit from the local aid post attendant a few days earlier. During his Well-Baby clinic in the village, "Dokta", as he is known, gave a talk on the causes of heart disease and diabetes and the benefits of eating locally grown and gathered foods versus eating the "white" food associated with diabetes: rice, flour, sugar, salt and junk foods. He also explained colostrum to the women and why it should be given to the newborn (see Figure 4). This, of course, is in direct contradiction to traditional thought that colostrum is semen-infected fluid in the breast that, if ingested, will cause the newborn to sicken and possibly die. A senior woman was adamant that the infant should not be given colostrum, but we were equally insistent that the child should have it. Finally, in exasperation, the senior woman left. Later that day, Mili did let the child nurse and obtain the beneficial colostrum (see Figure 1). If the baby did become ill or die, cause of death would be attributed to the child being fed colostrum.

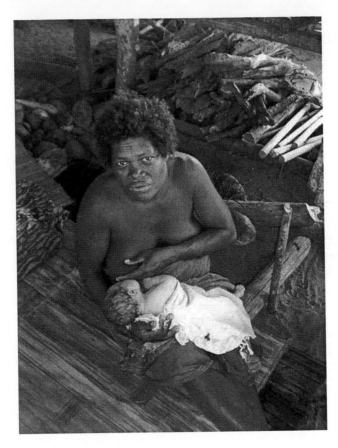

Figure 1. Mili and newborn daughter. Photo: © 2005 Naomi M. McPherson.

THE CHANGED SYSTEM OF REPRODUCTIVE CARE

The MCH facility implemented in 1982 at the Health Clinic and the 1995 VBA training project are the only services that are intended for the exclusive benefit of rural women. Indeed, these two government and non-government projects are the only contact women have with either the state or with NGOs and their attempts to improve the life of rural villagers. Both have failed. As noted above, in 23 years of its operation only 17% of Bariai village women present at the Health Clinic MCH due to lack of transport, food, time, fear of sorcery, dislike of nurses or because it violates their concepts of womanhood (for details, see McPherson 1994). The "walk-about" antenatal care clinic run out of the Health Clinic has always been sporadic. So, women are not getting any antenatal care or malarial prophylactics. The VBA training course was incomplete and those who were trained in phase one refuse to practice for lack of payment and village women are reluctant to call on the VBAs for lack of money to compensate them. These systems have not improved women's reproductive health, their experience of the birthing process, or the health of neonates. Indeed, I contend that they have done women a great disservice by denigrating women's knowledge, status, and role in the traditional reproductive care system then promising something in its place but not delivering on that promise. The ideologies of western biomedicine and Catholicism have had a tremendous mostly negative impact on women's reproductive lives.

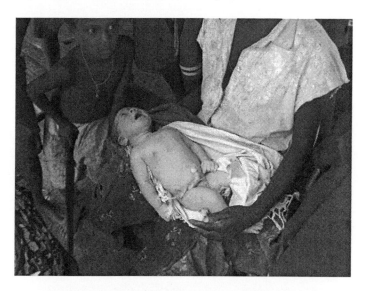

Figure 2. Mili's newborn daughter. Photo: © 2005 Naomi M. McPherson.

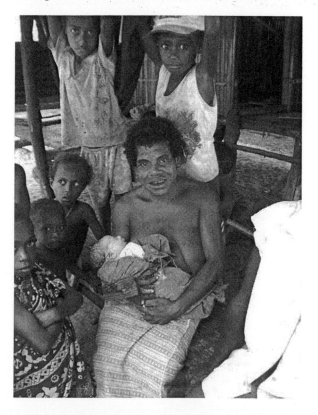

Figure 3. Mili's newborn, Aunt Agata and curious children. Photo © 2005 Naomi M. McPherson.

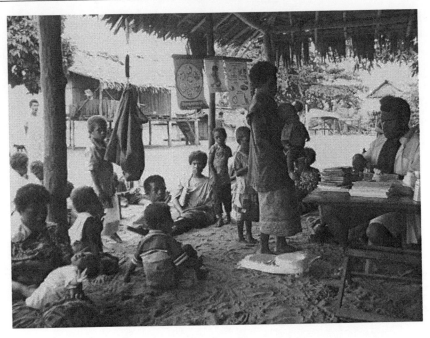

Figure 4. Dokta's Walk-about Well Baby Clinic, 2005. Photo: © 2005 Naomi M. McPherson.

WORKING MOTHERS

Compared to the 2.2 children per family noted by Haywood in 1959, my census in 2003 shows that the average number of pregnancies per woman is now 4.3 and that 40% of village women have had 5 or more (12 is the highest) pregnancies. As I have suggested, it is not better health care that is permitting women to have more children. Rather, more children are surviving into their own reproductive years due to child immunization programs, antibiotics and other services at the local aid post. Also, women are having more babies than in the past. Birth control methods are hard to obtain living in a Catholic parish and most Bariai are practicing Catholics who perceive birth control as a sin (despite women wanting to have fewer children). Most men desire many children and forbid their wives to use traditional or clinical birth control methods, although they never know if women are using traditional methods. Married men refuse to use condoms because of the stigma associated with condom use and birth control, with HIV infection, and illicit sex. The postpartum taboo that forbids a lactating woman to engage in sexual intercourse until her child is weaned is being ignored. The taboo operated to prevent nursing children from being polluted by semen entering its mother's milk. Women and men claim the taboo is now redundant because a child can be "cured" of the effects of semen pollution by western medicines (antibiotics). Although removal of the taboo on colostrum benefits the infant, it is not particularly beneficial to women. With the taboo, pregnancies were spaced at least two years apart, thus, siblings were spaced about three years apart or approximately 2 children in 5-6 years. Removing the worry of semen in breast milk has resulted in women are having two children in three years. Birth spacing is further compromised by the fact that the rule of residential sexual segregation has also collapsed and men no longer spend their days and nights in the company of other men in the men's ceremonial house. Married men are now living full time in the domestic household with their wives and children as a patriarchal nuclear family. Cohabitation permits more sexual access and, as dutiful Christian wives, married women are expected to "submit to their husbands" in all things including sexual needs. All of this adds up to more pregnancies, more children. Increasingly, mothers (and fathers) are finding it more difficult to feed, clothe and educate so many children. It is also a burden on women's bodies as the recuperative time between pregnancies is shorter and women's overall health declines, thus affecting her future pregnancies.

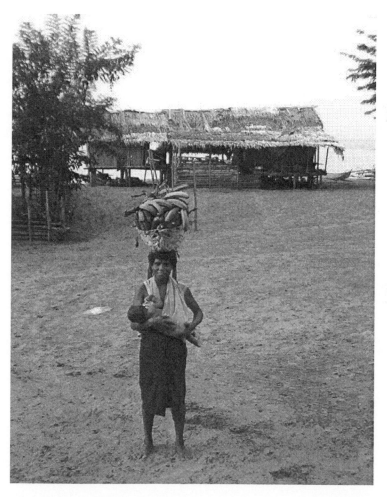

Figure 5. Mother nursing her eighth child while carrying produce home from her garden. Photo: © 2005 Naomi M. McPherson.

The increased onus on women as producers of food and money has also impacted on their reproductive health. Women are responsible for producing enough garden food to feed her family and to have sufficient garden produce to meet ceremonial feast requirements. Women are also responsible for feeding domesticated pigs—a fully-grown pig can eat as much as a fully-grown man (Sillitoe, 1998: 51). Besides garden production, women haul water twice a day, gather and store firewood as needed, prepare food, clean pots and dishes, do laundry and generally maintain the household and surrounding area (sweeping, cleaning up animal feces, clearing grass and weeds, and so on). With a larger number of small children to care for, older children in the family can relieve some of the burden from their mother by caring for their younger siblings. Children of both sexes learn how to care for children from a very early age, but the biggest responsibility usually falls on the eldest female child who is often kept out of school so that she can look after her siblings and do household chores and food preparation while her mother works in the garden or goes to market.

Women's productive labour has increased with larger families (and pig herds) to feed. In 1982, women went every second or third day to their gardens to bring home enough food to last until the next trip. In 2003 and 2005, women went to their gardens *every day* to weed, plant, and bring home a daily supply of food. In other words, a woman cannot carry home enough food to last the family for three days and must make the trek to the mountain garden plots each day to feed her family. Women's work has also increased from the necessity for cash income to pay school and medical fees and to purchase household items (e.g., pots, dishes, soap), food they don't produce—rice, tea, sugar, flour, oil, candies and treats—clothes, religious medals and books, and the list goes on. To access cash, women expand their gardens to grow "excess" food to sell at Cape Gloucester market to the teachers, health care workers, government workers, and others who live there but have no access to garden land of their own. They also smoke fish their husband's may have caught for them to sell. Several times a week for hours at night women collect *bêche de mer*, which they smoke dry and sell to travelling *bêche de mer* buyers. While women get relatively good money for their *bêche de mer*, it is a fraction of what these morsels sell for on the Asian markets. Women never curtail and rarely slow down their productive work when they are pregnant, working until the final stages of labour before giving in to the birthing process. The gendered division of labour and the day-to-day, heavy manual labour takes its toll on women's physical strength and health, and their quality of life.

CONCLUSION AND IMPLICATIONS FOR WOMEN'S HEALTH CARE

A key value (and privilege) of long-term ethnographic field studies is the opportunity it provides the researcher to view sociocultural change over time thus avoiding fixing peoples and cultures into a timelessness like bugs in amber. Under the influence of colonialism, missionization and the advent of the western medicine model of childbirth as the blue print for "developing" countries, the Bariai traditional reproductive system of care and women's reproductive lives have changed considerably. I have discussed how state and non-governmental projects and programs have focused on a western notion of childbirth as inherently dangerous, indeed, pathological. Thus, in order to prevent maternal and infant mortality rates, the technology and ideology of the western medical model of birth has been put into place. We see in Bariai maternal and child health clinics geared to erasing traditional knowledge and practices and inserting scientific and technological practices of birthing to reduce maternal mortality. I have provided statistical (however incomplete) information that suggests women have not and are not dying due to complications from gestation and delivery which are what the new system is set up to prevent. The maternal mortality rate is, as the patrol officer stated above, 'agreeably small'.

While the World Health Organization (WHO) speaks in global terms in its Millenium Development Goals (MDGs), the goal of Target Six is to reduce maternal mortality by three-quarters from 1990 to 2015 (WHO, 2003). The mechanism for achieving this goal appears *not* to be to label traditional systems dangerous and superstitious, or childbirth as pathological, thus, providing a rationale for funding and building more western-style technological birthing practices and facilities. MDG Target Six focuses on diseases—malaria, anaemia, and hepatitis—as major causes of maternal mortality.

WHO (2003: 4-5) states: "Targeted efforts to reduce incidence of these diseases in women should have the additional benefit of reducing maternal mortality rates". The mechanism for achieving this goal recognizes that maternal and infant mortality is more often a consequence of poor health and endemic disease than a consequence of traditional birthing techniques per se.

MDG Target Five is to reduce by three-quarters the under-five mortality rate from 1990 to 2015 (WHO, 2003: 4). Once again, the target does not focus on women's ability to deliver healthy babies and to care for and nurture their children. The focus is again on disease—malaria and tuberculosis—which during gestation can result in low birth weight and premature babies. With their immune systems compromised from birth, the chances of these children surviving malaria attacks, dehydration during fevers and fighting off other infections is significantly lowered. As the World Health Organisation (WHO, 2003: 4) reports: "It follows then, that treating these diseases in pregnant women will also help reduce the under-five mortality". Unfortunately, government and non-governmental attention has been focused on the mechanics of birthing (and whether traditional systems and women are up to the task) rather than the causes of maternal and infant mortality, namely, disease. The VBA training project probably shows a successful deliverable on its development project report, after all, *some* women were indeed trained to be VBAs. Follow up would show, however, that the development project to train VBAs has had a neutral if not negative deliverable for birthing women who, because birthing is commodified as a 'job' that requires payment, do not avail themselves of assistance for which they cannot pay. Pigg (1997: 233) puts this clearly: "few development projects ever work as imagined".

If one of the MDG indicators for progress in the reduction of maternal mortality is the "proportion of births attended by skilled health personnel", it would appear that the VBA program has failed and since my calculations show that only 17% of Kokopo women in a twenty year period delivered at the MCH facility, then the MCH must be deemed to have failed the women in this village. Granted MCH clinical services can save lives and the local Health Centre has saved women's lives. However, the bigger problem is disease, especially malaria, and eradicating disease is not being addressed. No efforts have been made in Bariai to teach villagers how to safeguard their environment in order to decrease malarial breeding grounds. There has been no provision of sleeping nets soaked in insecticides. There are no curatives for malaria attacks (such as artemisinin) available in the village or from health providers. Aid Posts and the Health Clinic are so severely undersupplied with even basic medications such as bandages, antibiotics and antimalarials that there is no hope of assisting pregnant women to deal with diseases that affect their health and impact on their pregnancies.

Finally, socio-economic changes are also affecting women's health and quality of life. Patriarchal ideologies inform men's desire to have many children, the Catholic ban on birth control, the demise of residential sexual segregation and the postpartum taboo, all result in women having more babies more frequently. Women are working harder with longer hours to produce food for larger families and they are working more hours to produce goods for the market place (vegetables, *bêche de mer*, smoked fish) in order to bring much needed cash into the household. Men do not produce anything to sell on the market and must leave the village for the urban centres in order to find paid work. Due to lack of skills, most men are not successful at obtaining paid employment and return to the village after several weeks or months of living with relatives in towns. Male search for employment and working in jobs away from their homes also contributes to women's burden in production, household maintenance and child caretaking.

At this point in my relationship with Bariai women and the Bariai district as a whole, I would recommend to government and international aid agencies that they not invest in programs of intervention geared to moving women out of traditional reproductive systems and into western biomedical systems (see Miller et al., 2003). These western biomedical systems require great expenditures of money for the appropriate facilities, technology and properly trained technicians, not to mention expensive drugs. Attention should be given to investing time and funds into eradicating the major causes of infant and maternal mortality— malaria, anaemia, and low birth weight. As the MDGs suggest, by treating disease (rather than the culture of childbirth), we should realize a decrease in the under-five mortality rates and in maternal mortality rates (WHO, 2003: 4-5).

REFERENCES

Batho, P.J., 1968-69, Patrol Report #8, Bariai District, March 10-16, 1969.

Copley, B.T., 1952-53, Patrol Report #5, Bariai District, August – September 1952. Microfiche of Patrol Reports for West New Britain Province, National Archives of Papua New Guinea.

Counts, D.A., & Counts, D.R., 1983, 'Father's Water Equals Mother's Milk: Conception of Parentage in Kaliai, West New Britain', *Mankind*, 14(1):46-56.

Dwyer, T., 1954-55, Patrol Report #6, Bariai District, September – October 1954. Microfiche of Patrol Reports for West New Britain Province, National Archives of Papua New Guinea.

Haywood, M.R., 1959-60, Patrol Report #1, Bariai District, June 16-27, 1959. Microfiche of Patrol Reports for West New Britain Province, National Archives of Papua New Guinea.

Haywood, M.R., 1959-60, Patrol Report #6, Bariai District, November 2-12, 1959. Microfiche of Patrol Reports for West New Britain Province, National Archives of Papua New Guinea.

Herdt, G. H., 1981, *Guardians of the Flutes: Idioms of Masculinity*, McGraw-Hill: New York.

Herdt, G. H., 1987, *The Sambia: Ritual and Gender in New Guinea*, Holt, Rinehart and Winston: Fort Worth, TX.

Jordan, B., 1993, *Birth in Four Cultures: a cross-cultural investigation of childbirth in Yucatan, Holland, Sweden, and the United States*, 2nd edition, Waveland: Prospect Heights.

Jorgensen, D., 1983, 'Concepts of Conception: Procreation Ideologies in Papua New Guinea', *Mankind*. 14(2): Special Issue, D. Jorgensen, Guest Editor.

Leabeater, T.J., 1950-51, Patrol Report #10, Bariai District, October 16-November 29, 1950. Microfiche of Patrol Reports for West New Britain Province, National Archives of Papua New Guinea.

McPherson, N.M., n.d., Tracing Tradition: Twenty-five years of Vernacular Architecture in Bariai, West New Britain, Papua New Guinea. Under review.

McPherson, N.M., 2001, *In Colonial New Guinea: Anthropological Perspective*, Pittsburgh, PA: Pittsburgh University Press,

McPherson, N.M., 1994, Modern Obstetrics in a Rural Setting: Women and Reproduction in Northwest New Britain. 'Urban Anthropology and Studies of Cultural Systems and World Economic Development', Special Issue: *Women and Development in the Pacific*, J. Dickerson-Putnam (Guest Editor), 23(1): 39-72.

McPherson, N.M., 1986. 'Childbirth: A Case History from West New Britain, Papua New Guinea', *Oceania*, 57: 33 – 52.

Miller, S., Sloan, N,m & Winikoff, B., 2003, 'Where is the "E" in MCH? The Need for an Evidence-Based Approach in Safe Motherhood', *Journal of Midwifery and Women's Health*, 48: 10-18.

Pigg, S., 1997, 'Authority in Translation: Finding, Knowing, Naming and Training "Traditional Birth Attendants" in Nepal'. In R.E. Davis-Floyd and C.F. Sargent (eds.), *Childbirth and Authoritative Knowledge: Cross-Cultural Perspectives*, pp. 233-262. University of California Press: Berkeley.

Sillitoe, P., 1998, *An Introduction to the Anthropology of Melanesia: Culture and Tradition*, Cambridge University Press: Cambridge.

Wright, N., 1962-63, Patrol Report #7, Bariai District, June 29-July 4, 1963. Microfiche of Patrol Reports for West New Britain Province, National Archives of Papua New Guinea.

World Health Organization, 2003, *'En-gendering' the Millenium Development Goals (MDGs) on Health*, Department of Gender and Women's Health: WHO.

In: Reproduction, Childbearing and Motherhood
Editor: Pranee Liamputtong, pp. 143-158

ISBN: 978-1-60021-606-0
© 2007 Nova Science Publishers, Inc.

Chapter 9

THE HOSPITAL AS A BIRTHING SITE: NARRATIVES OF LOCAL WOMEN IN NIGERIA

Chimaraoke Otutubikey Izugbara and Joseph Kinuabeye Ukwayi

INTRODUCTION

Disease, deformity, and death are terms popularly employed to describe the experiences of a vast majority of sub-Saharan African women during pregnancy and birthing (Harrison, 2001; Brookman-Amissah, 2004; WHO, 2004a). The bulk of African women are often viewed as highly at risk of infections, injuries, and death during pregnancy and the periods surrounding it. Much of the existing discourse focusing on the southern women's poor pregnancy and birthing outcomes is couched within a master narrative of modernity which treats maternal risks as the objective fallouts of women's refusal to seek and use hospitals for birthing. Often, women who risk acquiring a reputation of being ignorant, backward, and unwise because they do not seek or use hospitals for birthing are posited against progressive, modern, and wise women who do. This approach, which currently underpins the expert system of maternal risk analysis and management, has had the important role of prompting African governments to shore up investments in modern or hospital-based birthing services. But the expert framework is hardly the only narrative surrounding hospital births. One study after another continues to show that birthing and the sites in which it occurs provide rich spaces around which many discourses turn (Jordan, 1993; Davis-Floyd, 1996; Davis-Floyd and Sargent, 1997; Obermeyer, 1999; Janzen, 2002; Izugbara and Ukwayi, 2003, 2004; Izugbara and Brown, 2005). Discourses of the hospital (as a birthing site) concerned with female agency, power, and quest for culturally sensitive obstetric services exist alongside and sometimes challenge the medical, modernist narrative of the hospital as a safe and superior site for birthing (Obermeyer, 2000). Clearly, recent ethnographies of childbearing have demonstrated lay awareness of the dangers inherent in birthing, providing insights into how the choice of birthing sites connects with issues of danger, identity, power, and role-purpose among women. Izugbara (2000) has shown, for instance, that in many traditional Ngwa households, men leave decisions concerning birthing sites almost exclusively to women, the central reason being the belief that women knew better and thus were also more prepared to stake unapologetic claims to whatever became the outcomes of those decisions. If this evidence is anything to go by, it suggests, among other things, that in the imaginaries of local southern women, birthing sites go with risks and that local women's choices of birthing sites may as well be reflections of their views regarding these risks and how best to tackle them.

The central concern of this chapter is with lay representations and characterizations of the hospital as a birthing site among rural women. Taking its lead from more recent suppositions that far greater insights can be gained into the hospital through the windows of its limits rather than the thick armor of its capacities (Brown, 1998; Conrad, 2001; Mechanic 2001), the present study asks: How do hospitals feature as birthing sites in the imaginaries of local women and what patterns of obstetric care-seeking do lay narratives of hospital births authorize among local women? The chapter summarizes the results of a study of the discursive construction of hospital births among rural Ngwa women of southeastern Nigeria. The findings are expected to hone our understanding of issues and challenges surrounding local women's uptake of formal obstetric services in marginal areas of the world.

SAFETY LIES IN FORMAL HEALTH FACILITIES! THE MODERNIST NARRATIVE OF THE HOSPITAL

In the view of modernists, the hospital is a safer and more superior site for birthing than any other locations including homes, traditional birth houses, religious spaces and so on. Within this narrative, sub-Saharan Africa is often depicted as one mass grave of women dying from maternal causes owing primarily to poor or lack of modern obstetric services and continued use of traditional or informal birthing services by women. There is never a lack of damning statistics to support this viewpoint: Nearly two-third of all women who die annually from or are disabled by pregnancy and birthing come from sub-Saharan Africa (PRB, 2002; Ransom and Yinger, 2002): One out of every sixteen women in sub-Saharan Africa dies during pregnancy and birthing (UNICEF, 2001; WHO, 2001): For every African woman who dies during childbearing, 30 more suffer serious injuries, infections, and disabilities(Ransom and Yinger, 2002): If nothing is done to arrest the trend of high and growing maternal deaths in sub-Saharan Africa, there will be 2.5 million maternal deaths and 49 million maternal disabilities in the region over the next 10 years (UNICEF, 2001).

Proponents of this discourse often take pains to underscore the import of these alarming statistics: The bulk of women who die or are disabled during pregnancy and birthing are in the prime of their lives. Maternal mortality and morbidity thus deprive families of women's crucial role in household management and care (Parker et al., 1998; Kadoour et al., 2005), deprive newborns quality care (AGI, 2003; WHO, 2004b), cause an estimated annual global 8 million stillbirths and neonatal deaths (UNICEF, 1997, 2001), cost society its investments in the woman's education and skills (PRB, 2002), deprive the community a nurturer, a provider, care-giver, and productive member, and add significantly to the overall health burden of resources-poor African societies (WHO, 2001).

Within this modernist framework, the primary causes of this grim situation relate to the poor quality of obstetric facilities or and women's inability or refusal to uptake them (Thaddeus and Maine, 1990; Ondimu, 2000; WHO, 2001; Ransom and Yinger, 2002; UNICEF, 2002). The continent is usually described as hit by an exodus of medical personnel to oversea destinations, leaving the bulk of births in the region to be attended by unskilled personnel (Itano, 2002). The lean health budgets of African governments is also seen as often inadequate to deal with obstetric cases or and provide quality obstetric services to women who need them (Pang et al., 2002; Anonymous 2000; Oyowe, 1996). Further, modernists also blame ignorance and illiteracy on the part of health seekers for their inability to uptake formal obstetric services (Murphy and Baba, 1981; Kuti, 1998). One important source recently summarized the modernist discourse on the cause of the grim and unsafe childbearing and motherhood experiences in Africa thus: the unavailability of basic supplies and equipment, staff shortage and low morale, bad roads, and long distance between referral points, use of traditional birth attendants, and preference of mothers to deliver at home and in other informal sites (Ezechi et al., 2004). This narrative also basically suggests that pregnancy and childbirth will be much safer for women in Africa if they rely solely on hospitals for birthing. This framework urges the adoption of, and complete reliance on western-type health facilities, the promotion of interventions that will educate people, especially women on the importance of using modern obstetric services, and the elimination or at worst, modernization of traditional birthing services such as TBAs.

Important as the medical view of the hospital as a safe haven for child birthing is, many scholars (including McCormack,1982; Jordan,1993; Kaufert and O'Neil,1993; Obermeyer,2000) have argued that birthing and the sites in which it occurs provide a rich space around which many discourses turn and that efforts to address the challenges surrounding offering southern women greater access to hospital-based obstetric services will be enriched if we have insights into how women construct formal obstetric services. To this end, this study focuses on local Nigerian women's constructions of the hospital as a birth site and attempts to offer an analysis of the patterns of obstetric care seeking practices which such constructions authorize among them.

METHODS AND MATERIALS

To elicit local women's narratives surrounding the hospital as a birthing site, we specifically requested respondents to explain the pros and cons of the hospital as a birthing site, what they thought, knew, believed, and have heard about using the hospital as a birthing site and why they or other women may or may not use hospitals for childbearing purposes.

The original project, an ethnographic study of the socio-cultural factors in women's use of obstetric services, was conducted in four remote rural Ngwa-Igbo communities in Obingwa Local Government Area, Abia State, Nigeria. Going by available census figures, there is an average of 14,000 persons in each of these villages. Although the majority of people are Christians, there is also a handful of animists. Predominantly subsistence farmers, the people produce cassava, yam, and cocoyam. The people are also generally poor and many of them live in poorly built houses which are shared with livestock such as, birds, goats, and sheep.

Respondents in the original study include 13 TBAs, 23 women intercepted while presenting at the home of TBAs for pregnancy and birth-related matters, and 42 local women comprising mothers, grandmothers, and some local authoritative women. Key informants were employed to locate and identify one or more TBAs in each community. Each of the identified TBAs was individually met and interviewed. Permission to interview women presenting at their homes for services was also sought and obtained. Green and colleagues (2000) contend that service location intercept methodology relies on a purposive sample obtained by locating respondents or participants who would typically be difficult to locate in sufficiently high numbers through standard probability sample survey methods.

The data presented in this chapter were elicited in the course of interviews which relied on an open-ended in-depth, face-to-face individual interviewing schedule. This qualitative approach was adopted as it supports the generation of a rich pool of descriptive information. The interviews were administered in local language and the consent of the participants obtained to the audio-recording of their stories and responses. All participants were guaranteed confidentiality and anonymity of their responses. Audio-taped stories were later transcribed into English with the help of the field assistants and a few Igbo-speaking persons studying English language and linguistics at the University of Uyo. Samples of transcribed data were also independently discussed with sociologists and anthropologists in the faculty of social sciences, University of Uyo, Nigeria. They made useful suggestions that helped to refine, validate, and re-establish themes in the stories.

To analyze the data, we rely on the social constructionist perspective which favors direct articulations by lay people of their concerns, beliefs, thought, perspectives, and views through a range of narrative repertoires, including direct talk, stories, and discourses. This approach recognizes the capacity of ordinary people for lay authorship through language as well as the ethical and scientific salience of listening to and believing people's accounts and narratives. We, therefore, consider the data used (in this study) as critical aspects of the construction of maternal health and care-seeking in local cultures and as an invaluable source of insight into the thoughts, worries, views, wishes, fears, nay needs of local women which these stories embed as well as their significance for the planning and delivery of sustainable health care to marginal women and groups.

Yet, it is not our intention to imply that our current interpretation of the information gathered is incontrovertible or the only one possible. So, we do not consider our data as sacred texts or timeless truths. Rather, we are decidedly subjective, preferring to examine the potentials of the narratives to induce behavior, form knowledge, direct practice, produce discourse, and organize health-related reality. These narratives, for us, negotiate a complex semiotic and material terrain. Gagnon (2004) has admitted that by permitting us to infuse a certain amount of subjectivity and fluidity in how we read, examine, and interpret narrative texts, the constructionist framework provides the scholar ample room to mess about, albeit, fruitfully and authoritatively with textual materials.

This chapter, therefore, presents data on views about hospital deliveries circulating among local Nigerian women. While we merely aim to illuminate potential issues influencing women's perceptions and perhaps their use of formal obstetric care services, we agree with Manderson and Allotey (2003) that the specific context of health narratives may raise wide-ranging health services issues that connect with gender, change, globalization, resistance, identity, and class.

WOMEN, CHILDBEARING, AND SOCIETY

Local women in the study spoke of childbearing as a worldwide, natural, and normal function of women and considered it central to women's role purpose and identity. The ability to give birth was described as a unique attribute which nature has endowed on women only. "Men do not give birth, only women do", asserted one respondent. Although respondents were generally agreed that women were incapable of giving births without sexual contact with men, some noted that instances where women became pregnant without heterosexual contact exist. Children born without sexual contact with men were believed to possess unique powers. When we sought information on how they knew about this, we elicited responses alluding to folktales and the Bible. In one of the tales, a childless widow oppressed by in-laws and relatives goes into hiding in the forest and becomes pregnant without sexual intercourse with any male. She successfully gives birth without help. Her child, a boy, grows up exhibiting spectacular and rare powers such as foretelling the future, hypnotizing animals, and even being invisible at will. The boy finally grows up a hero who founds his own kingdom. It was also noted that evil spirits (*mmuo*) sometimes also entered women's womb. In such cases, the woman would think her husband was responsible. Such pregnancies, it was noted, could result in the women's death or the birth of a monster, wicked, or an abnormal child. Some women also believed that modern science can make woman pregnant without sexual relations with a man but that such children are usually less intelligent and smart than children born as a result of sexual contact with men. They were aware of hospitals where women go to have 'male sexual fluid' put into them but did not exactly know what the process involved. This, it was reported, occurred when the male sexual fluid was too weak to impregnate the woman or the woman' womb could not hold the man's sexual fluid when it comes through sexual contact.

Although respondents generally recognized that only women could give birth, they neither believed that all women could bear children nor did they consider all cases of childbearing to be appropriate. Respondents noted that there were women could not give birth and attributed it to nature, heredity, supernatural factors and accidents. Early childbearing and childbearing outside wedlock were viewed as inappropriate. Buttressing these points, one TBA noted:

> Although all women are expected to bear children not all of them are really able to. This may be the result of witchcraft, accidents, heredity, nature or other things. Sometimes women cause it themselves. We also know that if a woman indulges in witchcraft and kills children, eat up fetuses, or harm mothers she may suffer infertility... women who have engaged in abortion may also destroy their wombs or get the gods offended and have their wombs shut... While women are expected to give births, it should be also not be too early. Early childbearing can take a woman's life and also result in disability... It is also irresponsible and a sign of waywardness to bear children outside marriage. Our culture prohibits it. You are also not expected to give birth when you are too old or have become a grandmother.

Birthing was viewed as necessary for the continuity of the human race and it was widely believed that there would not be a next generation if there was no birthing. Children were viewed as tremendously important in the life of women, families and communities. They were spoken of in terms of guarantors of the future of the human race, sources of hope about the survival of family names and history, and as the key link between the present and the future. "The world will stop with us if we don't reproduce. When birthing stops the world also stops", asserted one pregnant woman. Inability to reproduce was viewed as the greatest calamity that can befall any society, community, household, family, man and woman. We were also told about local names in the community that buttressed the importance attached to birthing; *Uzoechi*, the lineage won't stop; *Amaechi*, the family name won't stop; *Ahamefula*, Let my name never get lost; *Azuka*, the next generation is important; Maduforo, there are still descendants; *Nwabike*, Children are a source of strength, *Nwabuechi*, Children are tomorrow, and *Azubike*, our offspring are our strength. Respondents noted that these names, which had been given for ages underscored the importance attached to birthing in their community.

Respondents associated birthing with women's role purpose and identity. Several of the respondents noted that getting pregnant and bearing children successfully accorded women higher status, cultural value, and honour. Despite associating women's honour and role purpose to the reproductive performance, respondents were nevertheless agreed that it was both wrong to limit the functions of women to birthing or to maltreat them when they were unable to do so. "All that women do isn't birthing, they have she's got other duties..." maintained one TBA. "If a woman can't give birth to children, nobody should maltreat her or taunt her for it... women do not deliberately shut their wombs up", she continued. Taunting or maltreating women who can not give birth was considered both inhumane and dangerous. To buttress this belief, one woman in the study told us a folk-story of how a crocodile, sent by spirits, swallowed up children who mocked an infertile woman. Although the crocodile later regurgitates the children out for their frightened parents, they were forced to swear to an oath never to taunt childless women.

CHILDBEARING AND BIRTHING SITES AS RISK

The fact that pregnancy and birthing were potentially risky was never far away in the narratives of the respondents. The periods were believed to put women at the crossroads of life and death, and were described as "journeys of uncertain outcomes", "risky businesses" "perilous asks", and "hazardous jobs". One TBA remarked that, during these periods women were never sure of their status. They were seen as half dead and half alive. Birthing was generally spoken of as laden with both risks and promises and its real outcomes were seen as often unpredictable. "A pregnancy may kill a woman, injure, or disable her. It may also be the basis of her survival, joy, happiness, and respect ... Childbearing is very critical... during childbearing women have one leg in the world and the other in the grave", offered one TBA. The periods of pregnancy and birthing were depicted as the most risky periods of women's lives. The women could not imagine any other event that put women at greater risk. They believed that childbearing and pregnancy have always been risky for women and did not believe that it was possible to eradicate all the risks that go with these periods of women's lives. Several of the women wished that it were possible for all the risks, which face pregnant and birthing women to be eradicated. The bulk of participants in the study did not believe that women's use of formal health services during periods of pregnancy and birthing made childbearing any less risky. Many commented that that even in big hospitals, women die during childbirth. We were told:

> Our own mothers faced risks and even had complications while pregnant or giving birth to us as did their own mothers while giving birth to them. It is the same with us, and our daughters may be no less different.

Respondents argued that pregnancy and birthing were not themselves threats to women's life and health. They were in fact viewed as good and desirable, and only made hazardous by the conditions surrounding them. It was noted that complications during pregnancy and birthing often resulted from supernatural, natural, hereditary, biological, or situational factors. Maternal complications were framed in terms of the negative outcomes that can result from pregnancy and childbearing Supernatural factors likely to cause complications during pregnancy and birthing were said to include witchcraft (*nsi*), spells (*ani*), curses (*ivu onu or igba akwukwa*), and falsely swearing to oaths (*idu isi ugha*). Others include infraction of taboos (*iru ala*), being disobedient to one's husband, elders, or and parents, extramarital sexual affairs (*ikwa iko*), and involvement in witchcraft (*igwo nsi*). Witches and wizards (*ndi nsi*) were spoken of as people who possessed special powers and could use such powers to visit problems and complications on women during pregnancy and child birthing. Witches and wizards can also cast spells on women to make them experience difficulties or even die during pregnancy and childbearing. Witches and wizards reportedly targeted pregnant women as pregnancy increased their susceptibility to witchcraft attack. Curses pronounced against women can also be a source of risk during pregnancy and child birthing. One participant told us:

> If her father or mother or an elder curses a young girl, it may work against her during pregnancy or child birthing. If my daughter offends me and I say, 'you bad girl, you will die during childbirth or you bad girl you will suffer in this world ...' it will certainly work. Curses are bad. That's why good parents don't curse their children ... Curses are powerful especially when pronounced by elderly people that one has truly or actually offended.

Evil children (*umu ojoo or ogbanje*) can also sometimes find their way into women's womb to cause them problems. Such children, often from the spirit world (*ala mmuo*) may be on a special mission to kill, torture, or cause complications for these women. Witches, wizards, and evil spirits (*umu mmuo*) were sometimes held responsible for sending evil children into women's womb. Women linked to the world of spirits as wives of deities, spirit beings, or other godlings also often make their spiritual husbands envious and angry when they (the women) marry human husbands. Spiritual husbands normally wait until when they (the women) are pregnant to seek revenge. Often, such women die at childbirth. Maternal complications also reportedly resulted from natural events such as lack of rest, poor nutrition, and violence against women, excessive use of alcohol, and excessive use of western medicine, poor personal hygiene, falls, malaria, and carelessness. A woman's biological characteristics could also put her at risk during pregnancy and birthing. Smallness of the womb and vagina and shortness of height were the frequently mentioned biological characteristics that put women at risks during pregnancy and childbearing. It was also observed that some of the complications women suffer during pregnancy and birthing were inherited. Some health conditions were believed to run in some families and sometimes transferred from parents to offspring. One informant puts it thus;

There are maternal complications that run among women from particular families … I know of a family in which the women often have problems expelling the placenta. Any woman from that family is at risk of this problem during childbirth.

Respondents dwelt long on the fact that birthing occurred in a number of places and sites in their community. They mentioned clinics and hospitals, homes of TBAs, home of mothers and their relations, shops of patent medicine dealers, and churches/prayer houses as the common birthing sites utilized by women in the community. There were also stories of women who had delivered in the farms with or without assistance. Respondents believed that no matter where it occurred, birthing remained inherently risky. One TBA noted that this was because every woman, every pregnancy, every birthing is different and may require special attention which may not be immediately available in a birthing site at a given point in town. Interviewees also noted that place of birthing and the people who attend to women during deliveries can make or mar the outcomes of birthing;

Pregnancy is a precarious thing. It can take the life of a woman. So care is needed in handling it. It is not just everybody that should touch a woman's stomach when she is pregnant and it is not just everybody that should come in when birthing in going on. In the hospitals, women are exposed to all kinds of people especially strangers and they can harm them under the pretence of helping them. The nurses or doctors that examine them are always strangers. Yet you don't know what they (nurses or doctors) have in their bodies. Some of them carry charms that are hazardous to pregnant women.

Generally, the women noted that it was often very difficult to predict the outcome of a birthing process as anything could happen at any time during the period. However, respondents believed that one of several ways women tried to negotiate the risks they face during birthing is by being choosy about where they go to have their babies. It was noted that decisions to use a particular birthing sites were often based on the concerns which women were interested to address during particular pregnancies. Women's choices about birthing sites were, therefore, reportedly fluid and not fixed, often shaped by the unique, real, and or perceived circumstances of a given pregnancy. As one of the women said, "A woman who has a homebirth today may decide to have a hospital birth next time, it depends on the issues she is trying to deal with or handle…"

NARRATIVES OF THE HOSPITAL AS A BIRTHING SITE

The hospital was recognized as one of the more popular birth sites used by women in the study community. Many of the women, however, noted that the hospital only emerged as a common birthing site among women in recent times. This view was most common among older respondents who maintained that it was only in the last two decades that hospitals became popular as birthing sites among women in the community. One of the women aged 58, observed;

When I was young woman hospitals weren't popular as birthing sites. I think hospitals around here only began to see their first pregnant women after the Nigerian civil war. Most women my age never went to hospital to give birth. We all delivered at home.

A woman, aged 36, informed us that her mother told her that in their own (her mother's) time, hospitals were not popular sites of birthing among women. Respondents of different generations were also agreed that despite its proliferation in recent times, hospitals were yet to become the ultimate site of choice for birthing among women in the community. The popular explanation for this was that local women did not actually consider hospitals any safer than other birthing sites. Hospitals were generally spoken of as having little or no advantage over other birthing sites. One of the respondents noted that "anything can happen anywhere... It's not the hospital that protects women during birthing, it is God. If God fails to intervene, what can the best doctor do?" Another respondent observed, "No birthing site is risk-free... In fact using the hospital as a birth site can even become a problem instead of a solution... There are instances where it will be safe to give birth in the hospital and there are situations it wouldn't be..." The question of hospitals as both risk-laden and as no less risky than other birthing sites was never far away in the women's accounts and narratives. It was popularly believed that the numbers of women, who die during birthing, suffer complications and disabilities, and whose babies die at birth were often higher in hospitals than in other sites. When we sought information on why respondents thought so, we elicited responses bordering on the fact the hospitals are only often able to deal with natural causes of problematic births whereas the supernatural factors are the more critical and common causes of problems associated with birthing. One of the respondents we spoke to told us that hospitals are often unable to help pregnant women facing issues related to the supernatural and asserted; "They can't do anything, because they can't deal with the impacts of factors like sorcery, curses, disobedience, taboos and witchcraft on the outcome of women's pregnancy... These are the issues women often face... There are providers who can handle such issues..." Supernatural factors were spoken of as an ever-present reality in the lives of women and many respondents confirmed knowing women who have died or who nearly died owing to supernatural forces, especially while giving birth in the hospital. We were also told, "If several persons are present when birthing is going, it is difficult to control the outcome ... I tell you if somebody crosses her/his leg near a woman in labour. She will have prolonged turbulent labour... In the hospitals, all kinds of strangers attend to women. You don't know who is a witch or wizard. They may appear to be helping the woman but may have other motives. It happens ... that's why many women die in hospitals while giving birth ..." Going to the hospital to give birth was also spoken of in terms of exposing oneself to risks of exploitation, maltreatment, sexual and physical abuse, and having one's baby stolen. When women go to hospitals to give birth they were reportedly subjected to all kinds of inhumane treatment by careless, greedy, and callous providers.

We elicited some negative stories about hospital based deliveries circulating among women in the community. In one of the stories, a woman goes to hospital to give birth. The family knew it was going to be a baby boy. Even the TBAs confirmed it. The family was happy as members anxiously waited for his birth. The husband was very happy and registered her in a big hospital in town with a large sum of money. He felt he was guaranteeing her safety and that of the unborn child. He was however seriously warned by his mother and wife's mother who preferred she gave birth at home where she could easily be monitored by experienced and careful hand. When her labor began, her husband took her to the hospital. She did not have troubles during delivery. And she actually had a baby boy. She wept with joy when she discovered it. However, the doctors and nurses injected her with a powerful sleep-inducer and immediately she fell asleep. When she woke up and asked for her boy-child, she was shown a baby girl. The hospital people had stolen her baby-boy and replaced it with a baby girl. The nurse later openly admitted that they were paid to do it.

In another popular story, a woman experienced labor very early in the seventh month of her pregnancy. So her family met and decided that she would need to go to a hospital. In the hospital, the doctors decided she would need to undergo caesarean operation. The family paid heavily for it. Then they cut her open and brought out the child. The child survived. But after bringing out the child the doctors forget their knives, scissors, razors, and needles inside the woman's womb. Several months after the operation, she began to feel ill and particularly felt heavy inside her body. She even thought she was pregnant again. Her aged mother examined her and confirmed something was inside her, but that the thing did not have life. She continued to experience abdominal pain, occasional vaginal bleeding, and other kinds of problems. Finally, she went to the hospital. The doctors examined her and found she had all kinds of metals in her womb. They cut her open again and all kinds of surgical implements were recovered from her womb.

In yet another story, a woman who went to hospital to deliver a baby had her birth fluid collected by hospital personnel and sold to ritualists. The new baby eventually got sick and died. She also became terribly sick. The family took her to several places for treatment without success. Several tests were conducted but did not reveal anything. Her condition continued to grow worse, until she was taken to a powerful traditional oraculist who accurately divined her problem and what caused it. The oraculist told her that the personnel of the hospital where she went to give birth had collected and sold her birth fluid to wicked ritualists for use in money making. However, the oraculist helped free the woman from the grip of the ritualists. There were also stories of women who, while uptaking hospitals for birthing services, were deceived into unnecessary caesareans, sexually abused by male doctors, and or enslaved by hospitals for not being able to settle her bills. The majority of respondents in the study generally thought these stories were true and part of women' s lived and true stories of using the hospital for deliveries. One of the respondents asserted, "All these stories of women getting killed, losing their babies, getting cheated, ripped off, and raped are true. They are not just rumors. Personally I believe them and most of the women here know they are true stories".

The powerlessness of women during hospital-based deliveries was also an issue that emerged in the narratives of the respondents in the study. The women spoke of the hospital as a place where women are ordered around, controlled, toyed with, infantilized, and forced to comply with rules. Respondents generally believed that when women go to hospitals to give births they are not often treated respectfully like adult. "Their views are never sought, they are insulted, bossed over, and maltreated; when they complain, they risk being branded as stubborn or even being punished by being asked to sweep hospital rooms, wash their own beddings or being refused attention", asserted one woman who claimed personally knowing a woman who experienced maltreatment while using hospital-based obstetric services. Another respondent also maintained that in the hospital, mothers risk being shoved up and down and forced to obey all kinds of rules. There were also mentions of women being exposed to strangers and people who they did not trust in the hospital setting. This, as one respondent noted, was often dangerous and contributed to the insecurity of the lives of women who used hospitals for deliveries. One TBA noted, "most of the women that I attend to are from this village. They know me and I'm trusted … I know their families and I am careful not to fail them. I give them prompt attention. When it is birthing time, I am careful not to fail them. I also make sure they deliver without being exposed to several persons. In the hospital, women are often not treated with respect".

Respondents in the study believed that women who use the hospital for birthing do so for a variety of reasons. They were agreed that women used hospitals when they were sure they would not be dealing with supernatural issues during birthing. It was noted that during the period of birthing, complications may arise for different reasons. When women were sure they would not suffer complications resulting from supernatural causes they reportedly preferred to use hospital services. Women also used hospital services when they and their households had enough money to pay for it. Hospital-birthing services were generally viewed as often very expensive and only affordable by the rich, and thus largely uptaken by women from well to do households. One of the respondents noted:

> Using the hospitals for birthing means you have enough money to pay for services. So whenever I get pregnant and hope to use the hospital for birthing, my husband and I always save enough money because you can never be too sure what you will be told to buy and pay for in the hospital. Also I am careful not to go to hospitals when I suspect I may have to deal with supernatural factors during the period of birthing.

Using the hospital for birthing was also viewed as a sign of modernity. Many of the women we spoke to viewed hospitals as mainly used by educated, modern women who were not strong enough for, or feared the pains of home-births. Respondents believed that women sometimes preferred to give birth in the hospital not necessarily because it was safer to do so but because it marked them as modernized women. They reported that giving birth at home has increasingly become associated with backwardness and poverty. There was also the belief that hospitals sometimes used medicines to lessen women's birth pains. Many women in the study viewed birthing pains as often helping to strengthen women and the newborn. They spoke of the purported use of medicines to lessen birth pains as often negatively affecting both women and their babies. Such medicines were viewed as likely to reduce women's fertility and to cause the newborn to be mentally-deficient. Quite a number of the respondents believed that children born in hospitals were less strong and survived less often than those born at home or other places where women are allowed to fully experience the natural pains of birthing. Many of the respondents, especially the younger women, noted they have used the hospitals and may also continue to if they can afford it. They were also generally more willing to recommend it to other women. Older women and TBAs were generally less willing to accept they would use hospitals for birthing were they to get pregnant again and also tended to be less willing to recommend it for other women. However, among the women interviewed, the popular belief tended to be that women should be careful in using the hospitals for birthing. They accepted that it was safest for women to use hospitals for birthing when the hospitals were near enough, their services affordable, and also when the users had trusted relations working in the hospitals they were using. Respondents noted the nearness to the hospital means easier physical access when labor begins. It also means that mothers can be coming from home after birth and save themselves the high cost of occupying hospital beds for extended periods. Utilizing hospitals where one's acquaintances and relatives worked was also believed to protect women from unfavorable circumstances and treatments in the hands of strange and potentially dangerous hospital staff. All in all, respondents spoke of the hospital as a site fraught with potentials to make birthing both safe and risky for women who use them. The hospital was primarily framed as an important birthing site but one that also often operated on dynamics that were at dissonance with women's cultural needs and expectations and which women must therefore be cautious to use.

DISCUSSION

Danger and risk are the popular terms commonly and currently used to frame the experiences of the bulk of sub-Saharan African women during pregnancy and the periods surrounding it. These women are often seen as highly susceptible to risks of infections, injuries, and death during pregnancy and the period of birthing. The modernist narrative which depicts maternal risks as primarily resulting from women's failure to seek and use hospitals for birthing has provided the main framework against which the poor maternal health experiences of women in developing societies have been understood and analyzed. In Nigeria, where the present study was conducted, the chance of a woman dying from reproductive health disorders and complications is put at nearly 1 in 12. Most of these deaths, disabilities, and infections are often said to be preventable if women received skilled care during pregnancy and childbirth. Currently however, a large number of women in Nigeria continue to use informal birthing services, which has been frequently blamed on their inability to conceive of the risks in using traditional health services. This chapter takes its lead from the persuasion that far greater insights can be gained on the issues surrounding southern women's infrequent use of formal obstetric care services by investigating how hospitals feature as birthing sites in local imaginaries.

Women in the study linked birthing to women's role purpose and identity and spoke of it as a very risky period in women's lives. The importance of birthing was elaborated to include ensuring the fulfillment of women and as a guarantee to the perpetuity of family names and communities. Current ethnographies of birthing (such as those by Jordan, 1984; Davis-Floyd, 1996, Izugbara, 2000, Janzen, 2002; Izugbara and Ukwayi, 2003) have suggested that their varying levels of development, notwithstanding, most human societies often have notions depicting pregnancy and birthing as precarious, which is an indication that ideas of obstetric risks are in no way a modern discovery. Obermeyer (2000) study among Moroccan TBAs and women show that they supported the opinions that 'during pregnancy women have one foot in the world and one in the other world' and that 'women's grave remained open for forty days after birthing'. Local women in the study offered insights into specific maternal risks and hazards and analyzed the scope, which biological, social, psychological, natural and mystical factors and conditions offer for the presence of these risks.

Respondents dwelt long on the fact that birthing occurred in a number of places and sites in their community. They mentioned clinics and hospitals, homes of TBAs, home of mothers and their relations, shops of patent medicine dealers, and churches/prayer houses as the common birthing sites utilized by women in the community. It is also clear from the narratives that the women believed that no birthing sites were risk-free or superior to others. Although local women recognized the hospital as one of the more popular birthing sites used by women in the community, they generally did not speak of it as having any advantage over other birthing sites. It was, thus, not viewed as a panacea to the risks which women faced during pregnancy and birthing. Hospitals were seen as only good at dealing with natural risk factors. Respondents in the study noted that women have their reasons for using the hospital for birthing. They were agreed that women used hospitals when they were sure they would not be dealing with supernatural issues during birthing. During the period of birthing, complications may arise for different reasons. When women were sure they would not suffer complications resulting from supernatural causes they reportedly preferred to use hospital services. Women also used hospital services when they and their households had enough money to pay for it. Hospital-birthing services were also viewed as often very expensive and only affordable by the rich, and thus largely uptaken by women from well to do households. Many of the women we spoke to viewed hospitals as mainly used by educated, modern women who were not strong enough for, or feared the pains of home-births.

There were also several negative stories about hospital based deliveries circulating among women in the community. These stories centered primarily on the high cost of formal obstetric services as well as the poor and weak moral positionality, untrustworthiness, carelessness, callousness, and unscrupulousness of hospital staff. There is reason to believe that these negative 'stories' of hospital births comment loudly on rural women's mistrust of, and lack of faith in medical services, how they want to be treated by medical staff, and the factors that could contribute to satisfactory hospital experiences among women. While accepting the view of scholars (such as Manderson and Allotey, 2004, Okafor, 2004) that hospital-related folklores are often fueled by the mismatch between the needs and sensitivities of users and the reality of hospital-based care, it is also noteworthy that these stories reflect local women's needs for obstetric services that are responsive to their cultural, economic and social sensitivities and draw attention not only to local women's expectations regarding what quality and responsive healthcare service entails but also to the factors that contribute to satisfactory hospital experiences for women.

All in all, rural Nigerian women's narratives surrounding the hospital reinforce, with details, the significance of making formal hospital-based obstetric services more responsive to local southern women's cultural needs and sensitivities. The narratives are critical commentaries on the urgent need and demand for healthcare systems that are sensitive to the needs of local women. Currently, hospitals do not appear to register in the imaginations of local women as a site where rural Nigerian women's search for risk-free birthing can be actualized. In this study, the hospital was largely spoken of as a setting where women are likely to meet unfavorable treatments and where maternal risks can be exacerbated. Local peoples' decisions to utilize particular healthcare services are often rational and based on their own considerations of how useful particular care services will be to their health needs and conditions (Mitchell, 1999). People generally tend to seek and use health facilities which they have faith in, and not those that they believe could worsen their circumstances. Women's views about hospitals as birth sites add validity to the need for a more public, academic-oriented discourse about the narrative production of health in local southern societies. Therefore, worthy of more scientific description is the connect between how local Nigerian women people understand hospitals and their willingness to uptake them for obstetric purposes. After all, recent research continues to show that health seeking practices are largely authorized by the way health services feature in the imaginaries of care seekers. Further, given that the way hospitals feature as birthing sites in the imaginaries of local southern women may not encourage their uptake by many women, there is need to shore up the quality of available hospital-based birthing care to be more responsive to the sensitivities and expectations of local Nigerian women. Indeed, to continue hoping that women will use birthing care services that do not meet their expectations, aspirations, and needs is a mistake that maternal health programme implementers in the global south have made for too long.

REFERENCES

Alan Guttmacher Institute (AGI), 2004, and UNFPA, 2003, *Adding It Up: The Benefits of Investing in Sexual and Reproductive Health Care*, AGI: New York.

Anonymous, 2000, 'Medical migration and inequity of health care', *Lancet*, 15; 356(9225):177

Brookman-Amissah, E. & Moyo, J.B., 2004, 'Abortion Law Reform in Sub-Saharan Africa; No Turning Back', *Reproductive Health Matters*, 12 (24 supplement): 227-234

Brown, P.J (ed.), 1998, *Understanding and Applying Medical Anthropology*, Mayfield Publishing: Mountain View, CA.

Conrad, P. (ed.), 2001, *The Sociology of Health and Illness; Critical Perspectives*, Worth Publishers: New York.

Davis-Floyd, R., 1996, 'The Technocratic Body and the Organic Body: Hegemony and Heresy in Women's Birth Choices', in C. Sargent and S. Brettell (eds.), *Gender and Heath: An International Perspectives*, pp. 123-166. Prentice Hall: Upper Saddle River, NJ.

Davis-Floyd., R., & Sargent, C. (eds.), 1997, *The Social Production of Authoritative Knowledge in Pregnancy and Childbirth*, University of California Press: Berkeley and Los Angeles.

Ezechi, O., Fasubaa, O., Obiesie, L., Kalu, B.K., Loto, O.M., Dubub, V.I., & Olomola, O, 2004, 'Delivery Outside Hospital after Antenatal Care: Prevalence and Its Predictors', *Journal of Obstetrics & Gynecology*, 24(7): 745-749.

Gannon, S., 2004, 'Crossing 'Boundaries' with the Collective Girl: A Poetic Intervention into Sex Education', *Sex Education*, 4(1): 81-99.

Goliber, T.J., 1997, 'Population and Reproductive Health in Sub-Saharan Africa', *Population Bulletin*, 52 (4): 1-32.

Green, E., Daniel, A., Rodriguez, C., & Romero,J. , 2000, 'A Study of Early Contraceptive Users in Mozambique', *African Journal Reproductive Health*, 4(2): 74-84.

Harrison, K., 2001, 'Maternal Morbidity and Social Economic Conditions with Particular Reference to Illiteracy and Poverty', *Sexual Health Matters*, 2: 50-54.

Itano, N., 2002, 'Condition Critical as African Doctors Head Overseas', *The Christian Science Monitor*, 324: 499-500.

Izugbara, C.O., 2000, 'Women's Understanding of Factors Affecting their Reproductive Health', *African Journal of Reproductive Health*, 4(2): 62-68.

Izugbara, C. O., 2006, *Did your Hear about the Woman Who?: Negative Stories of Hospital Birth among Rural Women in Nigeria*, paper presented at the 14th Annual Boston University Graduate Research Conference in African Studies, African Studies Centre, Boston University, Boston, March 17-18.

Izugbara, C. O., & Brown, A., 2005, 'Women, Pregnancy Risks and Birthing-Related Complications: Conversations with Traditional Birth Attendants', in R.E. Balin (ed.), *Trends in Midwifery Research*, pp. 167-184. Nova Science Publishers:New York.

Izugbara, C. O., & Ukwayi, J., 2003, 'The Clientele of Traditional Birth Homes in Rural Southeastern Nigeria', *Healthcare for Women International*, 24 (3): 177-114.

Izugbara, C.O., & Ukwayi, J., 2004, 'An Intercept Study of Persons Attending Traditional Birth Homes in Rural Southeastern Nigeria', *Culture, Health & Sexuality*, 6(2): 101-114.

Janzen, J.M., 2002, *The Social Fabric of Health; An Introduction to Medical Anthropology*. McGraw Hill Companies: Boston.

Jordan, B., 1993, *Birth in Four Cultures: A Cross-Cultural Investigation of Childbirth in Yucatan, Holland, Sweden, and the United States*, Waveland: Prospect Heights, IL.

Kadoour, A., Hafez, R., & Zurayk, H., 2005, 'Women's Perceptions of Reproductive Health in Three Communities Around Beirut, Lebanon', *Reproductive Health Matters*, 13(25): 34-42.

Kaufert,P.& O'Neil, J., 1993, 'Analysis of a Dailogue on Risks in Childbirth; Clinicians, Epidemiologists and Inuit Women', in S. Lindenbaum & M. Lock (eds.), *The Anthropology of Medicine and Everyday Life,* pp 32-54, University of Carlifornia Press: Berkeley.

Kuti, R., 1998, *Speech at the Opening Conference on Problems of Rural Dwellers in Nigeria*, National Institute of Policy and Strategic Studies: Kuru, Nigeria.

Manderson, L., & Allotey, P., 2004, 'Storytelling, Marginality, and Community in Australia: How Immigrants Position Their Difference in Health care settings', *Medical Anthropology*, 22: 1-21.

Mechanic, D., 2001, 'Changing Medical Organization and the Erosion of Trust', in P. Conrad (ed.), *The Sociology of Health and Illness; Critical Perspectives*, pp. 198-207. Worth Publishers: New York.

Mitchell, E., 1999, 'Delayed Access to EOC in Ecuador: Setting Priorities', paper read at the American Public Health Association Meeting, November: Chicago, IL.

Murphy, M., & Baba, T., 1981, 'Rural Dwellers and Health Care in Nigeria', *Social Science and Medicine*, 15A: 265-271.

McCormack, C., 1982, *Ethnography of Fertility and Birth,* Academic Press: London

Obermeyer, C., 1999, 'The Cultural Context of Reproductive Health: Implications for Monitoring the Cairo Agenda', *International Family Planning Perspectives*, 25: S50-S54.

Obermeyer, C., 2000, 'Risk, Uncertainty, and Agency: Culture and Safe Motherhood in Morocco', *Medical Anthropology*, 19(2): 173-201.

Okafor, B.C., 2000, 'Folkore Linked to Pregnancy and Birth in Nigeria' *Western Journal of Nursing Research,* 22(2) 189-202

Ondimu, K., 2000, 'Availability and Quality of Health Care Services for Safe Motherhood in Kisumu District, Kenya: A Situation Analysis', *African population Studies*, 15: 91-107.

Oyowe, A., 1996, 'Brain Drain: Colossal Loss of Investment for Developing Countries', *The Courier ACP-EU*, 159: 59-60.

Pang, T., Lansang, M., & Haines, A., 2002, 'Brain Drain and Health Professionals: Global Problem Needs Global Solutions', *BMJ*, 324: 499-500.

Parker, L.G., Rupta, R., Kurtz, K., & Marchant, K., 1998, *Better Health for Women:; Research Results from Maternal Health Care Programmes*, International Center for Research on Women: Washington, D.C.

Population Reference Bureau (PRB), 2002, *Women of the World Datasheet*, Measure Communication: Washington, D.C.

Ransom, E.I.& Yinger, N.V., 2002, *Making Motherhood Safer; Overcoming Obstacles on the Pathway to Care*, Population Reference Bureau: Washington, D.C

Thaddeus, S., & Maine, D., 1990, *Too Far to Walk: Maternal Mortality in Context, Fndings from a Multidisciplinary Literature Review*, Centre for Population Reference Bureau, New York.

UNICEF, 1997, *Guidelines for Monitoring the Availability and Use of Obstetric Services*, UNICEF: New York.

UNICEF, 2001, *Maternal Care: End Decade Database.* <http: //www..childinfo.org/eddb/ mat_mortal/index.htm>

WHO, 2004a, *Maternal mortality in 2000: Estimates Developed by WHO, UNICEF, UNFPA*, WHO: Geneva.

WHO, 2004b, *Reproductive Health Strategy to Accelerate Progress Towards the Attainment of International Development Goals and Targets*, WHO: Geneva.

WHO, 2001, *Maternal Mortality in 1995; Estimates Developed by WHO, UNICEF, UNFPA*, World Health Organization: Geneva.

PART THREE: CHILDBEARING EXPERIENCES AND IMMIGRANT WOMEN

In: Reproduction, Childbearing and Motherhood
Editor: Pranee Liamputtong, pp. 161-173

ISBN: 978-1-60021-606-0
© 2007 Nova Science Publishers, Inc.

Chapter 10

HARD LABOUR: MINORITY WOMEN, NURSES AND THE CHILDBIRTH EXPERIENCE

Denise L. Spitzer

INTRODUCTION

Approximately 200,000 immigrants and refugees enter Canada each year (Citizenship and Immigration Canada (CIC), 2005). Since the late 1960s, overtly exclusionary policies that reinforced the imaginary of a white Canada, conveniently erasing the presence of the indigenous population, have given way to immigration strategies designed to facilitate both family reunification and the demands of the labour market particularly in light of this country's declining and aging populace (Jakubowski, 1997; Anderson and Reimer Kirkham, 1998; Green and Green, 2004). Complemented by Canada's humanitarian commitments to admit refugees fleeing an increasing array of global disasters, newcomers have significantly altered the demographic profile of Canada. Currently, nearly one in five Canadians is foreign-born, making Canada second only to Australia in its ratio of foreign to native-born residents (Gold and Demeules, 2004; CIC, 2005). Migrants from the Asia Pacific comprise nearly 50 percent of newcomers to Canada followed by immigrants and refugees from Africa, the Middle East and Europe (CIC, 2005).

Cultural diversity, therefore, has become a prominent feature of Canadian identity—one that is reinforced by the official state discourse of multiculturalism. Public policies and public institutions, however, are generally oriented towards the needs of middle-class, white and often male clientele despite the adoption of gender and diversity analysis as a centerpiece of policy development in, at minimum, the federal level of governance (Anderson and Reimer Kirkham, 1998; Status of Women Canada (SWC), 2002; Spitzer, 2005).

Of interest to this paper is the health care system. The Canadian health care system is predicated on the five principles of universality, portability, accessibility, comprehensiveness and public administration (Wilson, 1995). While geographical location and the unequal distribution of human and technical resources—among other factors—can influence access to health services, the ability to pay is not regarded as a barrier to medical care. The capacity, however, to follow through with self-care regimens, therapeutic services such as physiotherapy and medications, is compromised among low-income Canadians—including many immigrants and refugees—who have limited access to workplace-based supplementary insurance coverage (Anderson et al., 1995; Steele et al., 2002; Lewchuk et al., 2003). Importantly, poverty in Canada often intersects with minority status in particular for migrants and Aboriginal Canadians[1] (Ross et al., 2000). Regardless of educational status, new Canadians, especially those from non-European countries, are more likely to be located among the ranks of the poor and are less likely to be upwardly mobile in subsequent generations than migrants of European origin (Kazemipur and Halli, 2001). Furthermore, migrant women are disproportionately represented among the lowest echelons of the workforce (Chard et al., 2000), as are Aboriginal women who also experience high rates of unemployment (Tait, 2000).

Given these dynamic demographic and social realities, hospital personnel working in three obstetrics departments in a large Canadian city[2] were interested in learning about their clients' perspectives of the services offered and requested that departing mothers complete a questionnaire. The returned surveys overflowed with narrative comments particularly from minority women prompting the hospital administration to commission this study in collaboration with a community based multicultural health organization to capture the experiences of this sector of their patient population.

METHODOLOGY

This research project was both exploratory and descriptive, and methods included ethnographic interviews and focus groups. The results of the discharge surveys and on-going experience prompted hospital staff and the community organization to target three communities for more in-depth investigation. Women who identified as South Asian (n=6), Vietnamese (n=5) or Aboriginal (n=5) who gave birth in one of the three hospitals were recruited to participate in the study. In addition, three low-income Euro-Canadian women partnered with Aboriginal men were included in a focus group. As nurses offer birthing mothers in hospital the most intimate contact, eleven obstetrical nurses were also interviewed. Four nurses were foreign born: two were from the Caribean, one was from the Netherlands, and another from the Philippines.

The research questions emerged from discussions with the key stakeholders and were based on their extensive experience with minority women. Co-researchers from the multicultural health organization aided in the recruitment of participants who were often known to them through their work in local health units, collective kitchens or other community activities. Their bi-cultural expertise helped ensure that the questions were culturally and linguistically appropriate (Neufeld, et al., 2001). Participants were offered an opportunity to partake in either group or individual discussions and were interviewed at the location of their choice.

---

[1] I employ the term "Aboriginal" to refer to First Nations, Inuit and Métis peoples.
[2] Due to confidentiality agreements signed with the institutions, the location of the research cannot be revealed. All names are pseudonyms.

Informed consent was obtained from participants after the project and the nature of consent was explained. Interviews and focus groups with the South Asian Canadian and Aboriginal women were recorded and transcribed—with a single exception. Transcriptions of focus group discussions and interviews were subject to theme analysis. The analysis was initiated by this author, but was commented upon and verified by the co-researchers.

SOCIAL AND CULTURAL CONTEXT

Both social and cultural contexts informed the development and interpretation of relationships between minority women, nurses and the institutional environment in which they operated. This research took place at the apex of health care reform in Canada. Propelled by globalization and the neo-liberal agenda, the resulting reduction of state intervention for public programs and increased fiscal restraint contributed to massive layoffs of predominantly female staff, closure of beds at health care institutions and the demolition of some facilities altogether (Armstrong, et al., 2002; Gustafson, 2000). Concomitantly, institutional care was increasingly off-loaded onto community-based services and the private household (Armstrong et al., 2002). Over a quarter of a million nurses in Canada experienced job loss or destabilization (Armstrong-Stassen et al., 1996). While the surviving staff were faced with increased work loads, they were also compelled to work with and reinforce new patient care guidelines including the use of an international classification system to account for their time and new policies such as the one that ensured new mothers were discharged from hospital between 24 to 36 hours after giving birth via vaginal delivery (Timmermans et al., 1998). The care of new mothers and their infants was shifted to home care nurses and to the family (Spitzer, 2000; Spitzer, 2004).

Health care institutions and nursing care are imbued with biomedical principles that presume a stable, universal body that can be treated in a uniform manner. Nursing education generally emphasizes the need to treat patients equally rather than equitably (Jackson, 1993; Spitzer, 2004). Under the conditions of health care reform, a new economy of care has been forged wherein "expensive" interactions—in terms of time—are avoided in favour of less costly ones. Notably, encounters with minority patients are often regarded as potentially time consuming and avoidance patterns can be read as racism by these new mothers (Spitzer, 2004). Furthermore, assumptions are made about the ability and willingness of patients to engage in self-care and what constitutes "common sense" about the body, childbirth and post-natal care that help reinforce the hospital setting as white space (Page and Thomas, 1994).

The response of minority women to their interactions with the institution and their representatives, nursing staff, is shaped by the historical relationship between their ethno-cultural community and dominant Euro-Canadian society as well as their cultural orientation. Experiences of systemic and personal racism have been common to all three of the communities engaged in this study. Exclusionary immigration policies that limited migration from non-European countries, the systematic dismantling of Aboriginal families through the forcible removal of children who were placed in residential schools, and inaction on indigenous land claims have the potential to trouble the image of state institutions in the eyes of many members of minority communities in Canada (Frideres, 1998; Jakubowski, 1997; Waldram et al., 1995)

Cultural distance further complicates these experiences. Despite their diverse heritage, Aboriginal women generally share a more holistic perspective of health than is offered in biomedicine (Waldram et al., 1995). Aboriginal women also begin childbearing at a younger age than the Canadian average. For instance, in this study the average age of Aboriginal informants was 20 years of age and at 24, the eldest participant was pregnant with her fourth child. Young Aboriginal women may also avail themselves of the support from extended family across rural reserves and urban locations. In South Asian traditions, pregnancy and childbirth are considered normal processes in the lives of women; however, depending on cultural community and other social factors, it may not be discussed openly nor should certain information be imparted to first-time mothers before it is deemed time-appropriate by female relatives and birth helpers (Woolett and Dosanjih-Matwala, 1990; Bhaskaran, 1993; Woollett et al., 1995). New mothers are supported through an optimally forty-day rest period where they are kept warm and fed nutritional foods (Spitzer, 2000). Vietnamese women also anticipate a rest period of thirty days following delivery (Spitzer, 2000). Pregnancy is also regarded as a normal process; however, pregnant women are encouraged to moderate their behaviours to maintain balance (Dinh et al., 1990; Mattson, 1995). Furthermore, childbirth is regarded as a female domain thus the presence of a male physician can create some discomfort (Mattson, 1995). Not surprisingly, many of these issues arise as points of misunderstanding or conflict particularly when cultural context intersect with class issues as will become evident in the discussion of research results.

THEORETICAL ORIENTATION

This work is informed by critical and feminist turns in research that highlight the intersections of gender and class within a political-economic framework. Both gender and culture/ethnicity are viewed as intersecting and performative identities that are discursively constructed and subject to both internal and external disciplinary regimes yet are also open to alteration through the effects of individual and collective agency (c.f. Butler, 1997; Bartsky, 1999). These identities, along with the hegemonic discourses of biomedicine, are informed by political-economic systems that demands attention to micro- to macro-social level relations of power, profit and oppression (Singer and Baer, 1995). Furthermore, as a feminist research project, the study highlights the lived experiences of women and contains participatory elements including engaging community workers as co-researchers and ensuring that research questions emerged from women's experiences (Reinharz, 1992).

RESULTS AND DISCUSSION

Prenatal Care

When birthing women arrived at hospital, their initial encounter with hospital staff generally involved an intake interview where they are queried about a variety of topics relating to their preparation for childbirth including attendance at prenatal classes. South Asian Canadian women, however, often refrained from participating in prenatal courses due to language barriers, embarrassment and the sense that certain types of knowledge about the body and childbirth process should not be revealed until the timing is appropriate (Bhaskaran, 1993). Neither were prenatal classes regarded as suitable for young Aboriginal women as well. Previous studies have identified lack of privacy, transportation problems and shyness with strangers as barriers to participation (Liu et al., 1994). Elder Aboriginal women generally counseled informants in this study to pay attention to their behaviour during pregnancy and childbirth as the fetus would absorb emotions and reflect maternal thoughts and actions. These young women, therefore, were often cognizant of the need to maintain a peaceful demeanour throughout their pregnancies and the birthing process. Moreover, they expressed discomfort with visual aids that depicted fetal development as the inner workings of the body were meant to remain concealed, and with the presumption that they were in a coupled relationship. Emily, an Aboriginal health educator explained:

> This video ... its strictly about different couples and how this man goes through all of this with the woman and three different types of labour, but still nothing that has anything to do with us as Native women. And this poor girl is watching and all you can see if the women in labour and they are whimpering and screaming and carrying on . . ."

As formal prenatal education is privileged in the context of biomedical management of pregnancy, when new patients acknowledged that they did not partake, hospital staff often presumed that little or no prenatal care was undertaken. This apparent lack of attention reinforced stereotypes about certain minority women as disinterested and uncaring mothers. Failure to participate in prenatal courses, however, did not equate to a lack of prenatal care. All of the informants in the study visited a physician on a regular basis and availed themselves of written materials and advice from female relations. Sometimes the volume of information was overwhelming and contradictory. Vien, a 34-year old mother of one who observed numerous births in Vietnam at the side of her midwife mother in Vietnam, remained unsure of what to make of this abundance of information. She said: "I read a lot of books and pamphlets. I think that they need to find a way to compromise Western and Eastern ways of doing things."

Incoming patients are also quizzed about their preparation for taking the infant home; however, in some cultures, such preparations would mean that a woman is over-confident in the outcome of her pregnancy, potentially tempting fate.

The Aboriginal health educator, Emily, offered this perspective:

> Well, there again, you know, it's a whole cultural thing of why is this woman coming in so unprepared, you know you're supposed to come in with your Samsonite luggage you know and be ready to take home baby and ours says, no, we don't do that. We wait. And then the clothing comes, after you know the baby's healthy.

Interactions with Nurses

Once admitted to hospital, labouring women's primary interactions were with nursing staff. Nurses provided comfort, support and advice and also served as the enforcers of policy and as liaisons between physicians and patients. Nursing staff also coped with the consequences of health care reform and the monumental shifts that occurred in the health care system. Reduced staffing occurred not long after infants and new mothers became cared for as a single dyadic unit effectively doubling the normal patient load of obstetrical nurses. Furthermore, as layoffs continued, senior staff was moved into hospital departments where needed sometimes displacing individuals with greater experience in that area who did not possess more years of service overall. Concurrently, changes were made to the distribution and food preparation systems within the institutions resulting in shortages of materials on the units and problems with food orders. Chelsea has witnessed a considerable shift in nursing since she graduated from nursing school in 1967:

> I guess basically you can't do the amount of teaching you'd like to do and that's frustrating because you're trying to determine the type of information the patient will need in a short period of time. And you have a short period of time and you're trying to decide what to decipher out of the whole issue. What else is frustrating? I guess many times too the supplies not being there. It's really frustrating to find things aren't there and have to wait such a long period of time.

Roxanne, a 16 year nursing veteran, went on to suggest that food issues can be particularly problematic for minority women who have just spent hours in intensive labour:

> If we have a Hindi woman in—she's vegetarian and she can't have meat or whatever. You know few consult the dietitian to see what kind of stuff she can have so that the kitchen can get it for her if she's in long enough, but if she's not, she gets peanut butter and jam, peanut butter and banana sandwiches instead of a healthy diet for a woman who is healing and nursing a baby!

Ranjit concurred. After her labour, she was given a cheese sandwich, when what she wanted was a "mountain of dhal and roti!"

The shift from institutional to home care and an average of 24 to 36 hour hospital stays meant that nurses were coping with rapid turnover and an even higher patient load. As nurses economized in their interactions with minority patients whom they presumed would require more of their time, informants were increasingly aware of the differential treatment they appeared to receive. Fifteen-year old Mariah who was having her first child shared this observation:

> For instance, like there was a white lady in there and she got everything. Everything she'd ask for they'd get her and, you know, she was just treated so well ... with me, or say any other Native lady was to, you know, ask for something, it would be like 'yeah, in a minute' What's so different between her and I? Nothing you know and sometimes that kind of upset me, too.

Language

Both new mothers and nurses cited linguistic barriers as major challenges. While hospital staff was encouraged to contact a regional interpreter service, the brevity of hospital stays for obstetrics cases often proved it improbable that contacts would be made. As a result, bilingual staff or family members were often pressed into service where possible although this was seldom regarded as an optimal solution. Even women who spoke English well encountered difficulty in expressing themselves when exhausted and in pain. Vien recounted an emotionally charged episode when her English vocabulary failed her:

> I pushed the button and she asked me what I wanted, I couldn't respond, so I just pressed it again and again until the nurse came. I tried to explain the catheter was really uncomfortable and I wanted it out, but we couldn't understand each other, so she took my baby away thinking it must be crying and bothering me! I just couldn't respond and I had to suffer the whole night.

Language barriers were also problematic for patients' families. A South Asian mother of two, Michelle began to hemorrhage after her delivery: "My own husband was there, but sometimes he misunderstands, too . . .They [her family] were sort of very upset. They were saying, I think, that for more than an hour and a half they didn't know what was going on, they were just panicking outside." Her sister Celeste went on:

> The health professionals as well, they were so much engrossed, they were running around trying to save her life rather than explaining. So if there were someone with communication skills calming them down, telling them "OK she's in the operating room, they're working on her and we'll have to wait. You go sit with the rest of the family and we'll come to talk to you." If there were time, to talk to anybody outside to say what is the procedure going on inside. Even during the childbirth, because when you are so much in pain, even you are fluent in English, you can't really say because it comes in your own mother tongue, in your own language.

Hospital Policies

Policies and procedures had been altered to reflect both the cultural diversity of hospital clientele and budgetary restraints. For instance, new mothers were allowed to retain their placenta for ritual purposes if so requested, to include as many visitors in the labour and delivery rooms as they wished, and to birth in alternate positions as they desired. Some women complained, however, that these policies were not regularly enacted. Nurses routinely asked visitors to leave, personal ceremonial music was confiscated, and placentas were discarded without approval. Pascale, an Aboriginal mother of three, had wanted to give birth in a squatting position, but had been unable to persuade staff to allow her to do so in previous hospital births. She said:

> with my third baby, that's when I told them right away. I kept going I want to squat this time. I want to squat. I made sure the nurses knew. I kept saying it repeatedly ... .

Aboriginal mothers in particular felt treated with disdain if they contravened policies, many of which had been implemented since previous hospital births. For instance, on prior occasions new mothers were supplied with items ranging from sanitary napkins to layettes for newborns; however, new regulations required women to provide their own materials and only a limited number were kept on hand for emergencies. When women availed themselves of these supplies as they had been instructed to do previously, they were accused of being thieves. Additionally, women were compelled to leave their rooms to make use of a limited number of telephones on the floor. Aboriginal women felt singled out for reprimand for "abandoning" their children even though their infants were left in the care of roommates.

Other nursing staff shared Chelsea's assertion that "East Indian women like to be treated like princesses." The discharge policy exacerbated these sentiments as nurses were charged with ensuring that the new mothers were mobile and self-sufficient within 24 hours following childbirth, yet South Asian, Vietnamese and other minority women who practice post-partum rest periods were counseled by family and tradition to remain in bed. Maya, a South Asian woman from Fiji, tried her best to comply with both her family and the hospital staff following her cesarean section birth:

> She told the other one [another nurse], she's supposed to go walk and she's not doing anything, she's just lying there. And you know I was having a big, great pain there and I can't stand up ... . But I always go to the washroom, right? I didn't bother any nurse to come and help me. But the way she said, it, it really hurt because I always have pain and I do it myself. I know they are busy, too.

Breastfeeding and Postnatal Care

During the brief period between delivery and discharge, nurses attempted to deliver "the Teaching." The Teaching consisted of a set of instructions for infant care centred on breastfeeding. Conveying the Teaching to new mothers exhausted from labour was already regarded as challenging; however, linguistic barriers and perceived cultural resistance often intensified nurses' frustrations with minority mothers. South Asian women in particular were chastised for seemingly foolish beliefs about the impurity of colostrum that resulted in delayed onset of breastfeeding. Rose, a Jamaican-born nurse, commented about the attitudes of some of her colleagues:

> We have some nurses who don't understand they're not going to put that baby to the breast until the milk comes in and then they get upset. Why get upset? Have you ever seen an East Indian baby out there looking starved? No, you never do! They have within their culture, they have this thing the grandmothers there or the other women in that family group that have had babies before take care of their own... . I usually say, how many of your East Indian, or whatever babies, that you have seen or heard of have been malnourished or ended up with impetigo? You usually see them as rosy little monkeys running around. Their children mean a lot to them, if you just help them... .I say, leave them. Leave them alone. You don't see those mothers coming back here with dirty bums; they don't come back here with infected bums. How many have you seen come back here?

Showering proved to be another site of struggle between nurses and minority women from some cultural communities. Lien, a Vietnamese Canadian mother of one, said:

> After delivery, a nurse wanted me to bathe and wash my hair. I couldn't communicate with her so I just followed her and took the towel, but I couldn't bathe. So I took a sponge bath. When the nurse saw that my hair wasn't wet, she started yelling at me and was quite upset.

Stereotyping and Racism

At times nurses' responses to this perceived resistance to comply with their directions was embedded in expressions of stereotyping if not overt racism. Sandra, a nurse for 20 years, remarked when we discussed showers: "And some women I don't know if they use deodorant all the time or not, because with the diet intake all the time of curry, their body order can be of curry and it can be quite strong." Carolyn, a licensed practical nurse from the Philippines said:

> You know a shower once a day is sufficient, you know like especially when you are having flow and this kind of thing. I find it also Native people sometimes that you know, they are not very compliant people. You know like when you tell them, like C-section, like OK, I'll take your dressing off today and may after lunch, I'll take you for a shower. They always have an excuse. They always say, "Oh, no later on." They like (sic) "My mum would bring and shampoo and you know like, I don't really feel like." But yet they will go down and smoke or whatever.

While Aboriginal women reported the most frequent racist encounters with nursing staff, observations that were reinforced by nurse informants who either shared their opinions that Aboriginal patients were most likely to be "drug-involved" or inattentive to their children especially as they seemed unconcerned about "sharing" them with an array of relations both in urban areas and rural reserves. Vietnamese and South Asian women also acknowledged receiving differential treatment. In particular, requests for analgesics or reports of pain were disregarded or not taken seriously making women feel at times as though they were invisible (Spitzer, 2004).

Supportive Interactions

Not all interactions between minority women and nurses were negative. All of the new mothers make mention of a particular nurse who offered encouragement, a gentle touch or who brought water without being asked. Indeed these apparently small actions were regarded as highly supportive and significant especially as respondents were acutely aware of the nurses' increased responsibilities and time constraints. Mina, a Vietnamese Canadian who offered support to other new mothers following her hospital experience, said:

> After delivery, a woman is in pain and exhausted. She needs someone to encourage her, someone with a soft voice to ease the pain. I remember I had a difficult labour, but a friendly nurse helped detract from the pain, encouraging me and making me feel like I'd done a good job.

Melissa, a Vietnamese Canadian mother of two who had a very difficult labour and post-partum period, still looked back fondly on one particular individual:

> There was one nurse from India, she was very nice, she helped me, it was like seeing my mom, she would say, Melissa, you push (stroking my arm), she really helped me.

Resistance and Resilience

While new mothers interviewed in this study, encountered often troubling circumstances, they also employed strategies to resist institutional control and to enhance their birthing experiences. Some women spoke about avoiding unwanted interventions by spending much of their time in the shower. Others literally fought back. One woman reported that she resorted to slapping a physician who refused to listen to her pleas to stop touching her in a painful area.

Most often though women located social resources to sustain themselves during their hospital stays. Often women affirmed their own strengths by both support seeking and support giving. Support networks included extended family, friends, members of volunteer agencies or their community, other new mothers, and health professionals with whom they had established a relationship. Experienced members of the support network helped reinforce decisions about appropriate behaviour, infant and maternal self-care, among other issues. Offering support to or advocating for others also helped women feel useful and empowered in face of the hospital bureaucracy. When Pascale saw another Aboriginal woman being ill treated, she approached her:

> I kind of made her feel comfortable and I'd sit and talk to her and have her show me how to use my moss bag properly... .

IMPLICATIONS FOR HEALTH AND SOCIAL CARE AND CONCLUSION

> Medical encounters are 'micro-level' processes that involve the interaction of individuals. These interpersonal processes, however, occur in social context, which is shaped by macro-level structures in society (Waitzkin, 1991: 11).

All women who enter a hospital to give birth are compelled to surrender to this often, totalizing institution as they are transformed by the patient role. In this environment, control over privacy, food intake, room temperature, visiting, and bodily integrity are relinquished to hospital staff who regulate the setting in an effort to maximize efficient and competent care. The ability however, to negotiate for greater control is dependent on access to power. Pappas (1990) states that: "Power is an aspect of relationships, as is manifest in the deployment of resources;" in context of biomedical institutions, these power relationships are most evident when viewed in terms of autonomy and dependency. In the context of hospital birth, women are dependent on the hospital for care, shelter, food and in some cases companionship. This unequal power relationship is also played out in terms of authoritative knowledge that has the ability to subvert and supplant embodied and traditional knowledge.

The institution of the hospital and the practice of biomedicine produce and treat a uniform, white subject (Jackson, 1993; Page and Thomas, 1994). With less access to social and cultural capital—reinforced by increased association with poverty—and greater cultural distance, minority women are more marginalized in this setting. Furthermore interactions between these new mothers and staff are conducted in compressed time and read through the lens of historical relations. All of the factors contribute to the hard labour that minority women in this study experienced.

To redress the imbalance, both sets of informants—nurses and minority mothers—suggested that cultural brokers, bicultural community health educators who could work as advocates and bridge institutional and program boundaries through relationship-based care, would be a welcome solution to this current crisis in care (c.f. Van Willigen, 1993). Mina offered:

> They [minority women] need company and emotional and physical support especially if they have small children at home. Small children want all the attention. I help baby-sit the children when mothers go to the hospital and often sleep over there. Pregnant women need support as they get close to the due date. Women can be frustrated because they can't trust someone to take care of their children while they're giving birth. Women need a program for prenatal and postpartum support.

By working with women and their families, cultural brokers not only gain trust, but they are able to provide the holistic care that is both desired and optimal. Cultural brokers could follow newly pregnant minority women, helping familiarize hospital and community health staff about the specific needs of individual women. Importantly these advocates can help redress the power imbalance between birthing women and hospital staff by aiding women in their efforts to retain or re-gain more control over their hospital birthing experiences with the view of transforming the sentence of hard labour to a joyful experience.

REFERENCES

Anderson, J., and Reimer Kirkham, S., 1998, 'Constructing Nation: The Gendering and Racializing of the Canadian Health Care System', in V. Strong-Boag, S. Grace, A. Eisenberg, and J. Anderson, (eds.), *Painting the Maple: Essays on Race, Gender, and the Construction of Canada*, pp. 242-261. University of British Columbia Press: Vancouver.

Anderson, Joan, Wiggins, S., Rajwani, R., Holbrook, A., Blue, C., and Ng, M. 1995, 'Living with a Chronic Illness: Chinese-Canadian and Euro-Canadian Women with Diabetes-Exploring Factors that Influence Management', *Social Science & Medicine*, 41(2): 181-195.

Armstrong, P., Amaratunga, C., Bernier, J., Grant, K., Pederson, A., and Wilson, K. (eds.), 2002, Exposing Privatization: Women and Health Care Reform in Canada, Garamond Press; Aurora, Ont.

Armstrong-Stassen, M., Cameron, S. and Horsburgh, M., 1996, 'The Impact of Organizational Downsizing on the Job Satisfaction of Nurses', *Canadian Journal of Nursing Administration*, 9(4): 8-32.

Bartsky, S., 1999, 'Foucault, Femininity and the Modernization of Power', in J. Kouranay, J. Sterba and R. Tong (eds.), *Feminist Philosophies,* pp. 119-141. Prentice Hall: Upper Saddle River, N.J.

Bhaskaran, H., 1993, *An Indo-Canadian Community Assessment Study,* Edmonton Board of Health: Edmonton.

Butler, J., 1997, 'Imitation and Gender', in L. Nicholson (ed.), *The Second Wave: A Reader in Feminist Theory*, pp. 306-316. Routledge: New York.

Chard, J., Badets, J., and Howatsen-Leo, L., 2000, 'Immigrant Women', in *Women in Canada 2000: A Gender-Based Statistical Report,* pp. 189-217. Statistics Canada: Ottawa.

Citizenship and Immigration Canada (CIC), 2005, "Facts and Figures 2004: Immigration Overview." <http://www.cic.gc.ca/english/pub/facts2004/overview/1.html> Accessed November 26, 2005.

Dinh, D. K., Ganeson, S., and Waxler-Morrison, N., 1990, 'The Vietnamese', in N. Waxler-Morrison, J. Anderson, and E. Richardson (eds.), *Cross-Cultural Caring: A Handbook for Health Professionals in Western Canada,* pp. 181-213, University of British Columbia Press: Vancouver.

Frideres, J., 1998, *Aboriginal Peoples in Canada: Contemporary Conflicts, 5th Edition,* Prentice Hall Allyn and Bacon: Scarborough, Ont.

Gold, J., and Desmeules, M., 2004, 'National Symposium on Immigrant Health in Canada', *Canadian Journal of Public Health,* 95(3): 13.

Green, A., and Green, D., 2004, 'The Goals of Canada's Immigration Policy: A Historical Perspective', *Canadian Journal of Urban Research,* 13(1): 102-139.

Gustafson, D., 2000, 'Introduction: Health Care Reform and Its Impact on Canadian Women,' in D. Gustafson (ed), *Care and Consequences: The Impact of Health Care Reform,* pp. 15-24. Fernwood Publishing: Halifax, N.S.

Jackson, E., 1993, 'Whiting Out Difference: Why U.S. Nursing Research Fails Black Families', *Medical Anthropology Quarterly,* 7(4): 363-385.

Jakubowski, L., 1997, *Immigration and the Legalization of Racism,* Fernwood Publishing: Halifax, N.S.

Kazemipur, A, and Halli, S., 2001, 'The Changing Colour of Poverty', *CRSA/RCSA,* 38(2): 217-238.

Lewchuk, W., de Wolff, A., King, A. and Polyani, M., 2003, 'From "Job Strain to Employment Strain: Health Effects of Precarious Employment', *Just Labour,* 3: 23-35.

Liu, L., Slap, G., Kinsmen, S., and Khalid, N., 1994, 'Pregnancy Among American Indian Adolescents: Reactions and Prenatal Care', *Journal of Adolescent Health,* 15: 336-341.

Mattson, S., 1995, 'Culturally Sensitive Perinatal Care for Southeast Asians', *JOGNN,* 24(4) May: 335-341.

Neufeld, A., Harrison, M., Hughes, K., Spitzer, D. L., and Stewart, M., 2001, 'Participation of Immigrant Women Caregivers in Qualitative Research', *Western Journal of Nursing Research* 23(6): 575-591.

Page, H., and Thomas, R. B., 1994, 'White Public Space and the Construction of White Privilege in U.S. Health Care: Fresh Concepts and a New Model of Analysis', *Medical Anthropology Quarterly,* 8(1): 109-116.

Pappas, G., 1990, 'Some Implications for the Study of Doctor-Patient Interaction: Power, Structure, and Agency in the Words of Howard Waitzkin and Arthur Kleinman', *Social Science & Medicine,* 30(2): 199-204.

Reinharz, S., 1992, *Feminist Methods in Social Research,* Oxford University Press: New York.

Ross, David P., Scott, K., and Smith, P.J., 2000, *The Canadian Fact Book on Poverty,* Canadian Council on Social Development: Ottawa.

Singer, M., and Baer, H. 1995, *Critical Medical Anthropology,* Baywood Publishing Company: Amityville, N.J.

Spitzer, D. L., 2000, 'They Don't Listen to Your Body: Minority Women, Nurses and Childbirth', in D. Gustafson (ed.), *Care and Consequences: Women and Health Reform*, pp. 86-106, Fernwood Publishing: Halifax, N.S.

Spitzer, D.L., 2004, 'In Visible Bodies: Minority Women, Nurses, Time and the New Economy of Care', *Medical Anthropology Quarterly*, 18(4): 490-508.

Spitzer, D. L., 2005, 'Engendering Health Disparities', *Canadian Journal of Public Health Health*, 96 (Supplement 2): S78-S96.

Status of Women Canada—Gender-Based Analysis Directorate (SWC), 2002, *Canadian Experience in Gender Mainstreaming,* Status of Women Canada: Ottawa.

Steele, L, Lemieux-Charles, L., Clark, J., and Glazier, R., 2002, 'The Impact of Policy Changes on the Health of Recent Immigrants and Refugees in the Inner City', *Canadian Journal of Public Health*, 93(2): 118-122.

Tait, H., 2000, 'Aboriginal Women', in *Women in Canada 2000: A Gender-Based Statistical Report,* pp. 247-268. Statistics Canada: Ottawa.

Timmermans, S., Bowker, G., and Star, L., 1998, 'The Architecture of Difference: Visibility, Control and Comparability in Building a Nursing Interventions Classification', in M. Berg and A. Mol (eds.), *Differences in Medicine: Unraveling Practices, Techniques and Bodies,* pp. 205-225. Duke University Press: Durham, N.C.

Van Willigen, J. 1993, *Applied Anthropology: An Introduction, Revised Edition,* Bergin and Garvey Publishers: Westport, CT.

Waitzkin, H., 1991, *The Politics of Medical Encounters: How Patients and Doctors Deal with Social Problems,* Yale University Press: New Haven.

Waldram, J., Herring, D. A., and Young, T. K., 1995, *Aboriginal Health in Canada: Historical, Cultural and Epidemiological Perspectives*, University of Toronto Press: Toronto.

Woollet, A., and Dosanjih-Matwala, N., 1990, 'Pregnancy and Antenatal Care: The Attitudes and Experiences of Asian Women', *Child Care, Health and Development*, 16: 63-78.

Woollett, A. Dosanjih, N., Nicolson, P., Marshall, H., Djhanbakhch, O., and Hadlow, J., 1995, 'The Ideas and Experiences of Pregnancy and Childbirth of Asian and Non-Asian Women in East London', *British Journal of Medical Psychology*, 68(1): 65-84.

Wilson, D. 1995, *The Canadian Health Care System,* author: Edmonton.

In: Reproduction, Childbearing and Motherhood
Editor: Pranee Liamputtong, pp. 175-194
ISBN: 978-1-60021-606-0
© 2007 Nova Science Publishers, Inc.

Chapter 11

THE EXPERIENCE OF CHILDBIRTH AND HOSPITAL STAY AMONGST ARABIC-SPEAKING IMMIGRANT WOMEN IN AUSTRALIA

Lina Nadia Abboud and Pranee Liamputtong

INTRODUCTION

Giving birth to a baby is part of the program that ensures the survival of our species. While this basic reproductive function has not changed, the cultural attitudes that surround reproduction have. Initially, people lived in small groups, hunting and gathering for food. Later, more complex societies developed in which people's life-styles and behaviour became quite different. Reproducing women have always been cared for and supported by other women. Very recently, men and the medical profession have become more involved and increasingly, partners and carers are depended on (Lipsett, 2004). The social structure surrounding birth has also changed dramatically. At the turn of the twentieth century, women were likely to think of labour and birth as part of a day's work. Women learned about labour and birth from their own mothers, sisters, and other women. Birth stories were an important medium for passing knowledge from one generation to the next. Most women laboured and gave birth at home, surrounded by their family, by other women who were knowledgeable about birth, and a midwife. The labouring woman was comforted, encouraged and supported throughout her labour and for days and weeks after the birth of her baby (Lothian, 2001).

The move from home to the hospital setting, and the change from midwifery care to the medical management of birth resulted in a dramatic shift in the activities and the thinking of birth. The experts, physicians, midwives and nurses became the storage of birth knowledge. The traditional ways of finding comfort and support were abandoned in favour of medication and new technological methods of intervention to the natural birthing process. Over time, the restrictions of the hospital environment and obstetric care practices limited women's ability to find comfort without the use of medication. As birth technology increased, and the interventions once reserved for complicated labours, such as intravenous lines, restrictions on eating and drinking, and confinement to bed, these became routine for many women (Lothian, 2001).

Birth has a very special significance for women, their partners, and families. The responsibility for birth is a shared one. This sharing role involves caregivers, individual women, and their families of which influence the experience of the pregnancy, childbirth and the hospital stay and its outcomes. The report of the Ministerial Review of Birthing Services in Victoria (Health Department Victoria, 1990) describes the models of care available to women giving birth in Victoria. The models consist of: standard public hospital care, specialist obstetrician care, general practitioner, obstetrician care, hospital birth-centre care, shared care, team midwifery care, home birth and free standing birth-centre care. Access to all these full range of models of care can be restricted by factors such as, geographic location of services, lack of knowledge about their availability, medical risk criteria, the social and cultural appropriateness of the services, and costs associated with care outside the public system. In most societies, it is recognised that following a pregnancy, labour, and the postnatal hospital stay, women need both emotional support and practical help. In Australia, the postnatal hospital stay is promoted as an opportunity for women to rest and recuperate. During her stay, it is intended that she would receive guidance, support and information on caring for her newborn (Yelland et al., 1998).

While in many respects the physiology of childbirth can be considered universally the same for all women, the meaning of childbirth is strikingly different. This event is influenced by cultural beliefs, traditional practices, spiritual beliefs, maternal age and education, socio-economic status, parity, personality characteristics, and influence from health care professionals such as birthing environment, feelings of control, support and knowledge sharing. The meaning of childbirth is unique within each culture and unique to each woman in a specific culture (Nichols, 1996). Cultural beliefs about and values associated with childbirth touch all aspects of social life in any given culture. Such beliefs and values lend perspective to the meaning of childbirth to the woman (Callister, 1995).

Some aspects of pregnancy are well researched. The experiences of pregnancy, labour, and the postnatal hospital stay of women from non-English speaking backgrounds, and particularly women from Arabic-speaking backgrounds, have not been targeted for research studies. There are few Australian studies that have specifically embarked on exploring what this community of women think about their maternity experiences including satisfaction with the caregivers, services, family, and friends. Research in this area focuses on the need to provide "woman-centred maternity services which take account of women's views and specifically address their need for choice, control and continuity" (Tinkler and Quinney, 1998: 30).

Exisitng literature suggests that pregnancy, birth and motherhood have different meanings and significance to women and the community from the "Arab world", and share the values and beliefs of the Arab culture. The focus of this chapter is on the women from societies where Arabic is the official language. The Arab world is made up of twenty-two countries who are members of the Arab League of Nations. This includes the countries of: Algeria, Bahrain, Comoros, Djibouti, Egypt, Iraq, Jordan, Kuwait, Lebanon, Libya, Mauritania, Morocco, Oman, Palestine, Qatar, Saudi Arabia, Somalia, Sudan, Syria, Tunisia, United Arab Emirates and Yemen. In defining the Arabic-speaking community, it is a cultural group sharing a common language, heritage, values and beliefs of an Arab culture (Kridli, 2002). The main countries of origin of Arabic-speaking immigrants to Australia include

Lebanon, Egypt, Syria, Iraq, Jordan, and Palestine. Both Christianity and Islam are important faiths for Arabic speakers in Australia.

We conducted a study to gain an insight into the experiences of pregnancy, birth and the postnatal period of women from an Arabic-speaking background who have given birth in Melbourne, Australia. We examined women's accounts of the pregnancy period, the labour, the hospital stay, and the time immediately after the birth. This study is an important research project because there are only a few studies conducted in Australia that explore some aspect of the birthing experiences of women from an Arabic-speaking background. There are also a small number of studies worldwide that target Arabic-speaking women and examine their experiences of birth either in their home country or after migrating to another country. Our study enables the investigation and exploration of the experiences and perceptions of the women as well as the variations of the women's experiences which can be attributed to age, religious beliefs, socio-economic and educational factors, language and patterns of migration within a similar group of women.

CHANGES IN CHILDBIRTH: THE AUSTRALIAN CONTEXT

There are many ways in which the present day Australia is different to how it was twenty or forty years ago. One of the biggest differences is the decreasing birth rate. The reasons for this are that women are marrying later, having children later and then having fewer children. While as for men, their role and involvement in childbirth has changed, it is largely due to women having a range of possible futures. They can be married or single, mother or not, have a career or just a job, study or not (Lothian, 2001; Stanley et al., 2005).

Before this century, newborns found themselves in the hands of women: mothers, grandmothers, aunts, and midwives. But now, newborns collide with doctors, typically male (Chamberlain, 1999). Giving birth to a baby has changed, particularly moving from the home to the hospital. There have been cultural, medical, and lifestyle changes. All of these factors influence the birthing experience (Lipsett, 2004). In a remarkably brief period, men have gone from being excluded from birth, to being admitted, then invited, and finally, expected in the delivery room (Reed, 2005). Birth has gone from having choices of natural or pain relief, giving birth standing, sitting or lying down, alone or with supporting persons, midwife or obstetrician (Devlin, 1995).

Throughout most of the nineteenth and twentieth centuries, fathers were excluded from birth. Men were recognised as making a small, though significant contribution to conception, but not throughout pregnancy, labour, and the delivery. The lore, rituals, and especially the biology of birth were a woman's domain. As Reed (2005: 10) puts, "women's discussion fell to hushed tones when a man entered the room; physicians asked fathers to leave during prenatal checkups, and hospitals barred fathers from watching the delivery of their own children".

Since the 1920s, the efforts of many individuals have led to the development of the methods now used to enhance relaxation, reduce stress, relieve labour pain, promote progress and strengthen early parent-infant bonds. History has provided changes to enhance each woman's birthing experience. One change came about from the work by *Dick-Read*, a British doctor who studied and promoted natural childbirth from the 1920s until the 1950s. His teachings stated that when a woman is afraid of labour, she becomes tense, and this thereby increases her pain. The more pain she feels, the more frightened she becomes. And the cycle is perpetuated and intensified. To interrupt this cycle, he advocated for education, relaxation and controlled breathing. Also, in the 1950s, *Dr Fernand Lamaze*, a French doctor, developed his psychoprophylactic method, which he adapted from methods used by Soviet doctors. This involved the use of distraction techniques during a woman's contractions to decrease the perception of pain or discomfort.

In the 1950s and 1960s, *Robert Bradley*, an American physician, promoted and refined Dick-Read's methods. His major contribution was to encourage husbands to participate as labour coaches (Morris, 2001). In the past, the men were restricted from the birth of their first child - for the good of the mother and baby, only to be expected at the birth of the later ones - for the good of the mother and baby (Reed, 2005). In the late 1970s, the public's interest in home birth, midwifery and patients' rights began to grow. The 1980s ushered in home-like birthing environments, including out-of-hospital birth centres and more attractive birthing rooms in hospitals. Also, the midwifery profession began to grow rapidly in response to women's demands. In the 1990s, some common obstetrical practices – such as routine episiotomy, routine intravenous fluids and routine repeat caesareans – decreased, while new methods of inducing labour, safer drugs and safer means to pain relief became widespread (Morris, 2001).

There have been many changes in Childbirth, particularly with the introduction of technology. With this, women often seem not to believe that they have within themselves the ability to give birth, breastfeed or mother their newborns without help from professionals. Despite the natural childbirth movement, the re-emergence of midwifery care, and the availability of home and birthing centre options for birth, the fear of "something going wrong" propels women into depending more and more on modern technology (Lothian, 2001).

METHODS

In this research, we used a qualitative approach to obtain information from the participants. Qualitative research allows the participants to speak of their subjective experiences. Hence, the information obtained is not biased by the researcher. As the childbearing and birthing event has emotional, cultural, spiritual and physical aspects, it cannot be described adequately and with understanding using a quantitative study.

The main focus of the interview was the woman's personal experience including the period of the pregnancy, the labour and the hospital stay. Also, the interview focussed on the experience and satisfaction with the health professionals and the services during the three periods being researched. Their choice of the model of care and the source of their information was also explored. One other main theme the researcher asked about was the type of advice women would give other women looking back at their overall experience. If during the conversations there were other themes that arose or more detail to a response would be beneficial, the researcher used probing questions. A probe is a follow-up question to elicit more information to fill in the blanks in a participant's first response to a question (Liamputtong and Ezzy, 2005).

In qualitative research the sample size is rather small. Sampling is based on setting a specific period of time and selecting mothers who during that time had a live birth. These women were recruited via word-of-mouth and the 'snow-ball technique'. Snowball sampling is when a researcher identifies one respondent and asks whether the respondent knows any other people who might meet the sampling requirements. The sample in this research is homogenous with respect to certain variables only – the birthing experience and having a similar ethnic background (Holloway and Wheeler, 2002).

The participants need to be selected to suit the investigated research topic. They are chosen because the researcher believes that they will provide the best information (Liamputtong and Ezzy, 2005). The researcher has to identify a sample of people who will be able to participate because they have personal experience of the phenomenon under study. This research focussed on 25 women from an Arabic-speaking background and living in Melbourne. Arabic-speaking background for this study means being of a nationality that is inclusive of 22 countries part of the Arab League of Nations. These are the member states: Africa (from west to east): Mauritania, Morocco, Algeria, Tunisia, Libya, Egypt, Sudan, Djibouti, Somalia and Comoros and Asia (from west to east): Lebanon, Syria, Palestine, Jordan, Iraq, Saudi Arabia, Kuwait, Bahrain, Qatar, United Arab Emirates, Oman and Yemen. The diversity of women from all these Arab countries may impact on the data as there are differences in the religious beliefs, cultural and social practices, health care systems and other factors which influence the lifestyle and decision making for the women. However, there are also similarities in their expectations of their birthing experiences and the support from family and knowledge and level of professionalism expected from health care providers.

These women experienced a pregnancy and a live birth within the three years. They would also have experienced some form of maternal service before, during, and after the pregnancy. There is no age restriction on the women willing to participate, which enabled the experiences of all childbearing women to be heard.

Each interview was held in an environment and place where the participant felt most comfortable and was able to respond freely. The location and time were decided by the participants, and most interviews took place at the participants' home. Each interview lasted between an hour and two hours and was tape-recorded for transcription and analysis. The interviews were analysed using a thematic analysis approach.

THE BIRTH EXPERIENCE

Just as each experience of pregnancy is individualistic and unique, every labour and delivery experience has those characteristics. There are many factors that influence and impact on these experiences as the women we interviewed demonstrated. Major factors are: the method of delivery, model of care utilised, relationship with carers, support systems, and expectations of the labour.

Expectation of Labour and Pain

All women were asked: 'What was your expectation of labour?' Multiparous women's responses showed that their expectations of the present birth were generally influenced by previous births. They made comparisons of how they were feeling and what they were experiencing in order to predict what the labour would be like. Most women described their expectation of labour pain for a natural birth from their own experiences although recognizing that each pregnancy and labour was different making it difficult to determine what was going to happen.

> ... My sister told me it was going to be hard and I should try to moan and try to remember the word of Allah. It's not called labour for the sake of it and it's true and it's hard work. It's the hardest thing a woman has to go through. You go through all the pain and agony but it's rewarding. At least you get something out of it that's worth it. You have this beautiful human being. (Jumanah)

Widad had been through her previous pregnancy and birth, however, the two were quite different experiences. With her first birth, she was offered pain relief. But, with the second pregnancy, the birth was natural, and she mentioned feeling the full birth and the pain associated with it.

> Severe, severe menstrual cramps. And that was pretty much what it was like... I guess you really don't know what to expect. I guess I didn't anticipate they'd be as sharp as they were sometimes and also that towards the end there would be less gaps between the contractions...um...so, I don't know if you really can ever sort of envisage what that will be like, and it's funny you have to go through it to know what it's like. (Widad)

Primiparae women, who experienced birth for the first time, spoke about their expectations and perceptions about what they thought childbirth would be like. The expectations and perceptions of labour and the pain of birthing was developed by reading books, watching documentaries, hearing stories from other women, and preparing oneself mentally for what was to happen. The pain of labour was the main aspect stated by women of not being able to fully understand and comprehend what it was like until having experienced it.

> Obviously I knew it was going to be painful particularly knowing that I didn't want to take any medication. I did a lot of reading and research on pregnancy and childbirth, as much as the reading I did, it was still not clear what it's like and especially the labour and what you go through. (Layla)

There were only few women who chose or agreed to have a caesarean section. Nadia, for example, chose caesarean birth as she would be able to be aware of the birth process and not having to go through labour pain. However, Manal described her unhappiness with caesarean birth, as she intended to have a natural birth. She remarked that the recovery after the operation was difficult, and she would not consider caesarean birth unless it was absolutely essential. Additionally, although most women intended to give birth without any pain relief, in reality, most would need certain pain relief to help them cope with the pain of childbirth.

Seeing and Holding the Baby after Birth

Most women expressed their intense emotions and feelings when they first sighted and held their newborn. Women reacted by crying, smelling their baby, and described the experience as being "the most beautiful thing in the whole world" and forgetting the pain once they were able to see their newborn baby and being able to hold them.

> The most exciting thing is when you see your baby and hold it then you forget everything. Then you don't remember the pain you just hold it. Straight after they gave me the baby and my husband cut the umbilical cord. It's an emotional moment... relieved that it's over and done with and then when you hold the baby and it's like 'Is that really mine?' (Maram)

Several women remembered and reminisced about first focussing on either the sex of their baby or the physical appearance of them though still expressing their happiness at holding their baby.

> When they took her out I could only see her head. I'm asking the anaesthesiologist 'is it a boy or a girl?' and he said 'you'll find out' and then I hear 'it's a girl' and then (husband) says she has blue eyes and I'm like 'what!?' (laughs) and then they brought her over to me and she was so hairy it was the first thing I noticed and I was like 'I've got a hairy baby'... And then they put her on me and I was so happy I just started crying and I remember (husband) was crying as well, it was so exciting at that time. (Fatinah)

While the majority of the women expressed their relief, happiness and joy at the experience of holding their newborn, Yusra talked about her dissatisfaction with the health care professionals and the impact they had on her experience.

> I couldn't even hold him when he came out. They slapped him onto me and then they slapped him off in like half a second and I didn't even get to see him I was in shock and they didn't even tell me if it was a boy or girl. I had to ask whether it was a boy or girl. It was the most horrendous experience. Had it been a natural one I would have held my baby and bonded with my baby and known if it was a boy or girl, they didn't even tell me. I can't believe they're a labour ward and they didn't have the audacity to tell me. (Yusra)

Role of Husband and Others during the Labour Period

Most women spoke about their husband taking an active role in childbirth by providing support and comfort, by holding their hands, getting a drink of water and putting a wet cloth on their faces. These actions were considered supportive and helpful to get through the stages and pain of labour. The husband was also described as being "very good" and "very strong" during this period and women acknowledged that having his strength helped. Nadia told us that:

> He was calming me and he was very calm as well and he was just supporting me and because I wasn't in pain we were both really excited when we saw the baby and first of all when they give him the baby he put it on my chest and he was holding me.

Other women focussed on the support they received from their husband and also from others in the delivery room including a midwife or friends. This included having a back rubbed, feeling secured and comfort because there was someone during the labour, having the support and positive thinking encouraged by people in the room, and being cared for by family members.

> They (husband, dad and mum) were all helpful, but my dad helped me the most because I would ask him to sing prayers to me so I could focus on them, and that helped me a great deal. It helped me to lose focus on the pain... He (husband) help me by thinking positive, by being beside me, supporting me, and also by holding my hand, and just by being in the room, I felt safe and secure by him being there, I knew nothing would go wrong. (Rana)

Although Abir and Rima had different methods of delivery (assisted natural and caesarean, respectively) both described the events that happened. Their accounts focussed more on the physical stages through labour, not so much on emotions, feelings and thoughts as much as other women, however.

> (Husband) was with me the whole time, although he was sleeping on the coach half the time. When they gave me the pethidine shot that's when they said there's probably at least whatever amount of hours later, but I would say anywhere from midday till three o'clock she was going to have the baby. So (husband) said he'd go down to call parents and get a coffee thinking we had hours to go. As soon as he left the room that's when my water's broke. It was eighteen minutes by the time I had her and he was gone for a total of ten minutes but that seemed like a lifetime because I refused to let her out and the midwives looking for (husband) and he made it about five minutes before and when he walked into the room that's when I did what they wanted and she came out. (Abir)

> He was actually being prepared to come into theatre while that part was happening. After that did happen they got him to sit next to me but he could actually see. As soon as they had pulled the baby they got (husband) to go and cut the cord and then start the weighing and those sorts of things. So he was involved in that part and he stayed with the baby right through while he was being washed up and cleaned up and he eventually bought the baby to me when I had gone back into the normal room. (Rima)

Kalila expressed her thoughts from the point-of-view of those in attendance (mother and husband), and how they would be feeling witnessing the birth.

> My mum was right there by my side. (Husband) was great. It was just such a big thing. I think it was worse for them than it was for me. I was in pain but they were hearing it raw and they could comprehend what was happening like when they were telling the father that this kid won't make it, if this doesn't work we have to take her up to caesarean, it's scary. And he'd been watching me, I can't see myself. I'd probably be frightened watching someone give birth than actually giving birth because it's just horrendous.

Health Care and Interaction with Staff

Women in private health care had positive responses about their relationship and interaction with their carer. The simple action of holding the labouring woman's hand was appreciated and supportive. The midwives in attendance were encouraging and informative by keeping women up to date of what was happening with the progress of the birth. They also informed the women about choices of pain relief and provided when the women asked for. The midwives attitude was a major aspect in contributing to the satisfaction of the women in this study.

> Well, as much as you can be satisfied when you're in pain, just with the level of support, with the encouragement that the...you know...they treat you...they don't patronise you and they treat you with respect and they help you through it just not only with their physical support but with the emotional and practical, like in terms of positive comments and encouragement. (Sabah)

However, Widad, who as in private care, expressed her frustration and dissatisfaction in having different information given to her by different people.

> With the first one well... I don't know... it was very frustrating because I was getting different information from different doctors like one would say that I was three centimetres dilated and one would say that I was seven and one would say that I'm one. So I don't know if you could go backwards and forwards but I felt like a bit like a yo-yo and being examined and also different nurses coming in all the time, being left alone some periods having just a student in there. With the first one no (not satisfied), but with the second one probably yes (satisfied).

Having chosen public care, multiparae women had mixed feelings about their interactions with the health care professionals, particularly when they compared previous birth experiences to the current one. The nursing staff were described as indifferent, not caring, and abrupt in their manner.

> Talking about the nurses, with my first pregnancy they took me up to theatre, knocked me out and I can still remember and it kind of put me off the hospitals. I was up stairs and I needed to hold a nurses hand and it was a chinese lady, and I asked her and she just took her hand away form me. I was really scared and no one was next to me and my husband wasn't next to me. All I wanted was a little bit of TLC. Someone to hold on to. And she took her hand away from me and then I was knocked out. And I woke up I was happy and sad. But that compared to my second pregnancy the nurses were fantastic. They were there all throughout it and came and told me what was available to me for the pain. (Jumanah)

There were a number of women attending the public system who responded positively about their experience. Women described being treated by midwives and nursing staff with respect, kindness, politeness, gentleness and understanding. They were seen as "good" and "supportive" and were attentive to the woman's needs. When the monitor beeped they would come in to check. If the woman needed to go to the toilet they would take the monitor off her to enable her to do so, as they were accommodating to the woman's needs.

A few women gave birth in a birth centre. Nida found it to be very positive and was happier at the centre than in a hospital setting. She had entered the hospital wanting a natural birth and was taken to the birth centre. After the birth she was transferred to the hospital labour ward as she was not booked into the birth centre and could not keep a suite there.

He (husband) can't stay overnight, you can't have as many visitors as you want if it's not private so that's the big difference but instead they were very comforting and they didn't care. They did end up moving me the next day because they had another lady wanting to have her baby and because I wasn't booked in, I had to go. And I was upset that I had to go because you get better care there I found. I enjoyed it. I was seen by midwives at the family birthing centre but then I had to go back to the team that I was assigned to with my antenatal classes that I had throughout my pregnancy. But had I booked the family birthing centre I would have stayed there. (Nida)

Yusra spoke about her labour and how she had made the decision for a natural birth through the birthing centre, which focuses on natural birthing. Her waters broke and a day and a half later after going to the centre. She had to leave because contractions had not started. And then she had to return to the centre, and she was "shuttled" to the labour ward because her contractions still had not begun. She spoke of her feelings during this time and how this impacted on her experiences and thoughts about her labour and the staff that she interacted with.

Because I was at the women's birthing centre and then gone down to the labour ward, I did not know who was a doctor, who was a student, who was a nurse who was a midwife, at one stage I had between 8 and 10 people in my labour room and I was in such a state I couldn't give a hoot who was who anymore I was just worried about getting the baby out the easiest way possible. I was in pain because I was induced and the contractions weren't my own contractions it was drugs and yes I was in pain even when I was being stitched up and I was in emotional pain, I was an emotional wreck knowing I'd been thrown out, I was just devastated. It was not part of the plan to be there. In my heart it always felt like I had geared up to it, I'd exercised, I'd worked, I'd meditated and I thought I was ready for a natural birth. And probably in fact I was ready for it but I wasn't allowed to have a natural birth. (Yusra)

Najwa talked about her experience with the carers during her labour and how distressing it was at a time when she was already in pain. She spoke about arriving at the hospital and being told by one nurse that she was four centimetres dilated and then being told that she was only 1cm dilated by the head nurse. She further described her experience as follows:

I was already 4 hours into having the pain, with me it would all come into the 4 hours with no breaks, and the midwife that was for three years trainee she said, you're not long to go your 4 cm dilated and the midwife looked at me and at the nurse and said 'nuh, your only 1cm.' she just really had an attitude and I thought from my ethnic background I really did, or I though maybe because I was Muslim because she did seem like she was a bit of a redneck. And the other one looked at me and my mum and said you're 4cm behind her back, but she said I can't do nothing she's the head midwife. (Najwa)

After considering what was being said to her and the time she had left of the labour she decided to have the epidural because she felt her body was too tired. She said she was "so dead set against the epidural" but she felt she needed it at that time. When trying to sit down to take the epidural she would be crying with the pain and as if "a pin was going up in my insides". The staff continually tried to sit her down after jumping up when she tried to do so and as she kept saying that she felt there was something wrong and "they would look at me like I was stupid".

> They tried three times and every time I would just scream, he said she just won't sit down I don't know what's wrong, he just walked out the door he goes I can't do it I won't risk it, he can't put the epidural so he just walked out. And I got very upset because the pain was just so severe and they said if I wanted to lie down, but I just froze and I don't know how later I got myself onto the bed, and the nurses looked and the head of my son was coming out and they were making me sit down on his head. So the training midwife was right and the head midwife wasn't. And what I sensed came true later. She didn't even say sorry, she didn't show pity, she was still very rude to me, later when the baby came out she just walked out and I didn't see her again. She was just plain rude, insensitive. I sense it was mainly because I was a Muslim or because or my background that she treated me this way. The other midwife was of European and she was just really nice. The next day she paid me a visit and spoke to me. I've had an old midwife before and she was great. (Najwa)

HOSPITAL STAY

All the women had spent time in the hospital after the delivery of their baby. That time would be influenced by contact with staff, the role of her husband, the presence of other children, family, friends and relatives. In this time of relief, rest and recuperation, most women responded either receiving or lacking understanding and support from the staff.

Contact with Hospital Staff

A few women in private care described how the staff impacted on their experience of the hospital stay and could mak e it either a positive or negative experience. The way in which nurses and doctors acted towards women and their attitude in helping them learn about caring for their newborn and their commitment to meeting women's needs were several factors of influence on the satisfaction of the hospital stay experience.

> They were really, really good, wonderful actually. Being a first time mum I guess they seemed to be sensitive to that. I remember having them trying to express the milk for me, you're sitting there, half undressed and here's some stranger trying to milk you. I had no idea how to do it. I guess if the nurses hadn't been so supportive and so understanding that would have been difficult to be but they were all lovely and sometimes there were fill-in nurses, nurses they got from agencies, who don't normally work in the hospital but they were just as lovely and understanding, and in the end they just gave you a different perspective on different things you had questions about. They had to check your wounds and again that would have been difficult to deal with hadn't the nurses been sensitive. (Rima)

Within the public hospital setting, women described mixed feelings while comparing one birth to another or comparing the treatment of one nurse to another and the impact each had on their hospital stay experience. There were women who recounted being given contradicting information and advice and then feeling confused and stressed and not knowing what to do. One woman whose baby would not settle spoke of being told by one nurse to feed her baby when she was hungry, but another nurse told her not to do so. To settle her baby they decided to give her a bath and when this did not help the nurse told the first-time mother to take care of her baby and walked out. The woman described how distressing and worrying this experience was as a new mother and not knowing what else could be done.

In a similar public hospital setting, women expressed their satisfaction with staff and the way they were treated after the birth. Women felt that their needs were important to the nurses and were happy that things were safely done in a "safe place".

> They were just so professionals, they were so gentle, so empathetic, they come with a sense of humour, one nurse came in for the night shift and she came in saying 'right, I'm your drug dealer for the night what do you want?' And it's true that's what every woman wants there. One's had a caesarean; everyone wants pain relief of some sort. And because I was getting headaches I needed to take tablets. The nurses were fabulous they just were under a very shabby system that's all. (Yusra)

Role of Husband

Women were asked, that while in hospital, what role their husband played during this time. Several responded that he would visit after work. This visit provided comfort, company and support of someone who was known and loved in a sea of unfamiliar faces.

> Actually the first couple of days he worked but he tried to leave early and come. It was just nice to have his company and if we had a lot of guests over I couldn't manage them all so it was nice to have him there. And if he came and had dinner with me it was nice rather than me eating on my own, which I had breakfast on my own, lunch on my own so it was nice to have some company for dinner. Really, just as a support for me. (Rihana)

Other women responded that their husband would visit and bring necessities such as bringing food and bath and baby items and women also had help with necessities such as bathing. Nadia and Hana mentioned having visits from their husband who also had to manage taking care of their other children while she was at hospital. At times it was necessary that the husband take time off work to care for their children, as there was no one else to care for them. The husband would be able to spend the day at the hospital while children were at school and went home later.

Having Visitors

Having visitors soon after the birth is a norm and understood with most of the women interviewed. However, women had preferences of the number of people visiting at one time and particularly when there was room sharing with another mother and her baby. Having a number of visitors immediately after the birth was rather overwhelming and tiring for women to deal with. Preferences were expressed to have immediate family members on the first day and other visitors the next day. There were several women who stated that they liked having people to visit. They were happy to see people and people were happy to see the new mother and baby.

> Yeah I did (get a lot of visitors). As soon as they left... I think it's just my nature, I love to be around people, I felt blessed when they were around and when they'd leave I felt lonely, I'd get scared, I didn't want to be by myself. (Kalila)

Although Rima's newborn was in an incubator, she expressed her desire to have visitors and how they helped her through the time at the hospital.

> Everyone was terribly excited. And obviously they couldn't see and pick up the baby because he was in the incubator. I found (husband) was a bit difficult at that time because he found them intrusive and he felt all these people coming to see his baby which I found difficult because I understand the people wanting to see our baby and I guess I just needed to have those people around me because it helped make it a little more real. I guess those people were visiting when (husband) had just come so he'd come and he missed out on time alone. Most of the time people came in the evening. It was difficult because you had set times when you had to express the milk so you kind of hoped it wasn't going to coincide with the time the visitors would start to come, but generally it worked out quite good. (Rima)

Room Sharing and Rooming-In

Several women found room sharing to be difficult and uncomfortable particularly in trying to establish a routine for herself and her newborn, sleeping and having visitors. However, this changed once they were given their own room and the difference in comfort and privacy was felt immediately. The women mentioned feeling more settled and relaxed when they could begin to develop a routine, such as turning on the television as they wished, and not having to worry if their baby cried as the crying would not be disturbing others.

> It was terrible. It was very crowded because, I mean, other than visiting times, she had her family with her, like her husband and she had another little girl so they'd be there most of the day, so there was always people talking next door. If you tried to sleep you couldn't and also when you're in hospital you're trying to get some sleep whenever the baby is sleeping, because you know, when the baby's up you're up. So like, my baby would be asleep, her baby would be awake and crying so I can't get to sleep. And then when my baby's awake her baby would be asleep and she wouldn't you know...so it was difficult for both of us. (Sabah)

Several women had a preference for their own room and expressed their dissatisfaction in not being able to have one. Sharing a room was uncomfortable and frustrating particularly when one baby would cry and "they all start crying".

Rooming-in has been a routine practice in Australian hospitals. The practice requires a mother to take active care of her newborn during hospital stay (Rice, 2000). Thana responded with a focus on rooming-in with her newborn and wanting that closeness whereas Rana found some relief in being able to be alone to rest for some time, as her baby was cared for.

> With me all the time in the room (baby). Except once I was that much tired and he kept crying and they took him, they wanted me to have a rest and I actually got out of my bed and I said 'please I want my son' and I started crying. And they bring him back to me. (Thana)

> I was well taken care of as well as the baby. They would take the baby to the nursery so I could get some rest and sleep. (Rana)

Feelings about Hospital Stay

Women were asked about their feelings about the hospital stay. Their responses ranged from very strong negative feelings as Yusra states, to Manal, for example, finding the stay in hospital to be "fantastic".

> There are a lot of little things that you could say I don't like her because of that, like with us being Lebanese a lot of visitors come after visiting hours and a lot of them come at once, some people get offended by nurses that say visiting times is up. That doesn't make them bad, they're just sticking by the books which is ok to me because I just want my rest time. Being in hospital is fantastic for me. It's away from the house, it's away from the work, my time with my baby and I love it. (Manal)

Thana was satisfied with her stay in the public hospital after the birth. She stated that it was "very clean" and they would clean the bathroom every day. Her mother would bring food to eat and in the evening her husband would join her. However, several other women were not too happy, were scared, upset and disappointed at their hospital experience. Women felt that they were rushed out of hospital "have a kid and shoo you out", and that they were not given enough time to settle with their baby and rest before taking the baby home. Women mentioned that to combat loneliness and being alone throughout the day, they tried to keep busy by doing various things in the hospital.

> The second child I had been two days in the hospital and I remember they said I have to leave tomorrow morning because you fine and nothing wrong. And I was supposed to leave one o'clock and they took me from the bed and it's 10.30, me and my baby, until my husband came and took me because they need the bed for somebody else. I was really upset because from 10.30 till finish breakfast til one o'clock, it's a lot and sitting on a chair. This time she ask me if I want to go tomorrow or you want to stay and I said I prefer to stay one more day because I don't have anybody at home. (Salma)

Kalila, a first-time mother, found several major factors had an impact on her experience at the hospital. She expressed her feelings of loneliness and lack of support in the few days stay. She was afraid of being on her own and did not want her husband to leave to stay alone in a strange environment. She stated being emotionally ruined and not knowing how to deal with being alone. However, as soon as visitors arrived she would be fine. "It was awful" being alone and crying.

Ready or Needing to Leave Hospital

Several women when asked what was the reason they left the hospital, they responded that they felt ready to go home and to take care of their newborn. They were excited, happy and confident to go home and take care of the baby. It was difficult being in the hospital even though it was an opportunity to learn new things and be cared for after the birth for several days. These women also had other children at home to care for.

> I was in hospital for 2 days and 3 nights. I just couldn't wait to get home. With my first one I enjoyed being in the hospital but with my second I couldn't wait because I wanted to see what my first son's reaction. I just couldn't wait to get home... I knew everything I was doing was right, the feeding was good, it was just going really well so I knew I was ready to go home. (Intisar)

Widad stated that her main reason for leaving the hospital was to take care of other children at home.

> Things were pretty bad at home. My daughter was... I think she was... I don't know... she was acting out a little bit. I think she found it hard with me being in hospital, she wanted to stay at her grandmothers all the time, she was not getting along with her father, not wanting to be with him and kind of I think... obviously missing me, I was absent, but not knowing how to express that. It was creating a lot of friction. And then mum saying 'leave her here' and [husband] saying 'no, I want her home' and she doesn't want to go home and screaming and... I thought in the end this is really annoying, I need to rest, and here in hospital I'm copping it from all sides so I went home. (Widad)

Abir and Layla, both first time mothers expressed wanting to go home and feeling lonely and having a dislike for hospitals. They felt that being at home was a better place to recuperate and be comfortable with the support of others. Nida made the choice to leave the hospital early than the discharge day, though later recognised that it was not the best decision to have made at that time.

> Stayed one night at the birthing centre and then they moved me to the wards. Stayed there two nights. I wanted to go home the second night. And mum's like why do you want to go home for? At least here you've got someone looking after you. And she was so right because when I came home... coming home was the hardest part. Because this baby would not stop crying and he wasn't eating. As a newborn he was very hard, he had colic, the first two months were difficult, the hard part till about five months because that's up until when he had colic but the first two months were the worst. (Nida)

DISCUSSION AND CONCLUSION

Although caesarean rates are increasing worldwide, from the sample of women in our study, it suggests that only several women preferred and elected to have a caesarean section. Women who gave birth by a caesarean section after a natural birth, and those who delivered naturally (with and without pain relief) preferred a natural birth. Most women, even among those who had experienced painful deliveries, mentioned that they would prefer having a natural delivery for subsequent births. Women made choices on the method of delivery according to time taken for recovery afterwards, convenience of knowing when the baby is due, previous experiences, advice and stories of other women, support from others and knowledge about those methods. Yet still, pain was a major contributing factor during the labour for women to change their preferences particularly with wanting pain relief. The findings suggest that women made this decision based on personal preference and benefits and only when there was risk attributed to the baby.

An Australian study (Turnbull et al., 1999) mentions also other factors that were important in making the decision for a natural or caesarean delivery within their sample. All women were likely to have been influenced in their decision by information by their doctor. Women who had elective caesareans were influenced by factors such as recovery and the ability to plan. In contrast, women who had an emergency caesarean were influenced by the physical stress of labour, and their partner's reaction in the labour room. Other factors included the consideration of pain and previous negative experiences of childbirth. A caesarean section delivery was more likely to be seen as an easier option and routine intervention by women speaking English at home than women who spoke a language other than English at home (Walker et al., 2004). In contrast, most of the women in our study had a good understanding of the English language, but they still expressed their preferences for a natural birth because they said women "have been doing it for years".

The postnatal period is a time where support for the mother-infant bonding and rest after the birth is essential. Women described having negative and/or positive experiences and being satisfied or unhappy and disappointed with the care they received. The three major themes emerging from the findings include the treatment by nurses and doctors, rooming-in, and initiating breastfeeding.

The time spent in the hospital after the birth, whether in public or private care, generated mixed reactions by the women in the study. Multiparae women assessed their level of satisfaction by making comparisons with their previous birthing experiences while primiparae women based their satisfaction on perceptions and expectations prior to the birth. Women with mixed feelings of their experience mentioned that "the nurses were fine but one". They were described as mean, annoying, and needing to be more considerate and careful of what they say. Being cared for by several nurses and having one nurse not treating them with understanding and empathy had tainted their experience of the hospital stay. Proportionally, there were more women who attended private care that were satisfied and happy with their postnatal care than women who attended public care. However, several women were also very satisfied with their choice model of care. The few women who chose the birth centre for their birth were very satisfied with the care by the midwives. Even though a few of these women were not able to deliver in the birth centre suite because of complications and needing to take pain relief, they still expressed their satisfaction with the care received there. Whether the treatment by the nurses was considered positive, negative or mixed, this assessment was based mostly on the nurse's attitude to the new mother.

In contrast, a study by Liamputtong Rice and colleagues (1999) of twenty-six Thai mothers in Australia found that the majority of women said they were satisfied with the postnatal care they received. Although, our women stated similarly, those women attending private care tended to be more satisfied than women in public hospitals. In a more comparative study (Kenny et al., 1993), women chose either home care after early discharge or hospital care until discharge after the birth, assessed the midwives interest and caring, education and information provided, their own progress with feeding and baby care, and their own physical and emotional health. The women who chose home care tended to rate their postnatal care more highly than women who stayed in hospital. In both groups of women, the majority gave positive responses. However, the women who had chosen home care gave extremely positive responses in all aspects. A notable difference was how rushed the midwives seemed. Almost all the women with home care felt the midwives 'always had enough time' to spend with them compared with thirty-five percent of the hospital group. We also found similar responses among women who used birth centre care: they stated it "felt like home". This suggests that women feel more comfortable receiving care in a home-like environment.

During the postnatal stay in hospital, the women participating in this study expressed their feelings about rooming-in with other women and their babies. Whether in private care or public hospitals, women were not content when they had to share a room with another mother. The main reasons given for feeling dissatisfied include babies crying at different times and waking up their babies, not being able to rest, the room getting crowded with visitors, not wanting to disturb other mothers, and not being able to settle into a routine with both mother and baby. Several women in private care, after moving into their own room stated, "I was more comfortable", and "it's much more different" and not having to worry about disturbing other mothers if her baby cried or she had visitors. Women in public care, although preferred having a room for themselves, expressed their dissatisfaction of not being able to do so.

As recommended by the World Health Organisation and UNICEF in 1989 (Svensson et al., 2005) that mother and baby should remain together day and night during the hospital stay, in many countries mother and baby are still separated after birth and rooming-in is not always practiced night and day. For example, in Lebanon as recently found, only ten of the thirty-nine hospitals in the study practiced rooming-in day and night. Rooming-in is practiced in most public maternity hospitals in Australia and entails the mother to care for her newborn while in hospital enabling the mother-infant bond to develop and strengthen leading to the early establishment and successful breastfeeding practices (Rice, 2000; Svensson et al., 2005).

Several women in this study specifically responded to rooming-in with their newborn. Some mothers were given the occasion to rest on her own in the room though one mother soon after became upset and requested that her baby be brought back as she stated that she felt the need to have her baby close by. The other mothers whose baby was taken to the nursery as she rested mentioned, "I was well taken care of as well as the baby". A few first-time mothers expressed a preference for the opportunity to have their baby in a nursery or being taken care of by the nurses to enable them some time for rest and recuperation that they may be better capable of taking care of their baby. The findings suggest that rooming-in with other women was a major issue, not the rooming-in with their baby, and a more flexible approach to maternity hospital care in the postnatal period with women given the option of rooming-in is needed. .

In support of these findings, an Australian research study conducted by Rice (2000) of 43 Asian women, reported that rooming-in can create conflict between new mothers and hospital staff. Women wished to observe cultural practices, such as 'good rest' and avoidance of physical activities, in order to regain health and strength after the birth of their baby.

However, these practices are in contradiction with rooming-in practices at the hospitals. These differences have led to dissatisfaction with hospital care in many of the women in the study.

The majority of multiparae women in the present research stated that a couple of days stay in hospital was an adequate period of time for them. They felt "ready" to go home particularly because they had the other children and had done it before. Primiparae women, although having given birth to their first baby, expressed their wishes to leave the hospital. Their main reason being that they had a dislike for hospitals and the loneliness felt in hospitals when the family and friends left after visiting. Generally, new mothers were satisfied to stay in hospital for as long as they could in order to gain as much help, support and education from the staff as was possible in the short period of time.

Our results are similar to findings in a study by Brown and Lumley (1997). Women who left in the first forty-eight hours after birth were more likely to be multiparous women, to have attended a public hospital, to have experienced a lower level of obstetric interventions, and to have a very low income. Whether women left after forty-eight hours or on day three or four, were not more likely than women who stayed five or more days to experience breastfeeding problems, low confidence about caring for their baby or depression six to seven months after the birth. Hence, women who stayed shorter days showed no adverse outcomes as indicated by this study and staying in hospital does not necessarily provide the support and rest and recuperating environment women required after the birth.

IMPLICATIONS FOR HEALTH CARE PRACTICE

There are several implications for health care professionals caring for pregnant and new mothers. Most importantly, it should be recognized that each woman's experience of pregnancy and birth is unique. Women have different expectations and perceptions of childbirth, which is strongly influenced and impacted on by many factors. Hence, throughout all stages of pregnancy, birth and beyond, carers and educators should ensure women have access to information and understand the options available to them. With this, communication needs to be an integral part of care.

The childbirth experience has the potential to affect either positively or negatively on a woman's self esteem and early interaction behaviour with her newborn. When caring for a woman during pregnancy, childbirth and postnatally, the variables that can influence a woman's perception should be assessed. In order to provide sensitive and expert care that will improve the childbirth experience for women, health care professionals must be knowledgeable about the factors that can influence a woman's perception of childbirth.

Health care professionals caring for pregnant women in a variety of settings across the span of the childbearing years can make a significant difference in the quality in the childbearing experience for the woman and her family. Gaining an understanding of and appreciation for the cultural and spiritual meanings of childbirth and recognising cultural coping patterns to the woman has important implications for nursing practice. Skill should be developed in cultural assessment to identify and understand the childbearing woman's attitudes, behaviours, values and needs. Carers with a more holistic focus will facilitate more culturally sensitive care for women thus increasing positive outcomes, including the promotion of feelings and self-actualisation in the woman, maternal role attainment, and fostering of positive relationship with others.

REFERENCES

Brown, S., & Lumley, J., 1997, 'Reasons to Stay, Reasons to Go: Results of an Australian Population-Based Survey', *Birth*, 24(3): 148-158.

Callister, L.C., 1995, 'Cultural Meanings of Childbirth', *Journal of Obstetrics, Gynecologic, and Neonatal Nursing*, 24(3): 327-331.

Chamberlain, D.B., 1999, 'Historical Perspectives on Pain', *The Journal of Prenatal & Perinatal Psychology and Health*, 14(1-2): 145-168.

Devlin, V. (ed.) 1995, *Motherhood: From 1920 to the Present Day*, Polygon: Edinburgh.

Health Department Victoria, 1990, *Having a Baby in Victoria: Final report of the ministerial review of birthing services in Victoria*, Health Department Victoria: Melbourne.

Holloway, I., & Wheeler, S., 2002, *Qualitative Research in Nursing*, 2nd edition, Blackwell Publishing Company: Oxford.

Kenny, P., King, M.T., Cameron, S., & Shiell, A., 1993, 'Satisfaction With Postnatal Care - The Choice of Home or Hospital', *Midwifery*, 9: 146-153.

Kridli, S.A.-O., 2002, 'Health Beliefs and Practices Among Arab Women', *MCN, Maternal and Child Nursing*, 27(3): 178-182.

Liamputtong, P., & Douglas, E., 2005, *Qualitative Research Methods, 2nd edition*, Oxford University Press: Melbourne.

Liamputtong Rice, P., Naksook, C., & Watson, L. E., 1999, 'The Experiences of Postpartum Hospital Stay and Returning Home Among Thai Mothers in Australia', *Midwifery*, 15: 47-57.

Lipsett, R., 2004, *No 'One Right Way': A Handbook for Parents*, Sea Change Publishing: Melbourne.

Lothian, J. A., 2001, 'Back to the Future: Trusting Birth', *Journal of Perinatal and Neonatal Nursing*, 15(3): 13-22.

Morris, D.J., 2001, *Pregnancy, Childbirth and the Newborn*, Hinkler Books: Seattle.

Nichols, F. H., 1996, 'The Meaning of the Childbirth Experience: A Review of the Literature', *The Journal of Perinatal Education*, 5(4): 71-77.

Reed, R.K., 2005, *Birthing Fathers*, Rutgers University Press: New Brunswick.

Rice, P.L., 2000, 'Rooming-In and Cultural Practices: Choice or Constraint', *Journal of Reproductive and Infant Psychology*, 18(1): 21-32.

Stanley, F., Richardson, S., & Prior, M., 2005, *Children of the Lucky Country? How Australian Society has turned its back on children and why children matter*, Macmillan: Sydney.

Svensson, K., Matthiesen, A.-S., & Widstrom, A.-M., 2005, 'Night Rooming-In: Who Decides? An Example of Staff Influence on Mother's Attitude', *Birth*, 32(2): 99-106.

Tinkler, A., & Quinney, D., 1998, 'Team Midwifery: The Influence of the Midwife-Woman Relationship on Women's Experiences and Perceptions of Maternity Care', *Journal of Advanced Nursing*, 28(1): 30-35.

Turnbull, D. A., Wilkinson, C., Yaser, A., Carty, V., Svigos, J. M., & Robinson, J. S., 1999, 'Women's Role and Satisfaction in the Decision to Have a Caesarean Section', *Medical Journal of Australia*, 170: 580-583.

Walker, R., Turnball, D., & Wilkinson, C., 2004, 'Increasing Cesarean Section Rates: Exploring the Role of Culture in an Australian Community', *Birth*, 31(2): 117-124.

Yelland, J., Small, R., Lumley, J., Liamputtong Rice, P., Cotronei, V., & Warren, R., 1998, 'Support, Sensitivity, Satisfaction: Filipino, Turkish and Vietnamese Women's Experiences of Postnatal Stay', *Midwifery*, 14: 144-154.

In: Reproduction, Childbearing and Motherhood
Editor: Pranee Liamputtong, pp. 195-208

ISBN: 978-1-60021-606-0
© 2007 Nova Science Publishers, Inc.

Chapter 12

Sensing Vulnerability, Seeking Strength: Somali Women and Their Experiences During Pregnancy and Birth in Melbourne

Paula Hernandez

The Importance of Mothering and Children: A Background to the Study

The importance of mothering and having children for Somalis cannot be underestimated. These are highly valued and profoundly significant providing women with a crucial element of their identity. The notion of fertility is centered on ideas about living enriched lives. For women in particular, the importance of having children lies in the belief that "children are our wealth": children cement a woman's link to her clan and provide security and sustenance, particularly in old age. To not have children was seen as living an impoverished life.

The significance of children and the important role and place they hold within Somali culture has meant that large families are very much desired. In Somalia, having ten or twelve children is the norm. Women marry at a relatively young age and begin to have children soon after marrying. In Australia, Somali women's experience of reproduction has altered significantly. At the same, however, the value of having children has remained. While women no longer have the large families they might have had in Somalia, women continue to have four, five sometimes up to eight children. Reproduction, however, is experienced in ways profoundly distinct from experiences within Somalia, revealing how the social landscape impacts on notions and practices of reproduction and in turn how these can alter women's sense of self.

The importance given to becoming a mother has meant that many Somali women have encountered the medical and social systems in place in Australia that regulate and take care of parenting – to some extent at least. In turn, these institutions have been confronted by Somalis' at times opposing and conflicting beliefs and attitudes towards pregnancy and birth that challenge both the efficacy of procedures and the often taken for granted ways of knowing relating to health, medicine and ideas of the self. My interest, therefore, is in exploring the ways Somali women's experience of pregnancy and birth has altered in the context of settlement in Australia.

Before commencing my research, my involvement in a volunteer home tutor scheme had exposed me to the lives of two Somali women. Like other Somali women, they had experienced motherhood at a very early age. They had also experienced motherhood under extremely hostile and difficult conditions: fleeing their war torn countries and being separated from family members. My relationship with these women became close and my doctoral research was inspired by their experiences of mothering in both Somalia and Australia. From these encounters, it became clear that the experience of pregnancy and birth in Australia had differed significantly from what women had experienced in Somalia. What also became obvious was the way in which women's own experiences and knowledge informed their understanding and encounters in Australia. The medicalization of pregnancy and birth has created one particular understanding of pregnancy and birth, yet it has not always been readily accepted. Rather, as many of the Somali women I have spoken to reveal, this model and particular way of knowing can be contested and negotiated on a number of levels.

UNDERSTANDING WOMEN'S EXPERIENCES: THEORETICAL STANDPOINT(S) ADOPTED IN THE STUDY

Throughout the world, pregnancy and birth have become highly medicalized procedures requiring specialized care and knowledge as western models of maternity have been introduced (Davis Floyd and Sargent, 1997; Liamputtong Rice and Manderson, 1996; Lukere and Jolly, 2002; Mallett, 2003; Ram and Jolly, 1998). This increased emphasis on the medical model of care, however, has attracted wide criticism, from various quarters, including feminist authors (see for example Martin, 1989; O'Brien, 1980; Oakley, 1984; Rich, 1977; Young, 1990). At the core of many of these critiques lies the notion that "the western medical model disempowers women" (Morton, 2002: 33). As Ginsburg and Rapp argue (1991: 318), the medicalized setting has been held responsible for "displacing or competing with indigenous practice [and] may disorganize or extinguish local forms of knowledge". The biomedical model's emphasis on specialized knowledge, what Briggitte Jordan (1993) terms "authoritative knowledge", has been seen to play a crucial role in displacing alternative ideas and practices around maternity where medical hegemony has assumed to account for all knowledge declaring others as "ill informed, ignorant or irrelevant" (Liamputtong Rice, 1999a).

As the ever-increasing anthropology of birth has revealed (see for example Kitzinger, 1978; Kay, 1982; Scheper-Hughes, 1992; Jordan, 1993; MacCormack, 1994; Davis-Floyd and Sargent, 1997; Liamputtong Rice, 1999a, 2000; Lukere and Jolly, 2002) contrasting practices and ideas around pregnancy and birth have persisted despite the pervasive nature of the medical model. In the west, feminist theories have also attempted to posit alternative understandings surrounding the experience of pregnancy and birth by challenging dominant models of interpretation and experience. In its place, women's own subjective experiences have become the focus drawing on the work begun by the anthropology of women in the early 1970s, which acknowledged the need to more critically analyze earlier assumptions made about women and their place in the world. There was a recognition that women's experiences varied where characteristics like ethnicity, class and religion, as well as personal experience, to name but a few variables, had a very real influence in shaping people's experiences of the world they encounter. Moreover, there was a realization that women's experiences of mothering and reproduction in particular could not be understood solely in terms of domination and oppression as was previously the case or as was espoused at times by the new wave of feminism of the same era. Rather, becoming a mother and all that this entails involves a complex range of elements that necessarily include emotional ties and not just aspects of what societal or cultural norms dictate.

My work, therefore, draws on a number of these theoretical standpoints, particularly in relation to how women themselves make sense of their experiences of pregnancy and birth and that of mothering given the experience of resettlement. This research has also drawn on ideas about the way in which differing and contrasting knowledge systems are interpreted and negotiated in new settings. For example, what determines which practices are accepted while others are discarded? How do women negotiate aspects of more traditional practices with more modern ones?

METHODOLOGY USED

As an anthropology student, I employed an ethnographic perspective to explore Somali women's experiences and attitudes of pregnancy and birth. Utilizing the methods of participant observation, descriptive analysis and interviews – both formal and informal, issues surrounding pregnancy, birth and early childcare were discussed and explored with participants.

Women were initially recruited through my continued contact with one of my Somali students. Most participants however were recruited through two Somali playgroups run in two municipalities in Melbourne through Maternal and Child Health Centres. This proved to be the most successful method for recruiting participants, as I was able to approach women with the help of the playgroup leaders.

Semi-structured interviews were conducted with twenty women. Numerous informal interviews were also conducted in various settings including the playgroups; some social events like birthday parties and home visits to women I considered had become close friends. Interview times often ranged from forty-five minutes to two hours with most interviews lasting one hour. Health professionals were also interviewed including Maternal and Child Health nurses and midwives both in community settings like community health centres and at a major public hospital. Other professionals were also consulted including social workers, community liaison officers, a kindergarten teacher, playgroup leaders, and Family and Reproductive Rights Education Program (FARREP) workers from two public hospitals. My aim was to explore the women's experiences from a variety of perspectives, particularly because it became clear from the women's interviews that some confusion and misunderstanding existed amongst the women about certain procedures during pregnancy and birth.

Given my interest in exploring the way in which women's experience of pregnancy and birth had altered, I had initially hoped to recruit participants who had given birth both in the

Australian context as well as in Somalia. The nature of Somali resettlement in Australia, however, meant that few women fell into this 'category'. As a refugee community with a high percentage of relatively young members, most women who arrived in Australia with children had either already given birth to several children and did not intend to have more, or had given birth in refugee camps rather than in Somalia although many of these women did intend to have more children in Australia. Furthermore, the high number of adolescent children that arrived in the peak period of Somali resettlement meant that their experiences of pregnancy and birth could not resemble the experience of their mothers. These demographic realities therefore meant that while a small group of women recruited did include those who had experienced birthing in both Somalia and Australia, the bulk of women interviewed often fell into the grouping of either a) women who had given birth in both refugee camps and Australia and b) women who had married in Australia and had therefore only given birth in Australia.

Interviews for this research were conducted in two time periods. Initially, a number of women were interviewed during the period from 2001 to 2002 with the remainder of the interviews taking place between 2004 and 2005.

SOMALIA: A HISTORICAL AND SOCIAL PERSPECTIVE

As its history reveals, Somalia has been subject to continued disruption and upheaval – largely due to its legacy of preferential clan representation and alliances and a history of colonial rule – but famine has also played a role. Although independent since 1960, the merger of the northern and southern territories of Somalia (former colonies of Britain and Italy), with their contrasting colonial rulers and clan differentiation, saw much unease resulting in the successful coup led by General Mohamed Siyad Barre of the Somali Revolutionary Council (SRC) on October 21, 1969. What followed, however, was an even greater emphasis on clan affiliation. Under Siyad Barre's rule, specific clan groups and individuals, such as intellectuals and religious leaders, were victimized so that instead of uniting regions and clans. As Hussein (1997: 171) explains, "Barre used the policy of divide and rule, magnifying clan distinctions for political ends".

The fall of Siyad Barre's regime in 1990, while long awaited, nevertheless resulted in much upheaval. Much of the infrastructure and public services such as electricity and water supply were destroyed. In the aftermath, clan differences continued to play a significant role – forcing thousands of Somalis to flee their nation. As opposing groups scrambled for power or sought retribution for past injustices, many Somali women, men and children were witnesses to or victims of looting, murder and torture. As a consequence, a large proportion of Somalis now living in Australia have encountered and experienced some form of trauma during the upheaval. Many women have recounted their experiences of trauma; others have acknowledged the presence of violence as they attempted to flee or find refuge in the aftermath.

The civil war in Somalia forced almost a million people to flee their nation. Initially, most made their way to refugee camps in neighboring Kenya, Ethiopia or Djibouti before being repatriated to other nations as part of humanitarian efforts. Australia accepted a large number of Somalis that included a significant intake of women and children accepted under the 'Women at Risk' program (Nsubuga-Kyobe and Dimock, 2000). This has meant that a large number of women have few or no extended family here. Furthermore, many Somalis have arrived without knowing the whereabouts of husbands, parents or siblings, creating much unease and anxiety in the community.

An estimated 5,000 Somalis reside in Victoria, with the bulk of the community living in the Northern and Eastern metropolitan regions of Melbourne including West Heidelberg, Kensington/Flemington, Carlton and Dandenong. This research was conducted in Northern region of Melbourne.

Traditionally, Somali women's experiences of pregnancy and birth in Somalia have been characterized by little medical intervention – unless complications arise. While hospital care is present and utilized throughout Somalia, home births have often been more widespread particularly in rural areas where traditional birth attendants assist the expectant and birthing mother, providing traditional medicines as well as using message techniques to assist the mother during birth. Births are not ordinarily rushed and women have spoken of having laboured for days with the assistance of traditional birth attendants and one or two close kin. While women who have given birth in Somali hospitals did receive more medicalised care, women birthing there often experienced similar conditions to women labouring at home. Little 'western style' pain relief was offered or sought and intervention was kept to a minimum unless obvious dangers arose for the mother and her child. Cesarean sections were rarely undertaken.

Throughout pregnancy and birth a woman is given wide-ranging support both in practical and emotional terms. Following the birth, the new mother is similarly supported. This period is marked by 40 days confinement during which time the mother is carefully supported and nurtured by close family and kin. The mother is given specially prepared foods and she is not expected to undertake any household chores as this time is intended as a period of rest and recuperation – her duties usually only revolve around breastfeeding her young infant.

SENSING VULNERABILITY, SEEKING STRENGTH: MAIN RESULTS OF STUDY AND DISCUSSION

While the main results of this research are only preliminary and require much more rigorous analysis, a number of themes and issues have nevertheless been revealed. In particular, women's stories regarding notions and practices of reproduction in the context of resettlement speak to ideas about bodily integrity and vulnerability as well as a sense of openness/exposure or fragility as they attempt to make sense of a whole array of practices and ways of thinking in a new setting. Many of these feelings in fact have mirrored what the women have experienced and felt in adapting to a new country. In the context of reproduction, however, these feelings have become embodied. They also speak of the way in which trauma experienced in fleeing a war torn country continues to impact on women's lives.

Altered Lives: The Experience of Resettlement

As I visited women during my fieldwork, women's stories were often initially marked by the way in which their lives had altered in Australia – at times quite dramatically – and it was during women's conversations about this change that they would begin to speak about their experiences during pregnancy and birth. During these encounters, women remembered their lives in Somalia with great fondness. They recalled the ability to freely roam the streets, of daily visits with kin and family – of a life where people could be relied upon. In contrast, life in Australia was often marked by a lack of extended family and by many responsibilities. As one woman recalled, "in Somalia, you always had to have food ready in your house in case people turned up. People were always visiting. Here in Australia it's not the same". Many women often remarked on the way in which "everyone is busy in Australia", revealing the way in which life had changed in Australia.

Many of the women spoke of great trauma and sadness at having fled their family and homeland often at extremely short notice or without being able to say good-bye. The sense of isolation and loneliness felt by women here as a result of this displacement was often at the forefront of the women's conversations – so too were the many attempts to sponsor elderly parents or relatives. At other times, women spoke about the great financial strain of regular remittances sent to family members still living in Somalia who had been unable to flee themselves. In her study of Somali women in Melbourne and their experiences of resettlement, Celia McMichael (2002: 172) explains "many [Somali] women experience loneliness, sadness, anxiety and depression due to the rupturing impact of war and exile and the exigencies of family separation and resettlement". For many of the women, these feelings of marginalisation in Australia often became even more apparent because of their Muslim religion, dress and skin colour. Women spoke about feeling removed from the wider community and vulnerable to opposing and contrasting values and practices. Such feelings were normally expressed when women spoke about how their children might become exposed to Western ideas and how this in turn could displace Muslim and Somali values inculcated by family. Women's concerns often meant that women did not feel confident to let children go out on their own, to the shops or to the park for example. During pregnancy and birth many of these feelings become more resonant. The sense of removal and isolation felt during resettlement as well as feelings of anxiety at having left family behind all come into play and impact on women's experience of reproduction and became discernible even in the very early stages of pregnancy.

Scrutiny and Bodily Integrity: Women's Experience of Medical Intervention

In Australia, pregnancy and birth are carefully monitored by a medical model of care. In this model of care, antenatal care in particular is utilized to ensure a healthy pregnancy and rule out any potential dangers or difficulties for both the mother and her child. But the 'scrutiny' and 'vigilance' given to women's body during antenatal care is not universally accepted or always understood.

For many of the Somali women this 'scrutiny' and 'vigilance' during antenatal care, often left women feeling exposed to practices and ways of thinking for which they had little grounding or understanding. While some women accepted the importance of these routine antenatal checkups, many more also felt that this scrutiny was often unwarranted and got in the way of other pressing issues. Women who had previously given birth in Somalia and refugee camps in particular were more likely to find these visits both unnecessary and time consuming, predominantly because of long waiting times at the hospital - but other factors also played a role. I was often told that in Somalia, pregnant women did not normally attend antenatal checkups unless they felt something to be wrong, or had reason to believe there was a problem. Hospital care was only required for the care of those suffering from an illness - pregnancy was not understood as an 'illness'. In the Australian context, therefore, a number of women missed appointments or arrived late because they did not feel these appointments would add anything of significance to their understanding of their pregnancies.

Other issues, however, also prevented women from attending antenatal appointments. In particular, women's lack of extended family and their large commitments to their immediate families, simply did not allow them the time to attend these visits especially if a choice had to be made between attending an antenatal check-up and perhaps attending an appointment to secure better housing. Others were prevented by the high incidence of depression found within the community. Speaking to a community midwife involved in a shared care program, I was told that numerous women suffered from depression arising either during a pregnancy or prior to becoming pregnant often because of the difficulties experienced in the resettlement process. This meant that women were often unable to attend an antenatal check-up even when they might have wanted to.

In thinking about these issues, I would argue that Somali women's experience of antenatal care in Australia has, in some ways, being detrimental to Somali women's experiences of pregnancy and birth in Australia. It has been particularly interesting to witness the way in which women's experience of pregnancy and birth is often one of anxiety and concern beginning with antenatal visits. Perhaps Somali women's exposure to this level of care has, at times, created more apprehension about the health and safety of infants as well as that of women's own well-being. Rather than alleviating concern, antenatal visits may have exposed women to possibilities that they may not have previously encountered or thought about. This may be partly due to women's lack of exposure to the concept of preventative health but also because Somali notions of pregnancy have not traditionally been centred on the idea that pregnancy routinely and inevitably requires medical scrutiny and attention. On the other hand, women have also spoken about how lucky and privileged they feel to have access to proper medical care – when required. I believe, however, that for a number of Somali women antenatal care has created some unease because it has exposed the women's bodies in ways that they have not been used to – particularly in relation to Female Genital Mutilation (F.G.M.)

The focus of this research was not centred around the issue of F.G.M. or female circumcision, as the women themselves refer to the practice. (I also prefer to use this term). As such, my questioning and conversations with the women initially did not actively pursue this topic unless women themselves expressed an interest in speaking about this. However, it has become obvious that female circumcision has played a large role in the way in which women have experienced pregnancy and birth within the medical setting and has revealed aspects of what I view as women's sense of vulnerability or bodily integrity.[1] (For a greater discussion concerning F.G.M. see for example Gruenbaum, 2001 and Babatunde, 1998.)

As a number of women have remarked to me, female circumcision in a sense provides 'wholeness' to a woman's body. The closing of the vagina during circumcision is often understood as a way to enclose or make whole those parts of the body that are seen to be 'loose' or 'rebellious'. From women's stories about pregnancy and birth in the Somali context, it would seem that woman's body are not normally subjected to the level of scrutiny women undergo in Australia. The vaginal area, in particular is not subjected to much inspection or examination. Only during birth is a woman's circumcision 'dealt' with when de-infibulation is required. It is important however to add that women's circumcision also becomes significant when women marry. Many find that they are unable to have sexual intercourse if the vaginal opening is too small. In Australia, however, women's circumcision often receives greater attention, which for a number of women is excessive and unnecessary attention.

During antenatal visits in Australia, women are queried and counseled about female circumcision and the choices they have regarding how best to deal with this. For women who might not have experienced birthing in the Australian context previously, this might be the first time that their circumcision becomes something requiring specialized care. This exposure and subsequent 'loosening' of the circumcision through de-infibulation either during pregnancy or at the birth, I believe, has left many women feeling quite vulnerable. Some women have spoken about feeling exposed once the circumcision is 'repaired' in Australia. Others simply do not like the way the vaginal area looks once its wholeness is spoilt. Many of these same women, however, also express a sense of relief as de-infibulation allows women to have a more fulfilling and pain-free sex life as well as making menstruation and urination easier.

Women's experiences of cesarean sections, I would argue, are often similarly understood. One of the striking findings in this research has been the way in which women have spoken about the possibility of undergoing a cesarean section during birth and the concern and anxiety this has provoked in a majority of women. Even when women have had no ground for such concerns, their conversations regarding cesarean sections reveal a deep-rooted anxiety. In fact, so much concern has been felt regarding the possibility of undergoing a caesarean section, that a number of women have been known to move between hospitals in order to avoid a caesarean section. In one example, a Somali woman, having been told she would

---

[1] According to Ellen Gruenbaum, 2001, it is estimated that approximately 98 percent of women born in Somalia have undergone some form of female circumcision. While the practice is illegal in Australia, it is difficult to know if any girls born in Australia have undergone female circumcision either in Australia or overseas.

Within the realm of what has been termed female circumcision there exist three main types of genital alterations (although forms that borrow from either 'clitoridectomy' or 'infibulation' will fall into different categories). The least severe form, according to Ellen Gruenbaum (2001), "are those where a small part of the clitoral prepuce ('hood') is cut away, analogous to the foreskin removal of male circumcision" (Gruenbaum, 2001: 2). This has been termed as the 'Sunna circumcision'. The "removal of the prepuce, the clitoris, and usually most or part of the labia minora, or inner lips" (Gruenbaum, 2001: 2) has been termed as "excision" or as "intermediate" forms of circumcision as it is a more severe form of clitoridectomy. The most severe form of circumcision, "entails the removal of all the external genitalia – prepuce, clitoris, labia minora, and all or part of the labia majora – and infibulation, or stitching together, of the vulva" (Gruenbaum, 2001: 3). This latter form of female circumcision leaves only a very small opening for urination and menstruation. In very severe forms sexual intercourse is impossible requiring the "cutting of the scar tissue around the opening" (Gruenbaum, 2001: 3). For birth, similar cutting of the scar tissue, or de-infibulation, needs to take place, but more extensively. The opening is usually re-infibulated after childbirth.

require a caesarean section, decided to leave that hospital and go elsewhere in the hope of finding a different outcome. Despite her endeavors, complications in her labor meant that there was little option and so the caesarean section went ahead. In another example, a woman's determination to not have a caesarean section, despite the advice from a number of doctors and midwives, almost resulted in the death of both her child and herself. In another case, a woman's refusal to have a cesarean section resulted in the death of the child – something which could have been prevented had she given permission for the procedure. While these cases are extreme examples of the outcomes of women's fears and anxieties, a majority of women have explained to me that they too would attempt to avoid a cesarean section, if only by remaining at home for as long as possible once contractions began and so going to the hospital only when absolutely necessary.

But, why is there such a concern about cesarean sections within the community? For many Somali women, there appears to be a well-established belief that they are over represented in cesarean sections performed. As one health professional explained, however, "there is no evidence to suggest that Somali women are being 'targeted' disproportionately for cesarean sections – rather it has been their perception that this is the case". Perhaps women's concerns have arisen because of their inexperience around medical procedures; maybe this resistance is based on women's lack of familiarity with the high incidence of cesarean rates found in Australia (see for example Lancaster and Pedisich, 1993; Nassar and Sullivan, 2001; Porreco and Thorp, 1996). For women who have had few dealings or exposure to such intervention, the high incidence found in Australia is viewed with alarm and apprehension. But part of the problem, I believe, has also arisen because of women's circumcision. Particularly during the early part of Somali resettlement in Australia during the mid 1990s, many Somali women felt that the high incidence of cesarean sections was intimately bound to health professionals' lack of knowledge about how to deal with female circumcision. Women felt that cesarean sections were being performed as a way to avoid the complexities surrounding female circumcision: how should the woman be 'cut'; what should happen once the circumcision has been opened; what level of re-suturing and 'repair' should be undertaken and so on. Many of these issues and debates have now been dealt with in the context of hospital care. In fact, health professionals attending Somali women during birth who have been circumcised have revealed that they prefer these women to give birth vaginally – stressing to them that cesarean sections should only be performed as a last resort. Despite these assurances, women's concerns have remained. But other issues have also created unease about cesarean sections.

As previously mentioned, the importance of large families within the Somali culture is undisputed. As a community deeply bound to communal and kinship ties, the importance of having numerous children is both highly valued and highly desired. In this context, any procedure that might limit the number of children women might have in the future is understood as something to be avoided. While it is possible to give birth vaginally after a cesarean section, women have at times been advised that to ensure the safety and well being of mother and child, it might be safer to not attempt a vaginal birth after a cesarean section. Somali women, however, are often unsure about just how many cesarean sections can be safely performed on a woman: some have cited three cesarean sections is considered safe, while others speak of women undergoing up to four cesarean sections. For many women, the prospect of having only three or four children may not be viewed as devastating. For Somali women, however, this restriction, if cesarean sections do restrict women's fertility, is acutely felt. Not only does it limit the number of children they could potentially have, but it also creates anxiety about who is controlling one's fertility. A sense of loss is, therefore, felt by women about their ability to choose the size of their families.

It has been the experience of a number of Somali women that the value and relish placed on having numerous children within the community has at times being viewed negatively and as inappropriate in the Australian setting. While few in the wider community have voiced such concerns publicly, women's conversations to me have often revealed the way in which non-Somalis have expressed such concerns at the shops, or on the street. Many women have told me how surprised non-Somalis appear when told they have four, five, sometimes up to eight children. Moreover, there appears to be a concern in the wider community about the women's financial and marital position and based on these whether they can or even should adequately provide for and allow for such large families. In this context, women's feelings about cesarean sections reveal a very real concern. It also reveals how a sense of vulnerability in the face of these opposing and contrasting values found in the Australian context could have emerged.

Resistance to caesarean sections, however, also reveals the way in which the sense of 'bodily vulnerability' or 'bodily openness' has impacted on women's perceptions. I would argue that in the same way antenatal visits and the scrutiny placed on the women's bodies there can displace their sense of wholeness and bodily integrity, cesarean sections do the same. This 'attack' on the body created through the cutting of body, may be viewed as something that jeopardizes women's ability to carry on as normal, but it also exposes women to unknown dangers and undermines women's confidence in their bodies. For example, women often spoke of the way in which cesarean sections required longer periods for recuperation and of the way in which the procedure impacted on a woman's health – particularly in relation to the possible side effects of an epidural or general anaesthetic and so on. Furthermore, as one health professional explained, women's resistance to cesarean sections could have arisen because traditionally "Somali women have a lot of confidence in their own bodies". For many Somali women, birth is understood as a natural process that does not normally require intervention preferring instead, as one health professional stated, "to do it [the natural] way". In this context, procedures like cesarean sections have the potential to jeopardize and undermine this understanding.

The 40 Day Confinement Period: Continuity and Change

These concerns about unknown dangers and possible side effects have become more resonant amongst the women because of the changes to the customary 40-day confinement period that normally follows the birth of a child. As previously mentioned the traditional 40-day confinement period provides a space for women to rest and recuperate. During this time, the mother is carefully cared for by close family and kin particularly because this period is felt to be a time of potential dangers for both mother and child given the experience of birth. In the Australian context, the 40-day confinement period has altered significantly. While women make attempts to recreate aspects of the 40-day confinement period, these are never perceived to be the same as what would have taken place 'back home' – in many ways it is almost impossible to mirror what takes place in Somalia. Again, the lack of extended family and altered way of life found in Australia has impacted on the women's lives.

Despite the significant changes to this period, women nevertheless attempt to help one another. Women's experiences of the 40 day rest period in Australia highlight the efforts women often go to following the birth of a friend's or family member's baby. They might deliver ready-made meals to families, often at great cost and effort to themselves. They might help out with the cleaning or shopping. If the mother has an unmarried sister or sister in law here, she might move in temporarily to assist the mother with the household chores. The assistance provided between family and friends in Australia, however, has become much more restricted and limited than what would have been provided in Somalia. For others, there is no semblance of the 40-day rest period. Women may have few extended family or where there is extended family present their own often-large family's responsibilities prevent them from providing extended support. As a result, women are forced to carry on as normal and as quickly as possible.

I would argue that women's inability to 'perform' the customary 40-day confinement period has been deeply felt amongst the women. It has prevented women from feeling that they are fully recovered after a birth. In so doing, the sense of fragility and vulnerability experienced by many has become more poignant, reinforcing the lost ties and connections taken for granted in the Somali context.

IMPLICATIONS FOR HEALTH AND SOCIAL CARE AND CONCLUSION

As previously mentioned, mothering and having children is an extremely important aspect within the Somali community. Women's identity is closely tied to becoming a mother. In this context, opposing and differing practices that may appear to challenge these values will be resisted and avoided sometimes with serious consequences – as in the case of cesarean sections. In addition, the pressures of the resettlement process and experiences of war and trauma suffered prior to arriving in Australia can increase women's fears and concerns as they come to terms with a new culture and new practices in a variety of situations and experiences, including those of pregnancy and birth.

It is also evident that the resettlement process can impact on women's lives in a variety of ways. While the resettlement process inevitably involves an adjustment period, this is not always necessarily simply about learning a new language, or learning new skills. As the Somali women I have spoken to reveal, resettlement can impact quite significantly on notions and practices relating to health and ideas of the self that may not be easily discernable.

In this context, the implications for health and social care resulting from this research speak about the need for health care providers to be sensitive to the way in which past trauma and experiences as well as the challenges of resettlement can continue to impact on women's lives. As Pranee Liamputtong Rice (1999b: 130) argues, attempts made to understand specific traditions and experiences can help "reduce misunderstandings and mismanagement in providing care to women". For Somali women specifically, however, is the importance of providing care that acknowledges the significance and value placed on having numerous children within the Somali community. In the case of cesarean sections, this might be achieved by providing women with better information about the possibility of giving birth vaginally after a cesarean section, thus, alleviating some of the concerns surrounding the number of children a woman might potentially be able to have.

Although traditions like the 40-day confinement period have altered markedly, women's conversations reveal that given the opportunity the ability to undertake some form of 'formal' rest period can significantly assist women in the period following a birth. While a number of maternal and child health services run by local councils as well as some shared care programs run in conjunction with large public hospitals have already implemented home visiting schemes other service providers could also be encouraged to implement such schemes. This could potentially alleviate a number of the women's concerns and feelings of vulnerability and fragility. The validation of important traditions in a new setting can also have a very positive affect on a community that may still be suffering from trauma as a result of war and marginalisation within a new location. Furthermore, the promotion and continued support of informal networks and groups as has been already been established through the formation of a number of community groups can, as Lenore Manderson and Celia McMichael (2004: 89) argue, "significantly benefit people's well being" in a number of ways. This has the potential to help a community settle more quickly and less traumatically into a new society.

For Somali women, the role and purpose of antenatal care has at times been daunting and puzzling. While large public hospitals have already put in place measures to better explain and promote the significance of preventative care, it might be worthwhile to review the way in which specific knowledge systems can continue to inform women's understanding and knowledge in the Australian setting despite educational programs in place. This might help alleviate some of the confusion experienced by health professionals in dealing with the women. Understanding the importance of wholeness in relation to the body for example might help bridge the gap that can sometimes arise between those caring for the women and the women themselves.

Many of the concerns raised by Somali women in the context of reproduction speak about the challenges they encounter regarding their reproductive choices in Australia. It also speaks to the persistence of women's strength and commitment to those elements they value. While I would argue women feel a sense of vulnerability and fragility in the Australian context, I would also contend that women's commitment to their families and the care given to them is a source of sustenance and strength for the women and as such needs to be considered and respected within the realm of health and social care. Moreover, the informal social networks that have been established within the community has ensured that continued support be provided to women despite the altered way of life found in Australia.

REFERENCES

Babatunde, E., 1998, *Women's Rites Versus Women's Rights: A Study of Circumcision Among the Ketu Yoruba of South Western Nigeria*, Africa World Press Inc: Eritrea.

Davis-Floyd, R., & Sargent, C.F., 1997, *Childbirth and Authoritative Knowledge: Cross-Cultural Perspectives*, University of California Press: Berkeley, California.

Ginsburg, F., & Rapp, R., 1991, 'The politics of Reproduction', *Annual Review of Anthropology*, 20: 311-343.

Gruenbaum, E., 2001, *The Female Circumcision Controversy: An Anthropological Perspective,* University of Pennsylvania Press: Philadelphia.

Hussein, S., 1997, 'Somalia: A Destroyed Country and a Defeated Nation', in H. M. Adam and R. Ford (eds.), *Mending Rips in the Sky: Options for Somali Communities in the 21st Century*, pp 169 – 175, The Red Sea Press: Larenceville, NJ and Asmara, Eritrea.

Jordan, B., 1993, *Birth in Four Cultures: A Cross-Cultural Investigation of Childbirth in Yucatan, Holland, Sweden and the United States*, Waveland Press: Prospect Heights, Illinois.

Kay, M. A., 1982, *The Anthropology of Birth*, F. A. Davis Co.: Philadelphia.

Kitzinger, S., 1978, *Women as Mothers*, Fontana: London.

Lancaster, P., & Pedisich, E. L., 1993, *Caesarian births in Australia: 1985-1990*, Australian Institute for Health and Welfare (AIHW) National Perinatal Statistics Unit: Melbourne.

Liamputtong Rice, P., (ed.) 1999a, *Asian Mothers, Western Birth – Pregnancy, Childbirth and Childrearing: The Asian Experience in an English-Speaking Country*, Ausmed Publication: Melbourne.

Liamputtong Rice, P., 1999b, 'When I Had my Baby Here!', in Liamputtong Rice, P., (ed.), *Asian Mothers, Western Birth – Pregnancy, Childbirth and Childrearing: The Asian Experience in an English-Speaking Country*, pp. 117-132. Ausmed Publications: Melbourne.

Liamputtong Rice, P., 2000, *Hmong Women and Reproduction*, Bergin & Garvey: Westport, CT.

Liamputtong Rice, P., & Manderson, L., 1996, *Maternity and Reproductive Health in Asian Societies*, Harwood Academic publishers: Amsterdam.

Lukere, V., & Jolly, M., (eds.), 2002, *Birthing in the Pacific: Beyond Tradition and Modernity?*', University of Hawai'i Press: Honolulu.

MacCormack, C. P., (ed.), 1994, *Ethnography of Fertility and Birth*, Waveland Press Inc: Prospect Heights, Illinois.

McMichael, C., 2002, 'Everywhere is Allah's Place: Islam and the Everyday Life of Somali Women in Melbourne, Australia', *Journal of Refugee of Studies*, 15(2): 171-188.

McMichael, C., & Manderson, L., 2004, 'Somali Women and Well-Being: Social Networks and Social Capital Among Immigrant Women in Australia', *Human Organization*, 63(1): 88-100.

Mallett, S., 2003, *Conceiving Cultures: reproducing people and places on Nuakata, Papua New Guinea*, University of Michigan Press: Ann Arbor.

Martin, E., 1989, *The woman in the body: a cultural analysis of reproduction*, Open University Press: Milton Keynes.

Morton, H., 2002, 'From Ma'uli to Motivator: Transformations in Reproductive Health Care in Tonga, in V. Lukere and M. Jolly (eds.), *Birthing in the Pacific: Beyond Tradition and Modernity?*', pp. 31-55. University of Hawai'i Press: Honolulu.

Nassar, N., & Sullivan, E. A., 2001, *'Australia's mothers and babies 1999'*, Australian Institute of health and Welfare (AIHW) National Perinatal Perinatal Statistics Unit: Canberra.

Nsubuga-Kyobe, A., & Dimock, L., 2000, *African Communities and Settlement Services in Victoria: Towards Best Practice Service, Delivery Models*, Department of Immigration and Multicultural Affairs: Melbourne.

O'Brien, M., 1980, *The politics of reproduction*, Routledge and Kegal Paul: Boston and London.

Oakley, A., 1984, *The captured womb: a history of the medical care of pregnant women*, Blackwell: Oxford.

Porreco, R, & Thorp, J., 1996, 'The caesarean birth epidemic: trends, causes and solutions', *American Journal of Obstetrics and Gynecology*, 175: 369-374.

Ram, K., & Jolly, M., 1998, (eds.), *Maternities and modernities: colonial and postcolonial experiences in Asia and the Pacific*, Cambridge University Press: New York.

Scheper-Hughes, N., 1992, *Death Without Weeping: The Violence of Everyday Life in Brazil*, University of California Press: Berkeley, Los Angeles.

Rich, A., 1977, *Of woman born: motherhood as experience and institution*, Virago: London.

Young, I. M., 1990, *Throwing like a girl and other essays in feminist philosophy and social theory*, Indiana University Press: Bloomington.

PART FOUR: MOTHERHOOD

In: Reproduction, Childbearing and Motherhood
Editor: Pranee Liamputtong, pp. 211-220

ISBN: 978-1-60021-606-0
© 2007 Nova Science Publishers, Inc.

Chapter 13

MOTHERHOOD AS A SCRIPT FOR NATIONHOOD[1]

Jamileh Abu-Duhou

INTRODUCTION

I have six children. Each of their birth has a story. As soon as I get pregnant, my husband gets arrest. And as soon as he is released, I get pregnant again. I had my son Ahamd while I was visiting his father in prison. I had Jamal, while his father was hiding (i.e. underground). Visiting my husband in hiding made me so stressed and I could not breastfeed Jamal, so I got pregnant during that time. Bearing children and the struggle have been our life. (Salema)

Since the 1980s, women's political struggle in the domain of reproductive rights and fertility control has been about the right to control over one's body, and the female body has been the primary site of such control (Petechesky, 1995). The female body becomes, as Susan Bordo (1989) notes, both a text of culture and a site of social control. Such control is embodied in a set of cultural assumptions about the appropriate embodiment, about womanhood and, in turn, motherhood (Hegde, 2001).

In contemporary Palestine, motherhood has been exalted both in the political and cultural texts, but only the right kind of mother is socially and nationally validated as the mother who can bear sons for the revolution. Traditional images of motherhood continue to circumscribe women's roles within the biological framework, devaluing women and reducing their maternal body to a machine for producing sons. Hegde (2001: 283) contends, "unpacking cultural constructions of motherhood and its emblematic status reveals".

This socio-cultural context is further reinforced by the political legacy of the Palestinian people. Women, like other Palestinians, have faced and lived with the hardships of the Israeli military occupation for many years, and the 1987 Intifada brought thousands of Palestinians including women into the streets. For women, such active participation added further complexities to their status (Abdo, 1999 not given in the Ref section - please add). While their

---

[1] This Article is based on the author's doctoral thesis 'Giving Voice to the Voiceless: Gender-based Violence in Palestine' (Key Centre for Women's Health in Society, University of Melbourne, Australia).

political participation exposed them to new ideas, values and challenges, the exposure did not increase their social freedom or reduce the traditional gender roles within the family.

Close examination of reproductive politics in Palestine, reveals a complex interplay between cultural and national meaning in the appropriation of women's bodies as reproductive instruments of the nation. According to Yuval-Davis and Anthias (1989: 8):

> They [Women] not only signify the nation but also embody it as subjects, as authors narrating the nation, as participant and leaders in nationalist struggle, and as those who bear and nurture children for nation-state projects.

In Palestine, the development of the specific ideological construction of women as national producers has had much to do with the specificity of the historical development of the Palestinian society as permanently under threat of war and political conflict. Particularly since the Israeli army deliberately targeted women, for instance women giving birth at a military checkpoint, preventing them from reaching hospitals or medical care, further humiliating them. Wick's (2002: 7), describes such experience as "a humiliating and dangerous experience for mother and a rude passage into this world for the newborn".

THE STUDY

The purpose of this research was to investigate gender-based violence (GBV) within the boundaries of the home, by analysing the hierarchical structure of gender relations in the society. This ethnographic study attempted to explore how cultural, social, religious, legal, and political issues related to the abuse of a group of married women in their reproductive age in the Palestinian society. The overall aim of this study was, to assess how the social, cultural, religious, and legal systems in the Palestinian National Territories (PNTs), coupled with the political environment affect women's experience of violence.

This study is an anthropological study of the Palestinian culture and society, it uses a range of qualitative methods to describe and analyse the socio-cultural setting, the religious, the legal and the political environments of the PNTs in order to understand the abuse that may be experienced by Palestinian women. This study used a range of qualitative methods namely: Semi-structured in-depth interview in order to obtain narratives from participants, key informants interview, to collect information about the socio-cultural setting, and the religious, the legal and the political environments of Palestine, in order to understand Palestinian women's experienced.

Recruitment for the study focused around five health service centres. These included two urban health centres, two health centres in nearby villages, and the only Women's Centre located in one of the refugee camps. While the choice of particular health sites in the rural areas, was based on the size of the catchment area of the health centre, and the social and economic diversity of the village, in the city the research was conducted in the only two governmental health centres.

The health centres were the most appropriate places to recruit married women of reproductive age (15-50 years), and the health centres were the most common places to find these women in all localities-urban, rural and camps-. In rural villages, health centres traditionally have served as a social gathering place particularly for these women, for whom social mobility is restricted by cultural and traditional systems. Thus, the act of going to the health centre for medical care either for a woman herself or for one of her children provided a legitimate excuse for her to leave the house and meet other women. And, by being the only medical and health services available in the rural areas, this meant that all women in a given area would have to come to the centre. Similarly, in urban areas, the Governmental Primary Health Care Centres are the only health services that offer immunisation and well-baby clinic services. Thus, most of the women of the targeted age would come to the centres. In refugee camps, the Women's Activity Centre provided me with access to a wide range of women from different age groups and socio-economic background, as the centres served as a place for social gatherings for most of the women residents in the camp.

RESEARCH SETTING

I arrived in the Palestinian National Territories to conduct my fieldwork research late October 2000. At that time, the political environment was not conducive for conducting research. In September 2000, the Palestinian National Territories (PNTs) began again to witness unprecedented levels of political violence, hence the political environment was and still is not conducive for conducting research. The political violence then and now could be translated into a widespread and a pervasive sense of loss of control for Palestinians in general and men particularly, which in turn would threaten women's ability to negotiate changes in their social status.

THEORETICAL FRAMEWORK

The theoretical framework of this research included both the structural elements and the socio-cultural factors that delineate women's status in the Palestinian society. The Palestinian case is unique in that the political environment drives activities within the society, as much as they are driven by all other systems (such as marriage and the family). Voice and experience were an integral part of this research, and the analysis was grounded in the empirical data and concepts that emerged from the interviews and the textual analysis of secondary document.

FINDINGS

The data I have gathered[22] has demonstrated that gender inequality is the crux of the gender socialisation process that enforces patriarchal control and gender inequality as well as the subordination of women through limiting women's life choices to marriage and through the repression of female sexuality. The formation and construction of gender identity have far reaching implications for women's status and role in society, and how masculine and feminine identities are perceived.

---

[2] Pseudonyms have been used to protect the identity of individual women.

Social Construction of Motherhood

> People call me Hajeh, although , I never went to Mecca for the pilgrim. See I am old, and I do
> not have a son to be called Umm (mother of). I have five daughters. My husband did not want
> to take a second wife for the son. He use to say 'This is the will of god to give us only girls
> and we should not question his will'. (Fatima)

In the Palestinian society, social and cultural conditions stresses the values and norms
associated with traditional ideas of femininity and motherhood, and the process of socializing
girls is aimed at enforcing traditional norms and values about femininity. To be feminine, a
girl is conditioned to be docile, submissive, discreet, modest and soft-spoken. Girls are taught
to be obedient, submissive and 'feminine'. The social and psychological pressure on girls to
adapt to their traditional female role, which starts so very early, increases with age and takes
concrete shape during adolescence. The behaviour of teenage girls is controlled even more
than during childhood. An adolescent girl must not have an opinion, must not show emotions
or have any aspirations. Girls learn that their social value is attached to that of their fathers,
brothers, and later to their husbands and their children, particularly male children. Rozario
2002: 45, writing on identity construction and adolescent women in Bangladesh argues that
"Marriage is still the only status available for adult women in rural Bangladesh... This is as
definitive for the adult identity of Bengali Christian women as it is for Muslim and Hindu
women". Similarly, in the Palestinian society, an adult unmarried woman remains a *binet*,
until married, and she remains socially a child. Her passage to adulthood is confirmed when
she bears male children, when she becomes *Umm* "the mother of" the male child. A married
woman with only female children is never called *Umm*, mother of, but rather is referred to as
the *Mara'h*, which literally means a married woman (Al-Khayyat, 1990). According to Nadia
her deliveries were near death experiences nevertheless, she continued to get pregnant:

> All my pregnancies and deliveries are very difficult. I always need to have an operation (i.e.
> Caesarean section). The birth of my first girl was the easiest. The birth of my second girl was
> difficult; I lost a lot of blood. The doctor told me not to get pregnant again. He said if you
> want to have another child wait a year or two. But I could not. See I had only two daughters
> and no sons. My husband and his family kept nagging me to have a son. My husband use to
> say, 'You want me to stay childless, you must bear me a son.' So I got pregnant again and
> again and again until my fifth pregnancy it was a boy, thank God. My third was very difficult;
> I almost died during childbirth. I was in intensive care for a whole week. Six months later I
> was pregnant again with my fourth girl, and the same story. (Nadia)

Her role in life is predetermined for her by the family and the society, not only as a wife
and a mother, but also as the kind of mother that bears male children. Palestinian parents in
general wish for a baby boy, especially if the firstborn is not a boy or the couple have too
many daughters already. During nine months of pregnancy the parents' expectations
concerning their future male baby differ from their expectations for a baby girl. Palestinian
parents in general wish for a baby boy. The delivery of a boy is celebrated with greater joy
than that of a girl. For instance, when a mother delivers a baby girl, she is consoled by well
wishers for her failure by a popular saying *"Allah Iwad Aileki bi el sabe"* which means
literally, "may God compensates you for your loss with the birth of a boy". Socially, this
means that the birth of a girl is treated as a loss, which only can be compensated by the birth

of a boy. The birth of the son is celebrated, while the birth of a daughter is mourned. Suha describes the birth of her daughter as

> I had my son first, and when he was born, my husband's family celebrated his birth with a party that lasted for a week. And when I had my daughter, everyone in the family including my husband had a long face. They did not even offer sweets for the people who came to the hospital. My mother cried and said to my husband "do not worry god willing she will bear you a son next time." My husband was so upset then, he even replied "if there is another time." (Suha)

In Palestinian society, the son not only carries the family name and passes it on to his own children, hence, securing the future existence of the family, but also inherits the family wealth, and carries the responsibility of caring for his parents and their economic survival. Even though a daughter may take care of her parents, she is not expected to secure the family income (Manasra, 1993; Taraki, 1997). Noura spoke of her pain, suffering and humiliation she had to bear for her failure to produce sons:

> I have to get pregnant again. I have been trying for two years now. I have three daughters but that is not enough. I must have a son. My daughters need a brother, a man to protect them. Everybody including my mother keeps nagging me about it. My mother says to me 'you need to have a son. Your husband needs a son to carry on his name or he will marry a second wife to bear a son for him. And if he does marry again, no one can blame him. Not even us your parents, you failed to bring him a son. (Noura)

In cultures such as Palestine where children are considered as a sign of a woman's social achievement, women become powerless and unable to control their reproductive life. According to Toubia and colleagues (1994, quoted by Abu-Hwaij, 1996: 5), "Gender and social roles which privilege men... women have little control over their own sexual and reproductive decisions". According to one Palestinian woman, it is too late to leave her husband because of her children. They are not only a symbol of her social status as mothers but also the only sign of her life achievements:

> I can't leave my children. And now it is too late to get a divorce, after I had a tubelugation. Now I can't have more children, suppose I get a divorce and remarried again, I can't have children, So I would have got out of the world nothing, I lost my children and I can't have any more children. (Nahla)

This social-cultural construction of motherhood as reflected by the prevailing cultural norms, values and practices, makes pregnancy, birth and motherhood an experience filled with anxiety and fear. Although, Palestinian women identity and passage to women hood is bond by their ability to reproduce and become mothers, however, their claim to motherhood maybe denied once they fail to reproduce sons.

Motherhood: Fertile Mother of the National Collective

> My husband is a fighter, he fights for liberation, he does his national duties. And I also must
> do my duties to Palestine and buy the price. I am a simple woman and the only thing I can do
> is to have children for Palestine. (Sarah)

Palestinian men and women, who have lived under the Israeli Occupation since 1967,
have equally joined the national struggle for freedom and independence. Many men and
women have been arrested, imprisoned and tortured (Sabbagh, 1998). While Palestinian
women have participated actively and equally in the political and national struggle with men,
the Palestinian nationalist narratives has continued to differentiate between masculinity and
femininity on the basis of traditionally constructed gender roles (Hiltermann, 1998).
According to Yuval-Davis (1997), nationalist narrative has tended to portray women as the
'biological' reproducers of the national collectives, while at the same time it has represented
men as the civil or 'military' reproducers of the nation, and in control of the decision-making
processes. This suggests that despite women's symbolic role as "mothers of the nation",
women are subordinated in the actual political processes of the national struggle or and in the
politics of nation building. For example, the Palestinian Basic Law limits the transition of
Palestinian citizenship rights from father to son, which signifies that the reproduction of
national identity is actually channelled through paternity not maternity (Massad, 1995).

A related image to that of 'mother of the nation' is also the image of being a 'fertile
mother'. This construction of the image of 'fertile mother' by the Palestinian national
leadership was motivated by Israel's definition of the conflict as a 'demographic one', in
which victory would be achieved by the side with the largest population. A popular
Palestinian saying, for example, boasts that "The Israelis beat us at the borders but not the
bedroom" (Abdulhadi, 1998: page number????). And as one Palestinian woman explained
how her husband who was a political activist insisted she bear more children particularly sons
to carry on fighting for the nation:

> As soon as I get pregnant, my husband gets arrested and I gave birth with him away in prison.
> And as soon as he gets released from prison, I get pregnant again. As soon as my husband
> come home from prison, in his the first night home, he would say 'you must get pregnant
> again. What if I get killed? I need many children, boys to continue to fight for Palestine'.
> (Randa)

The demographic struggle has always been a main feature of the Palestinian-Israeli
conflict. In 1931, there were only 58,000 Jews and 642,000 Palestinian Arabs in Palestine. In
1922, 175,000 Jews, and 861,000 Palestinian Arabs. On the eve of the 1948 war, the number
of Jews was 650,000 compared to 1,454,00 Palestinians Arabs (Farsoun and Zacharia, 1997).
Both Palestinian and Israeli leaders have always thought of the demography of Palestine as a
determining factor for victory in the conflict. While Israel has been trying to increase the
population of Jews inside Palestine by opening the borders to Jewish immigration from all
over the world, Palestinians have been trying to uphold their livelihood and resist their
uprooting from their homeland through various measures of resistance including the
maintenance of a high fertility rate. Hence the call for 'bearing children for the revolution'

has been heard repeatedly from the late PLO Chairman Yasser Arafat as he encouraged women to have no less than 12 children each (Najjer, 1992: 258). This national image of the fertile mother has precautions on the fertility levels. In practice, women continued to bear children for the revolution causing the total fertility rate to peak at 7.05 in the early 1980s, continuing at the high rate of 6.06 in 1995 (Palestinian Bureau of Statistics, Health Survey, 2000). As Samia explained,

> I married my cousin, he was a refugee in Jordan. We came back to Palestine to live in the refugee camp, so I can do a family unification for him. He said 'I want my children to be born here in Palestine. He wanted many children. He said 'I want sons, I want them Palestinians.' So soon as he got his papers (i.e. the unification papers) we started to have children not before. Thanks be to god, I gave birth to six sons and three daughters.

Massad (1995) argues that the Palestinian nationalist movement consciously signified the Zionist conquest of Palestine as 'rape of the land' and the Palestinians as the 'children of Palestine' and Palestine as 'mother'. In his word, Massad said that the 'rape' had 'disqualified' women from being able to legally reproduce the 'children of Palestine' – the Palestinians. This assertion by the national movement is reflected in construction of the Palestinian identity, as codified in the National Charter (Articles 4 and 5), and defined as:

> a genuine, inherited and eternal trait and is transmitted from fathers to sons. ... Palestinians are those Arab citizens who used to reside in Palestine until 1947 ... and everyone who born of an Arab Palestinian father after this date – whether inside or outside Palestine (Massad, 1995: 472-473).

In short, the Palestinian national agent is a masculine young male, and there is a complete absence of femininity and of women issues from the national discourse. Hence, Palestinian women's involvement in the national struggle has not resulted in significantly modifying their cultural-traditional motherhood role. The nationalist Palestinian movement worked to reinforce women's subordination through the mobilization of their reproductive functions in order to reinforce and reproduce the paternal identity of the nation. Hence, making the experience of motherhood a mere response to a national crisis and what was before a reference to women's productive function in the domestic realm is now elevated as gender characteristics that promotes women to the frontline confrontation with soldiers. As one narrate her life story under occupation

> I was the only one from my sibling that remained in our village with my parents. Our family all of them became refugees in Jordan after 1967 occupation, and my two brothers when they went to study at university in Lebanon, they joined the revaluation so they could not came back to the village, my three sisters married my cousins and went to live in Amman, and when it was my turn to marry, my father had told my uncle, he would not marry me off to his son, unless his son accept except to come and live in the village back in Palestine. So he did, I made a family unification papers for him. Now, it is up to me and to him to preserve the whole family right to Palestine. I gave birth to five children, three were girls, and one of the boys in prison for life. When I visited him last time, he asked me to bring him a brother, to fight for Palestine, because he can't now. I promised that I will give him a brother. I am young, I am only 39 years old, I was married when I was 16 years old, did not have a chance

to fight for Palestine. Now I can give birth to sons to fight for Palestine, it is my duty. I am not pregnant yet, but I am trying, *Insallah*. (Fatama)

In September 2000, the Palestinian Territories began again to witness unprecedented levels of political violence. Undoubtedly, these events would have dire implications on the state-building and democratisation of society, not least on women's efforts to promote a women's rights agenda in general, and reproductive rights in particular. The emotional needs of the Palestinian people, who are in a permanent state of war, when husbands and sons might get killed at any moment, play a much more central role than anything else in shaping the reproductive and motherhood experience of women, as described by *Umm* Sameer (Mother of Sameer, a Palestinian Martyr),

> I look at their pictures and read their notebooks. In all this I see how this violence and oppression took me children away from me. My older son looked forward to martyrdom. He wrote while alive that he would become a martyr. But my younger one did not see anything but revenge for his brother's killing. As if children are suppose to revenge the death of their loved one. I ask myself, why should this be the children's war and not the adult's war? Why should we mothers have to suffer the pain of losing our children? Look how Yassar wrote about martyrdom and how Sameer answered him back with revenge. (Umm Sameer)

As a result of this on-going loss of control and of lives, women's reproductive role as bearers of fighters and as mothers of the martyred becomes not only a symbol of the nation but also as a symbol of resistance (Johnson and Kuttab, 2001). Occupation itself was not within their power having more children was the only reaction available to them in the face of occupation., thus women were like factories increasing the production of ammunition during war. As Nahada said,

> Before this *Intifada,* we made a decision not to have any more children. We have three children, a boy and two girls, thanks to God they are healthy children. Now, my husband starts to say to me we must have another child, a boy,, he says if the Israeli, kill Ahamd, out son, we at least have another boy, besides, our generation could not win the fight for Palestine, maybe our children generation could, so it is our national duty to have children for Palestine. '(Nahada)

Mohammed Durra, became known to the world as the 12-year-old who was killed by repeated Israeli fire while his father's attempts to shelter him failed. Two years on, his mother was reported to have given a birth to baby boy and called him Mohammed. The case of Durra's mother, like that of many Palestinian women, suggests that the real dilemma for Palestinian women is not mothering sons, rather it is a more complex dilemma. Giving birth is seen by many Palestinian women as an act of defiance, an act of resistance and as a way of coming to terms with their terrible grief.

CONCLUSION

While, the prevailing cultural and social norms and values of the Palestinian society, giving birth to male children in the prevailing cultural and social norms of the Palestinian society legitimise the motherhood experience of women, at the same time such experience is seen as a form of Palestinian patriotism. They are the practical means of thwarting Israeli occupation policies that are designed to make life unbearable for Palestinians, in order either to drive them to migrate or to eliminate them altogether. What is more significant for Palestinian women is the need to resist and to survive this on-going violent oppression – needs which are strongly linked to the national aspiration of the Palestinian people. In any discussion of Palestinian women motherhood experience or their reproductive rights, we cannot afford to forget the connection between the right to motherhood and the national rights. Furthermore, this tension suggests that women are particularly caught in the tensions between the contradictory projects of nationalism and that of culture. Affirmations of national identity often entails control over women bodies and their reproductive roles.

REFERENCES

Abdulhadi, R., 1998, 'The Palestinian Women's Autonomous Movement: Emergence, dynamics and challenges', *Gender and Society*, 12(2): 649-73.

Abu-Hwaij, A., 1996, *Policy Implication for Reproductive Healthcare Delivery in the Rural West Bank*, World University Service and Union of Palestinian Medical Relief Committees: London.

Antonius, S., 1983, 'Fighting on Two Fronts: Conversation with Palestinian women', in S. Al-Khayyat (ed.), *Honour and Shame: Women in Modern Iraq*, Saqi Books: London.

Bordo, S., 1989, 'The Body of the Reproduction of Femininity: A feminist Appropriation of Faucault', in A. Jaggat and S. Bordo (ed.), *Gender/Body/Knowledge: feminist Reconstruction of Being and Knowing.* Rutgers University Press: New Brunswick.

Farsoun, S., & Zacharia, C., 1997, *Palestine and the Palestinian*, Westview Press: Boulder.

Hegde, R., 2001, 'Sons and Mothers: Framing the Maternal Body and the Politics of Reproduction in South Indian Context', in M. DeKoven (ed.), *Feminist Locations: Global and Local Theory and Practice*, pp. 282-303. Rutgers University Press: New Brunswick.

Hiltermann, J., 1998, 'The Women's Movement During the Uprising', in S. Sabbagh (ed.), *Palestinian Women of Gaza and the West Bank.* Indiana University Press: Bloomington.

Johnson, P., & Kuttab, E., 2001, 'Where Have All the Women (and Men) Gone? Reflections on gender and the second Palestinian Intifada', *Feminist Review*, 69: 21-43.

Manasra, N., 1993, 'Palestinian Women: Between traditions and revolution' in E. Augustin (ed.), *Palestinian Women: Identity and experience.* Zed Books: London.

Massad, J., 1995, 'Conceiving the Masculine: Gender and Palestinian nationalism', *The Middle East Journal,* 49.3: 407-90.

Najjer, O. (ed.) 1992, *Portraits of Palestinian Women*, University of Utah Press: Salt Lake.

Palestinian Bureau of Statistics, 2000, *Health Survey- 2000, Main findings*, Ramallah: Palestine.

Petechesky, R., 1995, 'The Body as Property: A Feminist Re-vision', in F. Ginsburg and R. Rapp (ed.), *Conceiving the New World Order. The Global Politics of Reproduction*, pp. 387-406. University of California Press: Berkeley.

Rozario, S., 2002, 'Poor and 'Dark': What is my future? Identity construction and adolescent women in Bangladesh', in L. Manderson and P. Liamputtong (eds.), *Coming of Age in South and Southeast Asia: Youth, courtship, and sexuality*, pp. 42-57. Curzon Press: Surrey.

Sabbagh, S. (ed) 1998, *Palestinian Women of Gaza and The West Bank*, Indiana University Press: Bloomington.

Taraki, L., 1997, *Palestinian Society: Contemporary realities and trends*, Women's Studies Programme, Birzeit University: Birzeit.

Toubia, N., Bahyeldin, A., & Abdel-Latif, H., 1994, *Arab Women: A profile of diversity and change*, Population Council: Cairo.

Wick, L., 2002, *Birth at the Checkpoint, the Home or the Hospital? Adapting to the Changing Reality in Palestine*, Institute of Community and Public Health, Birzeit University: Birzeit.

Yuval-Davis, N., 1997, *Gender and Nation*, Sage Publication: London.

Yuval-Davis, N., & Anthias, F., (eds.) 1989, *Women-Nation-State*, MacMillan: London.

In: Reproduction, Childbearing and Motherhood
Editor: Pranee Liamputtong, pp. 221-237

ISBN: 978-1-60021-606-0
© 2007 Nova Science Publishers, Inc.

Chapter 14

DOUBLE IDENTITIES: THE LIVED EXPERIENCE OF MOTHERHOOD AMONG HMONG IMMIGRANT WOMEN IN AUSTRALIA

Pranee Liamputtong and Denise Spitzer

INTRODUCTION

Motherhood – unmentioned in the histories of conquest and serfdom, wars and treaties, exploration and imperialism – has a history, it has an ideology, it is more fundamental than tribalism or nationalism. (Adrian Rich, 1992: 34)

If in Laos then I don't know, I may have about ten children, it could happen, because in Laos you need to have many children to be able to help you make the living on the farm. In this country, if you have many children, now it is ok, but when they grow older they will go to school and they will need to study and they will need money. I don't think that I will be able to provide for everyone if I have too many children.... Yes, it is the difficulty in raising children here. (A Hmong woman)

Studies concerning migrant women as a distinct category, Morokvasic (1983) argues, have not received much attention. According to Morokvasic (1983: 18), prior to 1970s migrant women "remain silent and invisible, present as a variable, absent as a person". Migrant women are, therefore, treated as "unproductive, and not worth investigating" (Liam, 1991: 31). Similarly, in her writing about motherhood, Bhopal (1998: 485) argues that existing literature on motherhood has been "ethnocentric and falsely universalistic. Motherhood has often been examined from a white, western perspective, neglecting divisions based upon 'race' and ethnicity." Bhobal (1998) suggests that it is likely that women from different ethnic groups may have different perceptions and experiences of motherhood. .

In this chapter, we attempt to address this issue by interviewing a sample of women drawn from a study with immigrant women who are now living in Melbourne, Australia. We attempt to answer how these immigrant women construct themselves as mothers and as migrant women and practise motherhood in a new homeland.

In Australia, as in most Western societies, studies on motherhood are primarily undertaken with women from Anglo-Celtic and middle class backgrounds (e.g., Harper and Richards, 1979; Wearing, 1984; Crouch and Manderson, 1993; Brown et al., 1994, 1997; Everingham, 1994; Maushart, 1997; Lupton, 2000; Lupton and Fenwick, 2001; Manne, 2005; Buultjens and Liamputtong, 2007). Studies of how women, from ethnic groups, view motherhood and how they experience being a mother have been few. Only in the last few years that we start to witness some writing of motherhood from non-White perspectives (see Liam, 1991, 1999; Liamputtong, 2001; Liamputtong and Naksook, 2003a, b; Liamputtong, 2006). Liam (1999) examined the experiences of Chinese first-time migrant mothers who come from different countries, and found that these first-time immigrant mothers have to encounter double transitions in their mothering roles and adjustment to motherhood. Becoming a first-time mother is overwhelming and with the burden of migration process, it makes the tasks of motherhood even harder for these Chinese migrant mothers. Similar accounts of migrant motherhood were also discussed in Liamputtong's (2001) personal account of being a mother in Australia. In this paper, Liamputtong demonstrates multiple marginalities of herself and several Thai women due largely to being an immigrant woman in a new homeland.

Motherhood is complex and multi-faceted (Bhopal, 1998). Just as the experience of motherhood varies according to class structure and family forms (Boulton, 1983; Sharp, 1984; Phoenix, 1988; Doyal, 1995; Liam 1991, 1999; McMahon, 1995; Maushart, 1997; Manne, 2005), ethnicity also has important effect on women's lives as mothers (Collins, 1994; Glenn, 1994; Bhopal, 1998; Liamputtong, 2001; Liamputtong et al., 2002, 2004; Liamputtong, 2006). Models of mothering, we contend, need to take into account ethnicity and class if the voices of many women, who wish to become a mother, can be heard.

THE HMONG IN AUSTRALIA

The Hmong in Australia are refugees from Laos. They left their country around the end of the Vietnam War in 1975; by and large in the same period as their counterparts who have settled in the United States. However, their resettlement in Australia has been slower. The Hmong first settled as refugees in Australia in 1976 (Lee, 1999), mostly in New South Wales. Between 1980 and 1991 there have been a small number of Hmong coming into Australia under the Family Reunion Program and the Community Refugee Settlement Scheme (Lee, 1999; Tapp and Lee, 2004).

There are about 250,000 Hmong living in the United States (Cha, 2000, 2003). In Australia, the number of Hmong is far less than in the US. It is estimated that there are about 1500 to 1800 Hmong in Australia (Stone, 1998; Lee, 1999; Liamputtong Rice, 2000). This number is based on an estimation of Hmong community leaders in Melbourne, as there are no official statistics collected on the Hmong *per se*. Officially, the Hmong in Australia are included under "people born in Laos".

According to Lee (1999), in 1986 there were 384 Hmong living in Sydney, Melbourne, Hobart, Adelaide and Canberra. However, the 1996 Australian census indicated 1420 "Hmong-speakers" in Australia; 603 in Queensland, 384 in Victoria, 272 in Tasmania, 126 in New South Wales, 29 in the ACT, and 3 in Western Australia. However, for those who defined themselves as having "Hmong ethnicity" the numbers are 1,603. These include: 748 in Queensland, 397 in Victoria, 257 in Tasmania, 161 in New South Wales, 28 in the ACT, 7 in Western Australia, and 5 in South Australia. In the last eight years, we have seen a secondary migration among the Hmong from the southeastern states to the far north of Queensland, mainly for economic reasons. This is the only area where they can do farming, and as Lee (1999) argues, the region's rain forests "remind them of their old home in the highlands of Laos".

In Victoria, where the study was undertaken, the Hmong live in close knit groups, mainly in high-rise public housing in an inner suburb and one outer suburb in the State capital, Melbourne. With new children being born into families, the number of Hmong in Melbourne, estimated in 1998 (Hmong Australia Society Inc, 1998), was 497. These included: 98 males and 96 females who are over 18; and 153 males and 150 females under 18.

Although more Hmong are unemployed relative to other Southeast Asian refugees in Australia, it is estimated that 35% of Hmong households now engage in small businesses. In addition, many Hmong now either have their own banana farms or work as hired labour for banana growers in northern Queensland around Cairns and Innisfail (Lee, 1999).

Most Hmong in Australia have not been converted to Christianity as their counterparts in the US have (see Cha, 2000, 2003). Although we have seen changes in Hmong life due to the need to adapt to a new environment, their culture has not altered greatly. Quincy (1995) states that Hmong children in the US speak little Hmong and more and more Hmong women exercise greater independence in the family. Our observations have not reflected the same trend among the Hmong in Australia, except for a few families which have done better or those who have settled for a longer period of time.

By and large, the Hmong in Australia try to maintain their cultural heritage, particularly among the first generation. They live relatively quiet lives, as most small minorities do. Health and illness are still interpreted within their cultural framework, but they have no hesitation in seeking Western health care if need be (Wang, 1998; cf. Cha, 2000, 2003. They still strive for freedom and resist being absorbed or assimilated into the host society, as has always been the case historically, but more so in Australia with its multicultural approach to migrant settlement (Tapp and Lee, 2004).

In general the Hmong are much poorer than other Southeast Asian refugees. Most Hmong are still unemployed, lack formal education, and many are still learning English. Culturally, the Hmong are animistic and follow Ancestor worship. They believe in reincarnation; the rebirth cycle. The Hmong are patrilineal and patrilocal. Family names follow the clan system (Cha, 2000, 2003). There are ten clans in Melbourne. The usual Hmong family is large.

Most Hmong women in this study described here have approximately four to six children and it is likely they will continue to have more children. Traditionally, the Hmong put a high value on having many children, particularly boys, since they could help in farming and continue traditional practices such as worshiping ancestral spirits, caring for their parents in old age, and carrying on the clan name. Such traditional customs are still practiced (see also Cha, 2000, 2003).

THEORETICAL FRAMEWORK

Gender, Identity and Gender Role Expectations

Gender, Croucher (2004: 179) suggests, "like ethnicity and nationhood, is a social and political construct. It is a category or mechanism of assignment and control as well as a source and site of belonging". While gender is generally allied along the axis of the dichotomous pairing of male and female, ethnicity, sexuality and class intersect to produce disparate and often multiple notions of gender (Cerulo, 1997).

Migration can further contribute to a re-conceptualization of gender identity and often necessitates a renegotiation of gender roles both within and without the realm of the family (Buijs, 1993). The fragmentation of kinship and friendship networks and changes in labour market participation compel immigrant and refugee households to reconfigure domestic responsibilities and to adjust to potentially different income generating roles and activities. These potential alterations in gender roles are further influenced by pre-migration experiences including preparation for, and decision-making about, leaving one's country of origin, linguistic capabilities, professional and educational background, and the disparities between the dominant culture in the country of resettlement and one's own ethnic heritage. Moreover, the historical and current linkages between countries of origin and resettlement through colonial and neo-colonial legacies, historical or contemporary conflict, and trade, will influence reception of migrants (Krulfeld and Camino, 1994). These matters may be reflected in the production of structural inequalities induced by admission criteria, the intensity of security concerns, the willingness to recognize educational and professional credentials, and expressions of personal racism. Thus, the ability of migrant women and men to participate in, and be accepted by, the host society is substantially informed by country of origin.

Crossing borders may also mean being transformed from being a member of a culture where most individuals in one's vicinity shared a common heritage to becoming a member of an ethnic minority. In this environment, newcomers ally themselves with a set of commonalities that create a sense of inclusivity while rendering others outside of these boundaries to establish communal identity (Hall, 1996; Gupta and Ferguson, 1997). While these "meeting points" provide the ground upon which to establish a multiplicity of identities (Hall, 1996), the repositioning of cultural identity in particular often requires members of minority communities to shore up the boundaries of ethnicity to prevent or reduce the threat of dissolution from the perceived onslaught from the dominant society.

As the meaning and boundaries of nations are embedded in cultural symbols and as women's bodies serve as some of the most potent symbols for demarcating these boundaries (Croucher, 2004), patrolling women's bodies and women's roles becomes increasingly important in sustaining ethnic borders in pluralist societies (Spitzer et al., 2003). Gendered responsibilities pertaining to care work, mothering and sexuality can be more intensely charged with moral valence in diasporic communities as women are expected to model "ideal" cultural behaviour and transmit these lessons to the next generation (Braun et al., 1996; Espín, 1999; Spitzer et al., 2003). Espín (1999) further maintains that efforts to preserve tradition that centre primarily on women's roles and controlling women's sexual and reproductive behaviour allows members of minority communities to assert a sense of moral superiority over the dominant racist society. Hmong motherhood in Australia, therefore, must be contextualized by the desire and need to sustain Hmong and Thai identity through social and biological reproduction.

Motherhood and Multiple Identities

Taking the symbolic interactionist perspective (Blumer, 1969), McMahon (1995: 15) argues that to better understand women as mothers, it is essential to examine the social processes whereby the women conceptualize themselves as mothers. Symbolic interactionism locates "meanings, identity, and experience of everyday life at the centre of its explanation of the social world. It conceptualized individuals as creative social actors whose conduct is oriented toward situations and objects on the basis of meanings these have for them" (McMahon, 1995: 16). As such, this conceptualization of identity implies the notion of multiple identities. As McMahon (1995: 24) puts, "a woman is never only a woman; multiple other social relationships of race, class, ethnicity, or sexuality shape the lived meaning of being female". We argue similarly that women are not simply just mothers. Rather, women have other interpersonal identities that are also salient to them and impact on their mothering roles. In the case of this study, it is the identity of being a migrant woman that is important for their motherhood and mothering (see also Liamputtong, 2006).

On becoming a mother, women seek out those who can significantly validate their valued identities. Children can be important "validators" for women's identity as a mother. Children, as McMahon (1995: 20) argues, "carry unique significance as validators not just of women's maternal identities but, by implication, of their characters as well". Accordingly, as we shall see, children's stage of being is essentially a major part of women's discourse on becoming a mother in their new homeland among the women in this study.

THE STUDY

This paper is constructed from the narratives of immigrant women in a qualitative study concerning reproductive health, including the experience motherhood, among 27 Hmong women in Melbourne, Victoria. The theoretical sampling technique (Liamputtong and Ezzy, 2005) was used to determine the number of women in the study. Put simply, the recruiting was terminated when no new data emerged. The women were recruited through different means. The Hmong women were contacted through a local community health centre and by personal contact of the bi-cultural researcher. At the first contact the women were told about the study and asked if they could talk about their experiences relating to the study. Once the women agreed to participate, an interview time was arranged to suit their needs. The women were individually interviewed in their own homes. All interviews were conducted in their native languages.

We utilize an open-ended interview approach in this study. Specifically for the issue relating to motherhood, each woman was asked to elaborate on becoming a mother in a new homeland. We open the conversation on this issue by the statement: "Please tell me what it is like to become a mother in Australia". From this, there are followed up questions that we prompted the women to elaborate further. These include problems and difficulties, happiness, what is to expect of the children, the wish to have more children and so on.

Each interview was tape-recorded. The length of the interviews varied, depending on the respondents' responses. For the motherhood section, each interview took between half an hour to forty minutes. Most women were interviewed once. There were, however, a number of occasions when we needed to obtain more information. Those women were then visited for a second time, and in some cases a third time. In addition, a participant observation method was used to allow observation and recording of the women's cultural beliefs and practices and their experiences in Australia more fully. The authors attended a number of ceremonies and participated in many activities during the fieldwork period. The initial interviews and participant observation were undertaken during 1994-1995 and follow up interview with several women was done in 1999.

For each woman, an informed consent was obtained after the information about the research and the nature of the woman's participation was clearly explained to her. Ethical approval was sought from and approved by La Trobe University Human Ethics Committee.

A thematic analysis approach was used to derive patterns in the women's responses (Miles and Huberman, 1994; Liamputtong and Ezzy, 2005). The transcripts were examined for the women's discourses related to motherhood. From these, several themes were derived. Our method of data collection (ethnography with participant observation) allowed "internal validity" (Bryman, 2001: 271) of our interpretations. In-depth interviews and participant observations conducted over a period of time allowed us to ensure a reliable level of "congruence between the concepts and observations". Women's names presented with their accounts in the paper were changed to preserve confidentiality.

THE WOMEN

The demographic characteristics of the women who participated in this study are summarised in Table 1.

THE CHALLENGE OF MIGRANT MOTHERHOOD

What does it mean to be a mother and a migrant woman at the same time? Being a mother in a new country presents certain challenge to the women's lives.

Reproduction plays a significant role in Hmong society. Without women, children may not be produced. Hence, this can threaten the Hmong society at large. Becoming a mother is, as perceived, an essential part of womanhood. Women internalize this gender role expectation through their socialization within the Hmong culture. But, how do they see it when they are no longer in Laos? Migration has changed many things in Hmong lives. Although there is evidence that the Hmong always resist change wherever they live, from China to Southeast Asia and now in Western countries like Australia (Cooper et al., 1995; Quincy, 1995; Tapp and Lee, 2004), we have also seen that the Hmong have to change their ways to some extent in a new land. Is motherhood affected by changes in a new living situation in a new homeland? We will examine this in the chapter.

Table 1. Characteristics of Hmong women in sample (n = 27)

Characteristics	No.	Percentage
Age		
20-30	9	33.34
31-40	8	29.63
41-50	4	14.81
over 51	6	22.22
Marital status		
Married	21	77.78
de facto	1	3.70
Widowed	5	18.52
Number of children		
1-3	7	25.93
4-6	15	55.56
7-9	1	3.70
10 and over	4	14.81
Level of education		
None	18	66.67
Primary	7	25.92
Secondary	2	7.41
Current activities		
Home duties	17	62.96
Learning English for migrants	7	25.93
Working	3	11.11
No. of years in Australia		
1-3	6	22.22
4-6	13	48.15
7 and over	8	29.63
No. of family members living in the house		
1-3	2	7.41
4-6	11	40.74
7-9	10	37.04
10 and over	4	14.81
Length of stay in refugee camp in Thailand (years)		
1-3	6	22.22
4-6	3	11.11
7-9	6	22.22
10 and over	12	44.45
Experience of childbirth		
In Laos only	5	18.52
In Thailand and Australia	15	55.55
In Laos, Thailand and Australia	2	7.41
In Australia only	5	18.52

The Meaning of Motherhood: Only for the Lucky Ones

Motherhood is seen as a positive part of life for women, as children look after them in old age and carry on essential rituals to send their soul back to heaven to be reborn.

> I think it is better to have children. For the Hmong, if you have children and when you get old, when you cannot support yourself, then your children can support you. So they will look after you in old age.

Only lucky women are able to become mothers, as one woman sums up: "according to Hmong tradition then I must have more luck than those who cannot have children." In addition, women's fortune and luck in having children is granted by a Hmong deity referred to as *Txoov Kab Yeeb* and they were given papers to bring to earth (their mandate of life) when they were born. Women see this as a gift for them.

> They say that having many children because heaven has given you the ability to do so. So it is a gift that the heaven has given you.

But, Hmong women also realise that conceiving, giving birth and raising children are not easy tasks for them. However, the rewards gained mean security in old age.

> It is a hard work to do but you also feel that you must have at least one or two children so that when you get older you do not envy other people who have children. If you don't have any at all then when you get older and you see other old people have children to love them, cook for them and look after them and that is when you start to envy them. But talking about when you give birth to children and bring them up it is very difficult for you. But when you get old it must be better for you.

Becoming a mother and having children also means that they will not be too lonely in old age since there will be many grandchildren around. One woman who has become a grandmother gives the following remarks:

> You have children and their children are with you and this makes you feel less lonely. You may not have young children anymore but your sons and daughters-in-law will have children and you look after their children while they go to work or go to school. The children may make a lot of noise but it won't make you worried at all. If you stay by yourself, or just the couple by themselves, how are you going to live day by day.

What then are the consequences of "unlucky" women who are not able to have a baby?

THE INFERTILE BODY: A CHILDLESS WOMAN

Infertility in Hmong society is seen as the woman's problem. Infertility not only affects the woman's identity, but also has a great impact on the identity of the "local moral worlds" (Kleinman, 1992) in which the woman lives; that is of the Hmong society. That the "infertile body" is the reflection of the "social body" in which it is located can be seen in the forms of where the blame is located and the expression of social control on the woman's body.

In all societies fertility and infertility are subject to social rules and cultural practices. These rules and practices are strictly observed and followed in traditional societies, which depend on having children to ensure the continuation of the lineage. Having children is crucial for the lives of Hmong people since it means that the lineage and hence the Hmong society will live on. It is perhaps even more crucial at present time due to a significant reduction in Hmong population due to successive loss of lives from fights with the Chinese in China prior to settlement in Laos and then the war in Laos in the 1970s (Cha, 2000; Liamputtong Rice, 2000; Tapp and Lee, 200). This has led to increased social pressure on the Hmong women. If they cannot have children they have to allow their husband to take in another wife to bear him children. Women, therefore, have to try by whatever means that are available to get pregnant and give birth.

Hmong women, not men, are blamed for being infertile. It is because of the malfunctioning of the woman's body, whether it due to her behaviour or the supernatural, that makes the woman childless. Hence, she is "socially subordinated" to her husband and provides a legitimate grounds for him to bring in a second wife to bear children for him, even though he may contribute to her childlessness. A childless woman has no say in this circumstance since she has shown to him and his family that she may endanger the continuity of the family line, which in turn threatens the reproduction of Hmong society.

Male infertility is rarely acknowledged in many societies, particularly in patrilineal societies (see also Chaper 1). The Hmong society is no exception. Men are thought to govern the Hmong world. Only men can perform important tasks and only men can carry on the clan name. The notion that men are infertile and therefore are unable to have their own sons (in particular) to continue their duties is seen as immoral and rarely acceptable. Similarly, Inhorn (1994b) argues that infertility is the challenge of men's procreation power. The creation of men's most important product is a child, and this provides a legitimate right of men to rule the world. If their wives are unable to produce the men's creation, it is the women who must have done something wrong, whether it is the fault of their own body, the interruptions of the social body or the interference of the body politic. Women are, therefore, the ones who nearly always bear the blame for not being able to bring a child into the "local moral worlds" of men. Therefore, male infertility is seldom recognised in Hmong culture, even though the women believe that their men can also contribute to their barrenness.

Being fertile is a crucial part of life for the Hmong. Fertility ensures the continuation of the clan, lineage group, and family; the three important pillars in Hmong world view (Yang, 1992; Symonds, 2004; see also Chaper 1 in this volume). Infertility, therefore, have great implications in Hmong society. Women are seen as bearers of children and they must have as many children as they can. Failure to do so, either through being infertile or lose of pregnancy, results in suffering both in this present life and the next. Similar to women in other patrilineal societies, Hmong women will try everything to ensure their fertility.

A woman who cannot bear children in the Hmong culture is known as one who has a difficult life. She is always seen as unfortunate, unlucky and unfulfilled, not only in this life but also in the next. She is also not regarded highly in the community: "Have no children!, if you have no children then other people look at you as an unimportant person". One woman sums it:

The ones that cannot bear children their husbands will not love them and the relatives will not treat them well either. They say that because they can't have children so their husbands should marry another woman and so later on in their life they will not be a respectable people.

The Importance of Children in Mothers' Lives

Children are regarded as the prosperity of the family, therefore, having children are highly desirable (Liamputtong Rice, 2000). Hmong women are expected to be able to produce many children. Ideally, to be a good woman she must bear at least as many children as her mother or mother-in-law. In Hmong culture, children are necessary for one's well-being, not only in this life but also the afterlife. If a couple do not have sons, nor daughters to marry out, there will be no one to look after them in old age. Sons are more important than daughters since they care for the family altar, feed the ancestors and carry on the *dab qhuas* (family spirit) to the next generation. This ensures the continuation of the family, lineage and clan. Without children, neither Hmong men nor women are perceived complete.

For the Hmong having a life together they must be able to produce one or more children so that when they grow older they will have support in that the children will look after them in their old age.

While Hmong girls and adolescents do not have equal social or familial status to Hmong boys and men, their status changes when they marry and are able to bear a child. The birth of the first child brings prestige to a Hmong woman. After giving birth to her first child a Hmong woman becomes known by the name of the child as its mother, e.g. "Blia's mother". She is no longer addressed as "my younger daughter" by her parents, nor as the woman of her husband as in "Mrs Lee Xiong" by others. Women gain respect and status when they produce children.

The high value of children is reflected in childrearing practices among Hmong women. We are struck by comments made by many women during the interviews when they say that whatever they do in raising children, it is important not to make "the child sorry". Although women's explanations are related to child health, we believe that it shows their love and care for their children too. For example, whatever ritual parents have performed for one child, all children will receive similarly. This is to show the children that they are all loved and cared for by the parents. One woman talked about her attempts to have a soul-calling ceremony (*hu plig*, a ceremony which is usually performed on the third day after birth for a newborn infant) performed for all of her children despite living in Australia.

With my family we choose to do it [*hu plig*] for all of them. When you do one then you have to do for the rest of the children. If you don't do that then the children will say that you love one but don't' love another. So the baby will bother you by becoming sick often even when they are not sick because they feel sorry.

The Health Consequences of being a Mother: The Down Side of Motherhood

As McMahon (1995) argues, motherhood has a paradox nature; motherhood brings joys but it is also a burden. One thing, which is a common perception of Hmong women, is that motherhood has its health consequences. Motherhood may give many rewards to them but it also imposes on their health (cf. Liamputtong and Naksook, 2003a; Liamputtong, 2006). Women believe the stress and strains of conceiving, carrying pregnancy to term and giving birth to children deteriorates their own health. The more children they bear, the worse health they will have.

> Talking about being a mother, I think that my health before having children is much better because when you haven't got any children you do not feel the stress and strains on your body. After you have children you feel these stress and strains. The more you have the worse the stress and strains on your body.

Despite the fact that in Hmong culture women practice the 30 day confinement rest after giving birth (Liamputtong Rice, 2000), women believe that they cannot completely rest since they still have to perform certain chores in their household as there is no one to support them. In addition, there are many prohibitions during the confinement period which they must observe in order not to cause ill health in old age, but sometimes they may do so without intention.

> When you have children during your confinement period you do not take a good rest and you might do some things which you should not do during the confinement. So when you are older you get sick. Even if you take a good rest you still have to do the house chores like cooking when there is no one to do it for your, you have to do it yourself. This contributes to that.

Women talk about ill health which has happened to them as something which they can not do anything about it. Hence, they just treat it as part of their life.

> With this health problem I don't know what to do about it so I just leave it alone. It is not a constant thing; I mean it just comes and goes with the change of weather. Some days when it rains I can feel that but when it changes to a sunny day I don't feel that much.

Due to this belief, it is not surprising to see that some Hmong women wish to regulate their fertility or stop their reproduction completely. When younger women were asked how many children they wished to have, most often they mentioned three or four if they had the choice. Some women mention that even if they still lived in Laos where they had to rely on many children for survival they would want to stop having as many.

> If I can do then I will not want any more children because if you have too many it is a very hard work. If I can control myself to not fall pregnant then I do not want anymore, but if I can't then I will have to have them. Even if I still live in Laos I would still say the same thing.

Nevertheless, some women still want to have as many children as they can. This is to fulfil the gender role expectation within the Hmong tradition. But, women also believe that they have been accepted in Australia as a refugee. They may have to return to Laos if they are no longer allowed to stay in a new country. Returning to live in their own tradition, they need many children in order to fulfill their needs and survival. Hence, to these mothers, while they are still capable of conceiving they may as well do it.

> Why do I want many children! It is because there are never enough children. Traditionally there are a lot of roles [tasks] to do so if you don't have enough children then the jobs won't be done. The children will have to help with the housework. And if we are not allowed to stay in this country and go back to Laos, we will definitely need the extra help for survival on the farm.... If the country [Laos] is back to normal, with no more war, and they said that that is your country and you must go back then we must go.

Women also talk about the emotional side of motherhood. Anxiety in rearing children, particularly the first child, is a common experience of many women. Will they become ill? Will they recover? Will they survive? These are common anxieties that women continuously experience. Having lived in a country where infant mortality rates were, and are still, high and being expected to make the child survive as a means for the continuation of lineage and society, women's anxieties are indeed legitimate and these place tremendous burden on their lives.

> You worry about the baby getting sick. When you have your first baby it will have the most sickness of all. With the Hmong, the first one is always getting sick and you will have to always *ua neeb* or *hu plig* almost all the time. You have one done and they say it is because of something else and you have to fix that too. You do it for 2 or 3 days then the baby will be sick again and you have to repeat the whole cycle again until the child grows a bit older. The ones after that first are not sick that often.... Hmong are always like that; the first one gets sick most often

Being an Immigrant Mother

Being a mother in a new country poses several uncertainties to many Hmong women. Despite living in a new country, most Hmong women still have the wish to see children carry on their traditions, but they also realise that this may not be possible in the future. Acculturation occurs rapidly among young people of immigrant backgrounds (Liamputtong and Naksook, 2003b; Liamputtong, 2006). For example, although traditionally children will look after old age parents, women are not so certain whether they will be taken care of by their children in their new homeland. This causes considerable anxiety among them.

> In this country, I don't know if I can manage my children. I am still doubtful if they will support me when they grow up. I am still very worried about this.... In my country I would not be worried about this. But being here the children take on the Western culture. I mean like when they go to school t hey go to learn the Western culture and I am very worried that they would not carry one our tradition. But then it depends on the children so you must try your best to teach them when they come home.

Many Hmong women continue to have children in their new homeland. Some do so as they believe they have not yet had enough children. Others do so because they fear that some of their children may not follow their traditions. One woman talked about having several children that:

> I don't know about the future but I think that I should have a few children so if one does not love me then the other one will. But I don't know about this in this country whether when they grow up they will love me or not. If they follow the Hmong tradition then if one does not love their parents then the other one will still love them.

However, for some women, when talking about the value of having many children, they are not so certain about it. This is largely due to their living situation in Australia where most households are unemployed and have to rely on Social Security Benefits. Having too many children may mean poverty for the family.

> I don't know about this in this country. But in Laos the ones with lots of children, they say that, it means lots of family member. This is greatly valued because the bigger the family the better the chance of survival since they are able to grow and harvest food. But I don't know about this in this country. I think it can be valuable, but sometimes I think that you will become poorer.

Migration has, therefore, had an impact on the way Hmong women see motherhood. There are numerous uncertainties in the process of becoming a mother and raising children. Most obvious, however, is their apprehension about the change of their traditions in future generations.

CONCLUSION

While motherhood is often essentialized and imbued with notions of maternal "instinct," the work of scholars such as Scheper-Hughes (1989, 1992) has begun to disrupt these idealized images by situating mothering within a political-economic context.

Clearly, the migrant women in our study deal with the double transition, or as McMahon (1995) proposes, "multiple identities", of becoming a mother and raising their children n a new country. This has marked impact on their lives as wives and mothers. According to Oakley (1986: 307), "becoming a mother is like travelling to a foreign county" since there are many profound adjustments that a new mother has to make. If this is applied to a mother who is at the same time is an immigrant, then we may say that she is travelling to two foreign countries at once. It is, therefore, not surprising that many mothers in the study feel the double burden of motherhood and living in their new homeland. As such, the lived experiences of the migrant mothers in this study situated neatly within the framework of "multiple identities" (McMahon, 1995) discussed earlier.

Women bear the primary responsibility for both the social and biological reproduction of a culture. Motherhood and the attendant expectations of mothers as socializing agents of their offspring are particularly charged responsibilities for migrant women as these roles are vital to maintaining the reputed integrity of ethnic boundaries. The efforts of Hmong mothers in Australia to fulfil these duties are challenged by the disparate context in which our informants find themselves. Thus, truncated familial networks and different patterns in economic activities, labour market participation, and domestic labour, have inevitably altered mothering and childrearing roles and practices. Moreover, the response of dominant Anglo-Australian society to the size of Hmong families can be troubling to mothers. These perceptions may further engender Us/Other distinctions contributing to the perceived need to stabilize the borders of Hmong ethnicity.

Investing in children may be an important way of ensuring the continuity of Hmong culture, yet, our women were also aware that the integrity of the borders they, as other migrant women, have been charged with upholding are in fact more fluid than are often acknowledged. While they may anticipate that their Australian-born children will forge new identities, Hmong mothers, too, negotiate multiple hybrid identities that Bhaba (1996) notes commonly emerge from the unsettling nature of migration and the fractured nature of diasporic cultures.

In conclusion, women's accounts reveal multiple identities of motherhood. Their narratives have shown that motherhood and mothering is complex and not easy, particularly when combined with migration. This is an important aspect if the discourse of motherhood is to be understood from a perspective basing on ethnicity. Only then can health services and care be made more meaningful to the many women who have decided to become a mother in their new homeland.

REFERENCES

Becker, H., 1960, 'Notes on the Concept of Commitment', *American Journal of Sociology*, 66: 32-42.

Bhabha, H., 1996, 'Culture's In-Between'. In S. Hall and P. du Gray (eds.), *Questions of Cultural Identity*, pp. 53-60. Sage Publications: London.

Bhopal, K., 1998, 'South Asian Women in East London: Motherhood and Social Support', *Women's Studies International Forum*, 21: 485-492.

Blumer, H., 1969, *Symbolic Interactionism*, Prentice Hall: Englewood Cliffs, NJ.

Boulton, M.G., 1983, *On Being a Mother: A Study of Women with Pre-School Children*, Tavistock: London.

Braun, K., Takamura, J., & Mougeot, T., 1996, 'Perceptions of Dementia, Caregiving, and Help-Seeking Among Recent Vietnamese Immigrants', *Journal of Cross-Cultural Gerontology*, 11: 213-228.

Brown, S., Lumley, J., Small, R., & Astbury, J., 1994, *Missing Voices: The Experience of Motherhood*, Oxford University Press: Melbourne:

Brown, S., Small, R., & Lumley, J., 1997, 'Being a 'Good Mother', *Journal of Reproductive and Infant Psychology*, 15: 185-200.

Bryman, A, 2001, *Social Research Methods*, Oxford University Press: Oxford:

Buijs, G. (ed.) 1993, *Migrant Women: Crossing Boundaries and Changing Identities*, Berg Publishers: Oxford.

Buultjens, M., & Liamputtong, P., 2007, When giving life starts to take the life out of you: Women's experiences with postnatal depression following childbirth. *Midwifery*, 23: 77-91.

Cerulo, K., 1997, 'Identity Construction: New Issues, New Directions', *Annual Review of Sociology*, 23: 385-409.

Cha, D., 2000, *Hmong American Concepts of Health, Healing, and Illness and Their Experience with Conventional Medicine*, unpublished doctoral thesis, Department of Anthropology, University of Colorado, Boulder.

Cha, D., 2003, *Hmong American Concepts of Health, Healing and Conventional Medicine*, Routledge: New York.

Collins, P.H., 1994, 'Shifting the Center: Race, Class, and Feminist Theorizing About Motherhood'. In: Glenn, E.N., Chang, G., Forcey, L.R. (eds.), *Mothering: Ideology, Experience, and Agency*, pp. 45-65. Routledge: New York.

Crouch, M., & Manderson, L., 1993, *New Motherhood: Cultural and Personal Transitions in the 1980s*, Gordon and Breach: Yverdon, Switzerland.

Croucher, S., 2004, *Globalization and Belonging: The Politics of Identity in a Changing World*, Rowan and Littlefield: Lanham, MD.

Doyal, L., 1995, *What Makes Women Sick: Gender and the Political Economy of Health*, Macmillan Press: Houndmills.

Espín, O., 1999, *Women Crossing Boundaries: A Psychology of Immigration and Transformations of Sexuality*, Routledge Press: London.

Everingham, C., 1994, *Motherhood and Modernity: An Investigation into the Rational Dimension of Mothering*, Allen & Unwin: Sydney.

Glenn, E.N., 1994, 'Social Constructions of Mothering: A Thematic Overview'. In Glenn, E.N., Chang, G., Forcey, L.R. (eds.), *Mothering: Ideology, Experience, and Agency*, pp. 1-29. Routledge: New York.

Gupta, A., & Ferguson, J., 1997, 'Culture, Power, Place: Ethnography at the End of an Era'. In A. Gupta and J. Ferguson (eds.), *Culture, Power, Place: Explorations in Critical Anthropology*, pp. 1-29. Duke University Press: Durham.

Hall, S., 1996, 'Introduction: Who Needs "Identity"?'. In S. Hall and P. du Gray (eds.), *Questions of Cultural Identity*, pp. 1-17. Sage Publications: London.

Harper, J., & Richards, L., 1979, *Mothers and working mothers*, Penguin: Ringwood.

Hmong Australia Society Inc, 1998, *A Report of Hmong Member in Victoria, 1998*, Hmong Australia Society Inc: Melbourne.

Krulfeld, R.M. & Camino, L.A., 1994, 'Introduction'. In L.A. Camino and R.M. Krulfeld (ed.), *Reconstructing Lives, Recapturing Meaning: Refugee Identity, Gender and Culture Change*, pp. ix-xvii. Gordon and Breach Publishers: Basel.

Lee, G.Y., 1999, 'The Hmong'. In J. Jupp (ed.), *The Australia People: An Encyclopedia of the Nation, Its People and Their Origin*, 2nd edition. Angus & Robertson: Canberra.

Liam, I.I.L., 1991, *The Challenge of Migrant Motherhood: The Childrearing Practices of Chinese First-Time Mothers in Australia*, unpublished master thesis, Department of Social Work, the University of Melbourne: Melbourne.

Liam, I.I.L., 1999, 'The Challenge of Migrant Motherhood: The Childrearing Practices of Chinese First-Time Mothers in Australia'. In P. Liamputtong Rice (ed.), *Asian Mothers, Western Birth*, pp. 135-160. Ausmed Publications: Melbourne.

Liamputtong, P., 2001, 'Motherhood and the Challenge of Immigrant Mothers: A Personal Reflection', *Families in Society*, 82(2): 195-201.

Liamputtong, P., 2006, 'Motherhood and "Moral Career": Discourses of Good Motherhood Among Southeast Asian Immigrant Women in Australia', *Qualitative Sociology*, 29(1): 25-53.

Liamputtong, P., & Ezzy, D., 2005, *Qualitative Research Methods, 2nd edition*, Oxford University Press: Melbourne.

Liamputtong, P., & Naksook, C., 2003a, 'Perceptions and Experiences of Motherhood, Health and the Husband's Roles Among Thai Women in Australia', *Midwifery*, 19(1): 27-36.

Liamputtong, P., & Naksook, C., 2003b, 'Life as Mothers in a New Land: The Experience of Motherhood Among Thai Women in Melbourne', *Health Care for Women International*, 24(7): 650-668.

Liamputtong, P., Yimyam, S., Parisunyakul, S., Baosoung, C., & Sansiripan, N., 2002, 'Women As Mothers: The Case of Thai Women in Northern Thailand', *International Journal of Social Work*, 45(4): 497-515.

Liamputtong, P., Yimyam, S., Parisunyakul, S., Baosoung, C., & Sansiripan, N., 2004, 'When I Become a Mother!: The Perceptions and Experiences of Thai Mothers in Northern Thailand', *Women's Studies International Forum*, 27(5-6): 589-601.

Lupton, D., 2000, 'A Love/Hate Relationship: The Ideals and Experiences of First-Time Mothers', *Journal of Sociology*, 36: 50-63.

Lupton, D., & Fenwick, J., 2001, 'They've Forgotten that I'm the Mum': Constructing and Practising Motherhood in Special Care Nurseries', *Social Science & Medicine*, 53: 1011-1021.

Maushart, S., 1997, *The Mask of Motherhood*, Vintage: Sydney.

Manne, A., 2005, *Motherhood: How Should We Care for Our Children?*, Allen & Unwin: Sydney.

McMahon, M., 1995, *Engendering Motherhood: Identity and Self-Transformation in Women's Lives*, The Guilford Press: New York.

Miles, M.B., & Huberman, A.M., 1994, *Qualitative Data Analysis, 2nd edition*, Sage Publications: Thousand Oaks.

Morokvasic, M., 1983, 'Women in Migration: Beyond the Reductionist Outlook'. In A. Phizacklea (ed.), *One Way Ticket: Migration and Female Labour*. Routledge & Kegan Paul: London.

Oakley, A., 1986, *From Here to Eternity: Becoming a Mother*, Pelican Books: Suffolk.

Phoenix, A., 1988, 'Narrow Definitions of Culture: The Case of Early Motherhood'. In S. Westwood and P. Bhachu (eds.), *Enterprising Women: Ethnicity, Economy and Gender Relations*, pp. 153-176. Routledge: London.

Rich, A., 1992, *Of Woman Born: Motherhood as Experience and Institution*, Virago Press: London.

Quincy, K., 1995, *Hmong: History of a People*, Eastern Washington University Press: Cheney, WA.

Scheper-Hughes, N., 1989, 'Lifeboat Ethics: Mother Love and Child Death in Northeast Brazil', *Natural History*, 98(10): 8-16.

Scheper-Hughes, N., 1992, *Death Without Weeping: The Violence of Everyday Life in Brazil*, University of California Press: Berkeley.

Sharpe, S., 1984, *Double Identity: The Lives of Working Mothers*, Penguin Books: Harmondsworth.

Spitzer, D.L., Neufeld, A., Harrison, M., Hughes, K., & Stewart, M., 2003, 'Caregiving in Transnational Context: My Wings Have Been Cut: Where Can I Fly?, *Gender & Society*, 17(2): 267-286.

Stone, D., 1998, 'When the Shaman Pulls the String', *The Age Extra/Features*, October 21, p. 5.

Symonds, P.V., 2004, *Gender and the Cycle of Life: Calling in the Soul in a Hmong Village*, University of Washington Press: Seattle.

Tapp, N., & Lee, G.Y. (eds.) 2004, *The Hmong of Australia*, Pandanas: Canberra.

Wearing, B., 1984, *The Ideology of Motherhood*, George Allen & Unwin: Sydney.

Weaver, J.J., & Ussher, J.M., 1997, 'How Motherhood Changes Life-A Discourse Analytic Study With Mothers of Young Children', *Journal of Reproductive and Infant Psychology*, 15: 51-68.

In: Reproduction, Childbearing and Motherhood
Editor: Pranee Liamputtong, pp. 239-251

Chapter 15

SIFTING OUT THE SWEETNESS: MIGRANT MOTHERHOOD IN NEW ZEALAND

Ruth De Souza

INTRODUCTION

At no other time in their lives do women get bombarded and overwhelmed with information and advice, often unsolicited, as when they are pregnant and have babies. As a nurse working on a post-natal ward many years ago, I remember meeting a vibrant and loving couple, who said their strategy for managing the mountain of advice, was to "sift out the sweetness." This sifting process is doubly significant for migrant women who have a baby in a new country. They must sift between their own cultural practices and those of the receiving communities. For many, it involves reclaiming long forgotten practices especially if they are separated from their traditional knowledge sources. In turn, there is an opportunity for receiving societies and their systems to sift through their practices and consider ones brought by immigrants to see if there are opportunities for improvement and innovation.

This chapter focuses on a study of women from the Goan/Indian community in Auckland, New Zealand and discusses how women manage the dual transition of motherhood and migration while separated from networks and supports. A brief history of New Zealand demographics, migration and policy is given, followed by an overview of Goan migration. A description of the study that took place follows including the theoretical standpoint and social and cultural context. The findings of the study are then discussed, focusing on how women negotiated their cultural identities. The chapter concludes with an overview of implications for social care and health professionals.

BACKGROUND

The Immigration Act 1987 ushered in an era of unprecedented ethnic diversity of migrants to New Zealand from non-traditional source countries. With this new diversity have come challenges for health and social services, struggling with the requirements of biculturalism and obligations to Māori (indigenous people of New Zealand) let alone the needs of other communities. Traditionally, visibly different migrant have been positioned as 'other', the following section provides an overview of the changing demographics of New Zealand.

Twenty three percent of New Zealand females were born overseas, predominantly in the United Kingdom and Ireland, Asia and the Pacific Islands (Statistics New Zealand, 2002). Goans make up a small minority of Indian New Zealanders, who are subsumed into the category 'Asian', an umbrella term that includes such diverse groups as Chinese, Korean, Filipino, Japanese, Sri Lankan, Cambodian, Thai, and other Asian ethnic groups (Statistics New Zealand, 2002). The most recent Census found that European/Pākehā (white New Zealanders) made up 67.6% of the population, followed by New Zealand Māori with 14.6 % people from the Pacific Islands 6.9%, Asians 9.2% and Middle Eastern, Latin American & African people 0.9%. The Census also found that 11.1% of people identified themselves as New Zealanders (Statistics New Zealand, 2006).

Census projections to 2021 suggest that Māori, Pacific and Asian populations will grow at faster rates than the European population but for different reasons. The Asian population is expected to more than double, mainly due to net migration gains, while the numbers of Māori and Pacific peoples will increase due to their higher fertility rates (Statistics New Zealand, 2005). This has significant implications for the development and delivery of health services to women. The Asian community has the highest proportion of women (54%), followed by Maori and Pacific (53% each) and European (52%) (Scragg and Maitra, 2005). Asian women are most highly concentrated in the working age group of 15-64 years compared to other ethnic groups, with only 4 percent of Asian females aged over 65 and 22% under 15 years of age. This is the result of migration policy that has led to Asian women migrating for study or work (Statistics New Zealand, 2005).

NEW ZEALAND CONTEXT

The settlement of Aotearoa New Zealand began after it was discovered by the great Tahitian Chief Kupe in 950AD. Tasman followed in 1642 and Cook in 1769, which led to contact with Europeans. Organised European settlement began in 1840, which was the same year The Treaty of Waitangi/ Te Tiriti o Waitangi was signed with Māori. Policies that favoured migrants of European descent resulted in their dominance and the marginalising of Māori so that they became 'others' in their own land. However, the treatment of visibly different migrants, such as Indians, Chinese and Pacific Islanders differed substantially from that of migrants of European descent. They became 'others' because of their physical appearance, religion or culture but without the status of the indigenous Māori (Du Plessis and Alice, 1998). The relationship with visibly different migrants has been ambivalent, on one hand they have been seen as desirable for being a willing labour force and on the other feared because of the potential to overwhelm or swamp the Pākehā population and 'way of life'.

Following World War Two, the notion of assimilation dominated. 'Invisible' migrants were seen as desirable and the goal was for migrants to 'fit in' rather than change the society they had entered and change was one-way. A philosophical shift in this policy occurred when Canada and Australia embraced multiculturalism during the 1960s, which held that people had the right to retain their culture and have access to society and services without being disadvantaged (Fletcher, 1999). Settlement was transformed into a two way process requiring change by both migrants and the receiving society. New Zealand policy made a strategic move towards multiculturalism in the 1986 review and subsequent Immigration Act 1987. This Act eased access to New Zealand from non-traditional source countries and replaced entry criteria based on nationality and culture to one initially based on skills and subsequently through the introduction of a points system. This policy emphasis on attracting highly qualified immigrants was similar to policy changes in North America and Australia (Pernice et al., 2000). The adoption of the points system in 1991 led to immigrants who had experience, skills, qualifications and money being selected for business investment in New Zealand (Ho et al., 2000).

Though Indians and Chinese had been migrating to New Zealand as sojourners since 1810, their numbers were relatively small until Asian migration began to increase in the late 1980s with the encouragement of foreign investment in New Zealand and the policy changes described above. There has been little discussion about the settlement of migrants because the last thirty years have been marked by the increased tension between Māori and Pākehā, particularly around grievances and claims relating to the Treaty (Pawson et al., 1996) and migration source countries (ie European) have shaped activities and concerns (Bartley and Spoonley, 2004).

GOAN CONTEXT OF MIGRATION

Goa is located on the south west coast of India and has an area of 3,701 square kilometres , with a primarily agrarian economy and more recently, a tourism and service industry (Mascarenhas-Keyes, 1979). Goa was a Portuguese colony from 1510 until 1961 and became the 25th state in the Republic of India (Newman, 1999). Opinion is divided about whether Portuguese colonisation catalysed Goans into becoming a mobile population, Mascarenhas-Keyes (1990) suggested that socio-economic factors such as land taxation to raise funds for Portuguese expeditions, appropriation of land from villagers leading to outsider control and the removal of people from their original source of livelihood were powerful contributors. Newman (1999) claims that what drove Goans to emigrate was that they valued a consumerist, bourgeois-capitalist society in Goa and sought more money, despite the relatively high incomes available at home. Historically, there has been a strong Goan ethos of moving up, caused by the small size of Goa and the inability to divide up communal land (Mascarenhas-Keyes, 1994).

THE STUDY

Little research has been undertaken into the experiences of 'ethnic' women with regard to their experiences of motherhood in New Zealand. The term 'ethnic' is used by the New Zealand Government to denote people who come from outside Māori, Pacific and Pākehā communities. This chapter is based on the findings of my previous post-graduate research regarding the experiences of Goan women who became mothers in New Zealand and goes some way to filling the gap (De Souza, 2002).

A qualitative approach was used to expose the concerns of Goan women. Internationally, research with migrant mothers has tended to focus on pathology, deficit or risk rather than strengths (Aroian, 2001). Such an emphasis can mean that the innovative and resourceful strategies that migrant women use to enable survival and wellness are invisible, unrecognised, unarticulated and un-legitimated. I was committed to following Mirza's (1998: 81) dictum of having "an overt and political commitment to the researched, as well as a commitment to doing non-hierarchical, reciprocal, negotiated, emancipatory and subjective research" as I was keen to avoid the reproduction of pathologising, universalising and marginalising constructions of migrant women who are 'other mothers'. Furthermore, as a member of this community I was aware that I would have relationships with the women in the study beyond the life of the study and that my conduct would also have an impact on my extended family (for further discussion see De Souza 2004a).

The study took place in Auckland, New Zealand among women of the Catholic Goan community. I had attempted to include the experiences of Hindu and Muslim Goans but was only able to recruit Catholics, who form a significant majority within the Goan community in New Zealand. A purposive sampling technique was used and selection criteria limited participation to women who self-identified as Goan. Having 'emic' or insider status made entry easier into the Goan community and facilitated dialogue with new Goan mothers. All participants had migrated to New Zealand from outside of Goa highlighting their history of multiple migrations. Data collection involved the use of in-depth semi-structured interviews conducted in English. Data analysis occurred alongside data collection and involved repeated reading of the interview transcripts and open coding similar to a grounded theory approach where a label is assigned to certain data (Strauss and Corbin, 1990). Codes were then reduced grouped into categories and given a name. These categories were then compared and contrasted with those in the literature. The following section focuses on how Goan women managed to maintain their culture during the perinatal period.

FINDINGS AND DISCUSSION

This section discusses the main findings in the context of the ante-natal, labour and delivery and postnatal periods, these are shown in Table 1 below:

In the antenatal period participants who would have heavily on a network of family and friends to advise them were faced with the loss of knowledge resources who would have prepared them creating a "vacuum of knowledge" (Liem, 1999: 157).

Table 1. Summary of findings

Period	Antenatal	Labour and delivery	Postpartum
Theme	An empty bowl; A fresh start; Vacuum of knowledge	Disappearing traditions; changing roles	Reclaiming the old; strengthening the new; on your own
Gains	Privileging of expert knowledge (scientific basis), birth as natural	Fathers more actively involved, Expectation of taking control of birth	New peer networks, new ways of doing things
Losses	Birth as sacred and preciousness	Loss of extended family and peer group	Bring in family, both ways of doing things, assimilated, choosing between current and traditional practices\

My idea of pregnancy or knowing anything about children was someone else's and you just cuddled them and give them back kind of thing so I was totally unprepared (Rowena).

This vacuum of knowledge about childrearing needed to be filled and many participants became eager to acquire knowledge of the experiences of mothers from the host country. The breaks in knowledge provided them with choices that extended beyond those of their own communities and also provided them with freedom from fear based and taboo views of birth. Lorna and Rowena were liberated from old ways of doing things, particularly advice from well-meaning family friends and 'old wives tales' that seemed to have no logical basis and replace them:

No certain things they would say Oh don't eat it but I really didn't pay much attention to it because sometimes I think they are just old wives tales and superstition. Sometimes you know they have a good reason behind it. They said don't eat too much of chilli because your child would have a lot of hair on them and I'd said if you eat too much of chilli you feel sick the next day (Rowena).

Initially, this knowledge of the West displaced and became more valued than that of women elders who traditionally would have been the 'experts'. The new experts were disembodied objective 'knowers' and the authoritative status of dominant ideologies (for example evidence based practice) had a powerful influence and were privileged over 'traditional' beliefs which were rendered irrelevant or pathological. This space or break in knowledge provided women with the opportunity to envisage having a baby as a natural event rather than one with taboos and fear. Their expectations were raised by the discourse of naturalness and taking control of their births that dominated midwifery discourses.

What I experienced here was that child bearing is natural, that natural factor was a great thing (Lorna).

However, this natural discourse also presented women with the burden of carrying on normally with their pregnancy rather than viewing it as a sacred time. Migration provided an opportunity for the participants to take control of their birth experience. This discourse, which positions western women as educated, liberated, modern, agents of choice who have control over their own bodies and sexualities (Khoo, 1996) can lead to distress. Given that it creates expectations about the degree of control that women can exercise in childbirth that cannot always be met. Many women ended up depending on their husbands more as their family members and peers were unavailable during labour and delivery. Fathers became more active participants in the birth and child rearing process unlike in India where it may have been peripheral. Flora's midwife ensured that Flora's husband could be involved in a way that he hadn't been able to in India:

Yeah, like he never saw the delivery for Cedric and here, the midwife involved him. Chris used to come with me for all my check-ups and she used to explain (Flora).

Lorna's husband's role changed so that he took on roles that he might not have been able to in India where family members would have stepped in:

No, not really because he is by nature caring and a family man so I would have got a shock if he didn't lift a finger. The extent to which he went about was great because as you say the typical Goan male, husband, father is not very involved in child rearing. They don't really take a very active part (Lorna).

The lack of family support was ameliorated to some degree with having supportive lead maternity carers who were nurturing, In Flora's case, the way her fear was managed and the inclusion of her son Cedric and husband Chris in the whole process from pregnancy to postpartum, were polished off with nurturing and the reinforcement of her femininity after labour:

I was not scared, you know on the day it really happened. Yeah and she was there throughout, even after the baby was born she gave me a sponge and she dressed me up. My God it was like in India I was left there in the Labour ward. Here immediately after the delivery she really gave me like a bath sort of thing and she opened my suitcase and she said come on I'll put your nice night-dress. You know what she did, she sent Chris home 'Chris go bring Cedric' and he said 'no, no I'll bring later' 'no I want you to bring Cedric now, because you know she involved Cedric during the whole pregnancy and she said 'no I am sure Cedric would want to see his brother immediately.' So she was sending Chris away. She said, before Chris comes I want to dress you up. So by the time Chris came she had me presentable. You know wee small things which were thoughtful of her. Yeah the thing is with my Midwife because she knew I had nobody here (Flora).

The postpartum period provided the greatest challenge with women struggling to manage the transition with the resources they had available to them. Many women brought over their mothers or mothers-in-law, developed new support systems in particular formal rather than natural supports and developing new peer groups. By far the greatest challenge was attempting to be bicultural and grasp the best of both worlds and hold parallel beliefs, traditional and new, in a world where only the new was supported. Participants resisted and contested the discourse of assimilation but found that they were often forced to choose between home culture and host culture.

A study of South Asian women by Dobson and Homans (cited in Woollett et al., 1995) found that the women held parallel beliefs rather than having beliefs that clashed. They maintained some traditional practices but valued Western medical care. Attempting to carry over traditional rituals into the dominant culture created some challenges for Rowena:

> Here they wouldn't believe in massaging baby as such you know. Just bath the baby and change, wrap the baby up. Even in India you'd have baby sleeping with you in your room, whereas here they just say you know, have the separate rooms for the baby. We were flatting by then; we were sharing a big house, so we didn't have the luxury of having the upstairs rooms and all that kind of things. Marita stayed in a cot in our room, it was a big room but yeah and I used to just do things. Like I still remembered massaging her with oil and I used to see women do that all the time in India. They said it was good for them. I just went ahead.

Rowena's example shows how care providers privileged their ways of knowing above Rowena's by universalising dominant group standards or 'appropriate' ways of parenting that included a separate room for the baby. Rowena resisted such 'appropriate' and commonsensical dominant discursive practices by doing what was culturally appropriate for her.

Other clashes identified were the tensions between current practice that encourages women to be independent and mobile as soon as possible and traditional practice that supports the woman to have a period in which to recuperate while being attended to by family. These are acutely articulated in Muriel's story:

> It's such a different situation out over here. Mum says oh, it's so cold in this country, don't give a bath here. The midwife says give a bath every day, when hardly a week, the baby is born the midwife says why don't you take her for a walk, it's a sunny day, you know why don't you go out? In India you wouldn't go out for 40 days and things like that. So many conflicting kind of things, which was very difficult and it's really different (Muriel).

Muriel's example uncovers how migrant women are challenged between choosing one set of beliefs over another. Furthermore, it is more likely that 'traditional' ways will be lost as the resources and structures that are available to support Muriel in her role as a new mother are geared towards the philosophies and practices of the majority culture. Migrant women can be caught between their new culture that holds their aspirations while working hard to fit into their traditional culture representing their past and the values that have shaped who they are. Muriel's experience resonates with Liem's (1999) findings in a study of Chinese first-time mothers who gave birth in Australia. Liem argues that migration exposes new mothers to other ways of thinking and they then have to decide not only what is best for them and their baby but also who not to offend or embarrass, new or old authority figures.

IMPLICATIONS FOR WOMEN'S HEALTH CARE

The increasing diversity of New Zealand presents an opportunity for New Zealand health services to go beyond the perception of migrants as a risk and problem to migrants as a catalyst for developing innovative responses to diversity of people. In the following section, the implications of these findings are discussed and how they can be implemented into the health system is outlined. It is suggested that further research is necessary to evaluate the cultural frameworks of health professional and migrants and to evaluate the effectiveness of cultural safety versus universalism. Secondly, an expansion of philosophy and practice is called for, that acknowledges multiple identities and the diversity of ethnic communities and broadens the bicultural agenda to incorporate multiculturalism and inter-culturalism. For me, the findings raise more questions than answers, such as:

1. How well is what we already have (Cultural Safety and biculturalism) working? Are health professionals effective?
2. What is missing? Is there any evaluation of the effectiveness of service delivery from the perspective of migrant women?
3. Where are spaces for new developments and roles? Such as Link workers, cultural workers?
4. How can changes occur so the onus is not on the outsider to fit in within the existing assimilatory paradigm? How do we promote wellness and resourcefulness? How is settlement being considered as a part of the total health and wellness experience?

By all accounts, migrant motherhood provided research participants with the opportunity to become bicultural. They were able to involve their husbands and felt cared for by health professionals in the labour and delivery period. Antenatally, women noticed gaps in their knowledge but this also proved to be an opportunity. The area of most concern was in the post-partum period when women were caught in an assimilatory health system. Health services are largely still monocultural with the occasional concession to difference in the form of parallel services for Māori and Pacific people. The US Department of Health and Human Services, National Healthcare Disparities Report (2003, cited in Giddings, 2005) suggests that health disparities are sustained through the institutionalisation of policies and practices in the health arena.

The concept of cultural safety in the health context is well understood in New Zealand. However, it is largely only applied to the relationship between Māori and the health system. In the next section of this chapter, I will explore some of the limitations of cultural safety and attempt to propose some ways forward, such that the notion of cultural safety might be usefully applied to other ethnic groups.

In New Zealand, biculturalism and cultural safety have been institutionalised since the 1980s and challenge previously monocultural and assimilatory institutional practices. Biculturalism is derived from The Treaty of Waitangi/ Te Tiriti O Waitangi and has the following objectives (Durie, 2005):

1. Acknowledge things Māori;
2. Make State operated facilities more responsive to Māori;

3. Foster Pākehā engagement with Māori culture;
4. Provide specially for Māori in institutions;
5. Combine elements of both cultures to forge a common national identity.

Cultural safety developed by Māori nurses, has become a compulsory part of nursing education in New Zealand for over ten years. It is made up of both a conceptual framework for understanding the power inequalities that structure the relationships between New Zealand's Māori or Tangata Whenua and health professionals and practical strategies that can be utilised (Nursing Council of New Zealand, 2002). It requires that all human being receive care that takes into account their uniqueness (culture, gender, religious backgrounds) and rather than being a checklist of customs or practices, its focus is on the nurse as a culture and power bearer. New Zealand expects all nurses to practice cultural safety and it is their actions which are under scrutiny rather than the diversity of clients, thus their client defines whether the care they have received is safe. Simply put "unsafe practitioners diminish, demean and/or disempower those of other cultures, whilst safe practitioners recognize, respect and acknowledge the rights of others" (Cooney, 1994: 6).

Cultural safety has two fundamental assumptions; one is that by understanding oneself, the rights of others and the legitimacy of difference, the nurse should be prepared to work with all people who are different from themselves (Nursing Council). Secondly, that by focusing on oneself one can understand one's own culture and theory of power relations. The nurse always operates from her/his own cultural mindset which influences how she/he relates to those she/he cares for and therefore every health care interaction is influenced by the cultural context in which it occurs (Nursing Council of New Zealand, 2002). Cultural safety is based on four principles that are summarised as follows:

1. Improving the health status of New Zealanders (Treaty, access, health gain of marginalised groups).
2. Enhancing the delivery of services through a culturally safe workforce (power relationships, empowering users, understanding diversity in own context and the impact of that, going beyond tasks to relationships).
3. Broad application recognising impact of context (inequalities as a microcosm, impact of history, employment etc, legitimacy of difference, attitudes as barriers, quality improvement and rights).
4. Close focus on individual nurse (culture bearer, power relationships which favour providers, balancing power differentials, moving towards equitable delivery and minimising risk to marginalised) (Nursing Council of New Zealand, 2002).

Cultural safety has been broadened to apply to any person or group of people who may differ from the nurse/midwife because of socio-economic status, age, gender, sexual orientation, ethnic origin, migrant/refugee status, religious belief or disability (Ramsden, 1997). However, critics argue that its focus has been on Māori rather than other groups (DeSouza, 2004b). Giddings (2005: 225) proposes that it has created a hierarchy of 'isms' and marginalised "other cultural differences and related social injustices such as sexism, heterosexism, and classism," while Jeffs (2001) suggests that it has focused on education providers rather than the practice setting. There is a need for research to investigate the effectiveness of cultural safety in multicultural populations from the point of view of ethnic consumers so that the whether it prepares nurses and midwives for working with ethnic communities is established. Safety is defined by the recipient of the care given, so this appears a vital strategy.

Develop Multicultural Policy

To some extent, the lack of development of multicultural policy has come about as a result of a statement by the New Zealand conference of churches in 1990 at the sesquicentennial anniversary of the signing of the Treaty (Bartley and Spoonley, 2004). Proponents of the statement claimed that biculturalism should take precedence and subsequent arrivals to Aotearoa needed to negotiate a primary relationship with Māori (Bartley and Spoonley, 2004). Multiculturalism would eventuate as a result of completed bicultural negotiations, however a no process has ever been suggested or developed (Bartley and Spoonley, 2004).

Develop Intercultural Skills

Not only are health care consumers becoming increasingly diverse, New Zealand's health workforce is becoming more diverse as a result of migration and workforce shortages. The proportion of nurses from the dominant Pākehā culture is decreasing, there is a need for nurses to develop intercultural skills.

Health Care Workers as Settlement Resources

As shown in the previous section, migrant women from Goa were faced with the loss of resources throughout the perinatal period. There is a lack of knowledge about the settlement process among health workers. The notion of settlement has only recently been operationalized with the development of an Immigration Settlement Strategy for migrants, refugees and their families. The strategy's six goals (New Zealand Immigration Service, 2003) are for migrants and refugees to:

1. Obtain employment appropriate to their qualifications and skills;
2. Are confident using English in a New Zealand setting, or can access appropriate language support to bridge the gap;
3. Are able to access appropriate information and responsive services that are available to the wider community (for example housing, education, and services for children);
4. Form supportive social networks and establish a sustainable community identity;
5. Feel safe expressing their ethnic identity and are accepted by, and are part of, the wider host community; and
6. Participate in civic, community and social activities.

This suggests that the role of the health and social services professional needs to be widened to one of resource broker and to be participants in realising the vision.

Recognition of Multiple Identities and Diversity within Communities

Migrants tend to be defined in terms of belonging to communities that are homogenous, bounded and static and whose meanings are interpreted in a universal way (Salih, 2000). Of more value is the notion of postmodern identities, which are unstable, diverse and subjectively identified group interests. There is a danger in privileging any of those identities over the other (race, class, ethnicity, gender).and ignoring the ways in which they intersect Identity must be seen as subjective, socially constructed, contextually dynamic and historically specific and embedded in multiple sites of oppression (Musisi, 1999). Furthermore, differences within groups can be as significant as between groups (De Souza, 1996).

Developing Innovative Practices

The model of assimilation, which requires that migrants reject their own ways in order to fit into the receiving culture, whilst the latter remains unchanged is predominant in the health care system. An implicit expectation is that those who enter the health setting must give up their power to be a 'good patient.' However, migration provides an opportunity for health systems to allow themselves to be changed and invigorated.

CONCLUSION

Migrant women are transformed by migration and motherhood. In turn there is a need for the receiving community's institutions to be transformed to meet the needs of diverse groups of people.This mutual transformation process extends to 'sifting out the sweetness' in the cultural practices of both health services and professionals as well as migrants and their families Existing strategies, such as cultural safety, have largely focused on the needs of Māori and ensuring that Treaty of Waitangi obligations are met, but the health system remains largely assimilatory. With the increasing diversity of New Zealand society, there is a need for a more responsive system where health professionals are both informed and interculturally skilled. Migration creates new possibilities not only for migrants but for health services to become more vibrant and responsive offering new possibilities of care. Approaches that are cognisant of the settlement process are promising as well as those that expand the notion of cultural safety beyond indigenous Māori to encompass a multicultural or intercultural approach. Further research is needed that takes into account migrants views of the services they utilise and whether cultural safety is working.

REFERENCES

Aroian, K. J., 2001, 'Immigrant Women and Their Health', in D. Taylor and N. F. Woods (eds.), *Annual Review of Nursing Research: Women's Health Research (Vol. 19)*, pp. 179-226. Springer: New York, NY.

Bartley, A., & Spoonley, P., 2004, 'Constructing a Workable Multiculturalism in a Bicultural Society', in M. Belgrave, M. Kawharu and D. V. Williams (eds.), *Waitangi Revisited: Perspectives on the Treaty of Waitangi, 2nd edition*, pp. 136-148. OUP: Auckland, NZ.

Cooney, C., 1994, 'A Comparative Analysis of Transcultural Nursing and Cultural Safety', *Nursing Praxis in New Zealand,* 9(1), 6-12.

De Souza, R., 1996, '*Transcultural Mental Health Care',* paper presented at the Caring and culture, culture and caring ANZ College of Mental Health Nurses Conference, Auckland, NZ.

De Souza, R., 2002, *Walking Upright Here: Countering Prevailing Discourses Through Reflexivity and Methodological Pluralism,* unpublished MA thesis, Massey University, New Zealand.

De Souza, R., 2004a, 'Motherhood, Migration and Methodology: Giving Voice to the "Other"', *The Qualitative Report,* 9(3), 463-482.

De Souza, R., 2004b, 'Working with Refugees and Migrants', in D. Wepa (ed.), *Cultural Safety,* pp. 122-133. Pearson Education New Zealand: Auckland, NZ.

Du Plessis, R., & Alice, L., 1998, *Feminist Thought in Aotearoa/New Zealand.* Oxford University Press: Auckland, NZ.

Durie, E., 2005, *The Rule of Law, Biculturalism and Multiculturalism,* paper presented at the ALTA Conference, Hamilton, NZ.

Fletcher, M., 1999, *Migrant Settlement: A Review of the Literature and Its Relevance to New Zealan,.* New Zealand Immigration Service: Wellington, NZ

Giddings, L. S., 2005, 'A Theoretical Model of Social Consciousness', *Advances in Nursing Science,* 28(3), 224-239.

Ho, E., Cheung, E., Bedford, C., & Leung, P., 2000, *Settlement Assistance Needs of Recent Migrants.* University of Waikato: Hamilton, NZ.

Jeffs, L., 2001, 'Teaching Cultural Safety the Culturally Safe Way', *Nursing Praxis in New Zealand,* 17(3), 41-50.

Khoo, T. L., 1996, 'Who are We Talking About? Asian-Australian Women Writers'. *Hecate,* 22(2), 11-32.

Liem, I. I. L., 1999, 'The Challenges of Migrant Motherhood: The Childrearing Practises of Chinese First-Time Mothers in Australia', in P. Liamputtong Rice (Ed.), *Asian Mothers, Western Birth,* pp. 135-160. Ausmed Publications: Australia.

Mascarenhas-Keyes, S., 1979, *Goans in London: Portrait of a Catholic Asian community.* Evans of the Kinder Press: New Mills, UK.

Mascarenhas-Keyes, S., 1990, 'Migration, Progressive Motherhood and Female Autonomy: Catholic Women in Goa', in L. Dube and R. Palriwala (eds.), *Structures and Strategies: Women, Work and Family in Asia,* pp. 119-143. Sage: New Delhi, India.

Mascarenhas-Keyes, S., 1994, 'Language and Diaspora: The Use of Portuguese, English and Konkani by Catholic Goan Women in Goa', in P. Burton, K. K. Dyson and S. Ardener (eds.), *Bilingual Women: Anthropological Approaches to Second Language Use,* pp. 149-166. Berg Publications: Oxford, UK.

Mirza, M., 1998, 'Same Voices, Same Lives? Revisiting Black Feminist Standpoint Epistemology', in P. Connolly and B. Troyna (eds.), *Researching Racism in Education; Politics, Theory, Practice,* pp. 55-67. Open University Press: Buckingham.

Musisi, N. B., 1999, 'Catalyst, Nature, and Vitality of African-Canadian Feminism: A Panorama of an Emigre Feminist', in A. Heitlinger (ed.), *Emigre Feminism, Transnational Perspectives*, pp. 131-149. University of Toronto Press: Toronto.

New Zealand Immigration Service, 2003, 'New Zealand Settlement Strategy outline'. www.immigration.govt.nz/community/stream/support/nzimmigrationsettlementstrategy/>.

Newman, R., 1999, 'The Struggle for a Goan Identity', in N. Dantas (ed.), *The Transforming of Goa*, pp. 17-43. The Other India Press: Goa, India.

Nursing Council of New Zealand, 2002, *Guidelines for Cultural Safety, the Treaty of Waitangi and Maori Health in Nursing and Midwifery Education and Practice*, Nursing Council of New Zealand: Wellington, NZ.

Pawson, E., Bedford, R., Palmer, E., Stokes, E., Friesen, W., Cocklin, C., et al., 1996, 'Senses of Place', in R. L. Heron and E. Pawson (eds.), *Changing Places: New Zealand in the Nineties*, pp 347-349. Longman Paul: Auckland, NZ.

Pernice, R., Trlin, A., Henderson, A., & North, N., 2000, 'Employment and Mental Health of Three Groups of Immigrants to New Zealand', *New Zealand Journal of Psychology*, 29(1), 24-29.

Ramsden, I., 1997, 'Cultural Safety: Implementing the Concept - The Social Force of Nursing and Midwifery', in P. T. Whaiti, M. McCarthy and A. Durie (eds.), *Mai i rangiatea*, pp. 113-125. Auckland University Press: Auckland, NZ.

Salih, R., 2000, 'Shifting Boundaries of Self and Other: Moroccan Migrant Women in Italy', *European Journal of Women's Studies*, 7, 321-335.

Scragg, R., & Maitra, A., 2005, *Asian Health in Aotearoa: An Analysis of the 2002-2003 New Zealand Health Survey*, The Asian Network Incorporated: Auckland, NZ.

Statistics New Zealand, 2002, '2001 Census: Asian People'. <www.stats.govt.nz/people/communities/asianpeople.htm>

Statistics New Zealand, 2005, 'Focusing on women'. <www.stats.govt.nz/analytical-reports/children-in-nz/growing-ethnic-diversity.htm>

Statistics New Zealand. (2006). QuickStats National Highlights: Cultural diversity. Retrieved 21 December, 2006, from http://www.stats.govt.nz/census/2006-census-data/national-highlights/2006-census-quickstats-national-highlights.htm?page=para006Master

Strauss, A., & Corbin, J., 1990, *Basics of Qualitative Research, Grounded Theory Procedures and Techniques*, Sage Publications: Thousand Oaks, CA.

Woollett, A., Dosanjh, N., Nicolson, P., Marshall, H., Djhanbakhch, O., & Hadlow, J., 1995, 'The Ideas and Experiences of Pregnancy and Childbirth of Asian and Non-Asian Women in East London', *British Journal of Medical Psychology*, 1995(68), 65-84.

In: Reproduction, Childbearing and Motherhood
Editor: Pranee Liamputtong, pp. 253-267

Chapter 16

ACCESSING MARRIAGE AND MOTHERHOOD: THE EXPERIENCE OF WOMEN WITH DISABILITY IN RURAL CAMBODIA

Alexandra Gartrell

INTRODUCTION

Of the 600 million people with disability worldwide, 400 million live in the Asia Pacific region and it is estimated that 70-80% live below the poverty line making them one of the largest disadvantaged groups among the so-called vulnerable groups in the world (Ilagan, 2002). The World Bank estimates that about 20% of the poorest of the poor are people with disability (Elwan, 1999). Paralleling these global trends, people with disability are one of the poorest groups in Cambodia (Disability Action Council (DAC), 2001, Cambodia MOSAVLA, 1996), and face considerable structural inequalities and barriers to claiming their human rights as equal citizens (Gartrell, 2004).

Women and girls with disability experience multiple layers of disadvantage in their daily lives. The Gender and Development Network Cambodia (2006) note that women with disability face discrimination at all levels of society; they live in isolation, marginalised from mainstream society and without equal access to opportunities. Women with disability are more likely than men with disability, and their able-bodied counterparts, to be living in poverty, denied the right to a decent livelihood (Elwan, 1999; Ilagan, 2002; Takamine, 2003; Gartrell, 2004). Stigma, discrimination, invisibility and loss of voice characterize the lives of many women with disability. Furthermore, the literature shows women with disability have considerable reservations about finding a partner; they are less likely than women without disability to marry, are more likely to marry later and to be divorced (Franklin, 1977). Images of women with disability typically represent them as alone (Asch and Fine, 1997).

The exclusion of men and women with disability in society has been paralleled in academic discourses. Scholars have been slow to take up the examination of the multiple social processes underpinning the marginalization and impoverishment of people with disability, and particularly those unique to women with disability (Asch and Fine, 1992;

Wendell, 1996; Morris, 1996; Thomson, 1997). Studies on disability in non-western societies are even scarcer, although there are some exceptions (Groce and Scheer, 1990; Estroff, 1993; Ingstad and Whyte, 1998; Stone, 2005). When disability has been written about, the medical model has been the dominant analytical perspective, which Oliver (1996: 21) refers to as the ideological hegemony of 'personal tragedy theory'. Medical explanations individualize and de-politicize the social inequalities experienced by people with disability and do not further our understanding of the multiple forms of oppression and injustice that produce and reproduce disablement in gendered and culturally specific ways. By focusing on the experience of women with disability in rural Cambodia, this research contributes to filling the knowledge gap on the gendered construction of disability in non-western societies. More specifically, this chapter identifies the cultural processes that construct women with disability as unable to be reproducers and nurturers.

In their research in the United States, Asch and Fine (1997) argue that cultural stereotypes of disability reinforce images of women as dependent, compliant and good natured – attributes suitable to the 'good wife'. They ask that if this is the case, why then do women with disability struggle to find men who pay them any attention, let alone want to marry them (Asch and Fine, 1997: 243). Examining the views of people without disability towards those with disability is insightful. Disability is rarely viewed positively (Shakespeare, 1994), and in Cambodia is popularly associated with moral transgression and poor karmic status (Gartrell, 2004). Additionally, men and women with disability are seen to be useless, without value and dependent on the labour power of others. They are expected to passively accept their karmic fate, objects to be pitied and cared for by others; women with disability are not expected to be wives, mothers and workers.

METHODOLOGY

This chapter is based on ethnographic research conducted in one village in north-west Cambodia in the non-monsoon period for nine months in 2000-2001. The aim of the research was to understand the daily lives of men and women with disability and by doing so identify the key factors shaping the experience of disability. The narratives of men and women with disability were placed within the changing material and cultural circumstances of Cambodia, following Michael Oliver's (1996) research framework. Several research methods were employed, including participant observation, a survey of all households in the research village (n=492), qualitative semi-structured and in-depth key informant interviews. Multiple interviews with 34 people with disability, 15 women and 16 men, were conducted. In-depth case studies and life history interviews were completed with 11 of these women. A further 25 interviews with government and non-government representatives working in the disability sector were undertaken. Analysis is interpretative, drawing upon the cognate disciplines of human geography, feminist theory and anthropology.

Most households in the research village - Daəm Dooŋ (a pseudonym) - engage in a combination of activities to meet their needs, such as rice farming, marketing gardening, fishing, labouring or running small businesses; a few villagers combine these with government employment as teachers, court or Commune officials. In the study village, only 17.5% of households have sufficient food all year, with 40% having no rice in store at all.

Almost half (44%) of the villagers are landless; a further 39% own barely enough land to achieve subsistence levels of rice production. Landless households have to continually work to buy their daily rice. They have no safety net and live hand to mouth. As a Commune official describes:

> When people lack food, they try to work in other areas harvesting or labouring or they find fish and other food. They will find food in the morning and store it until the evening. This is the situation of the general population (fieldnotes, 5 March, 2001).

In Daəm Dooŋ village 52.5% of the population are women; 34% of households are female headed and 19.2% of household heads are widows. There has been an increasing trend toward the abandonment of wives and children and the taking of second wives. Poverty, drought and floods are forcing people, particularly men, to travel to other provinces in search of work. As time away from home gets longer, men take second wives at their place of employment and return to the village either intermittently to give their first wife money or not at all. Women's vulnerability is being accentuated by these poverty related factors.

Of the 11 case studies, three were married and one had a disability at the time of marriage; two were separated; two were women in their early twenties living with their families, and the remaining 4 were women living alone or with extended family who had never married (2 women had polio as children and were 35 and 45 years old; one acquired a mobility disability when she was 25 and was 54 years old, and the other was in her early 60's and had acquired a mobility impairment two years ago).

In this chapter, I use the terms 'people with disability' or 'women with disability' as opposed to 'disabled people' or 'disabled women' to highlight the oppressive social relations that impose 'disability' on people with physical and/or mental impairments. Although in the Khmer language this differentiation is meaningless, the term 'people with disability' is more commonly used in western countries, and has been followed in the English discourse of government and non-government organisations in Cambodia (see for example DAC, 2001), as a means of emphasising the person. By using the term 'people with disability', I focus on the power relations at work in the subjection of people with impairments to the social practices of exclusion, oppression and marginalization. It is these processes that are primarily disabling, not solely differences in physicality. This chapter draws on social models of disability (Finkelstein, 1980; Oliver, 1983). I now turn to discuss the context of contemporary Cambodian society and economy.

CONTEMPORARY CAMBODIA

Cambodia's recent history of civil war, genocide and international isolation has left the population traumatized and impoverished, and much of the country's physical, social and human capital devastated. The breakdown of basic economic and social infrastructure as a consequence of the Khmer Rouge Regime (1975-1979), in which between 1.5 and 2 million people died due to starvation, disease and mass killings (Ledgerwood, 1992: 7), and two decades of civil war, has led to chronic malnutrition, poor sanitation and living conditions, all of which increase the risk of disablement and compound the difficulties women, particularly women with disability, face meeting their daily needs. Cambodian health status is among the worst in the Western Pacific Region (Cambodia, MoH and MoP, 2001), and the most severe health problems are caused by the socio-economic and physical environment (UNICEF, 1990: 61; Annear, 1998).

Despite Cambodia's integration into the regional and global economy since the Paris Peace Accord (1991), Cambodia continues to have some of the worst human development indicators in the world with just over a third of the Cambodian population (36%) living below the poverty line (UNDP, 2001). Cambodia is one of the poorest countries in Asia, with an estimated per capita income of US $315 in 2003 (UNDP, 2005). Poverty is predominantly rural: in 1999 per capita income in Phnom Penh was US $691, compared with a rural per capita income of US $197 (Hughes, 2006). Furthermore, more women are living in poverty than men (UNIFEM et al., 2004). Despite achieving growth rates of above 5% per annum in almost every year since 1994, inequality appears to be increasing (ADB, 2005; Hughes, 2006).

Cambodia has the lowest level of gender equity in Asia (ADB. 2005), and women's vulnerability has increased in the last two decades (Gorman et al., 1999). Gender gaps are becoming more entrenched as new opportunities and resources flowing into the country are distributed according to underlying cultural assumptions about gender and power relations. The Cambodian Ministry of Planning (MoP, 2002: iii) observe that women have less access to education, paid employment, land ownership and other property rights, and are more disadvantaged than men by the lack of adequate health services, largely because of risks associated with pregnancy and maternity. Women are more likely to be landless or have significantly smaller plots of land than men and are more vulnerable to losing their land in the event of economic shocks (UNIFEM et al., 2004), such as illness and injury.

It is widely accepted that Cambodia has one of the highest per capita rates of disability in the world and an estimated 21% of this population are children (DAC, 2004). Gleaning a precise picture of the prevalence of disability in Cambodia is difficult. However, estimates range between 1.5 to 3 percent of the population (MoP, 1999, 1997; DAC, 2001); more recent estimates are as high as 9.8% (MacKinley, 2004). Despite the perception that disability due to war, conflict and landmines are the most prevalent, the data shows that illness and disease are the most common, particularly for women (MoP, 1997). This pattern of disability causation is indicative of the low level of primary health care services, malnutrition, chronic food scarcity, and the multiple barriers to accessing what services are available (van de Put, 1992; Annear, 1998). Disability is symptomatic of the structural deprivation, inequality and poverty that characterise Cambodia, rather than its cause (Gartrell, 2004; MacKinley, 2004). As DFID (2000) note, people with disability are caught in a vicious cycle of poverty and disability, each being a cause and consequence of the other. Disability is both caused by and a result of limited access to health services, education and employment, economic and social disadvantage.

Women with disability encounter specific institutionalized disadvantages from birth. If girls with disability survive, they are likely to face discrimination and possible rejection within the family, receive less care and food, and be excluded from family interactions and activities (Elwan, 1999). They have less access to health care, educational and employment opportunities (Elwan, 1999; Gartrell, 2004) and are more at risk of physical and mental abuse, sometimes by those within the household, and their families are often stigmatised for having a daughter with disability. Girls with disability grow up lacking a sense of self worth and confidence and are denied roles as women in their communities (Takamine, 2003). Women with disability in developing countries are twice as prone to divorce, separation and violence as able-bodied women because of perceptions of dependency, an inability to contribute to household chores or to the household economy (UNDP, 1995).

MULTIPLE STRUCTURAL AND EMBODIED VULNERABILITIES

Rena is a 32 year old mother of three children who was recently injured when returning from work in the paddy fields several kilometers from her village. It was dusk. Suddenly, Rena and the other village women she was with, saw bandits on the road up ahead. They were stopping motorbikes as they passed by, taking at gunpoint whatever money or gold villagers had with them. Rena remembers hearing a shot being fired and finding herself on the ground wondering what happened. She had been shot in the hip by a random bullet. Rena describes the series of events her injury and subsequent mobility impairment sparked:

> After my accident, it [her marriage] changed. My husband threw me away. I don't know why his heart changed.....if he stayed with me he thought we had no future as we can't work...so he left. He didn't pity me.....he was ambitious with pretty girls....we had no safety together. There was always conflict. When we have a disability, we can't make money so they don't want to live with us....it is different from when we have legs and arms...before I could do business more successfully than men. My husband was different after my disability...he thought I couldn't work, that I had no value....now I struggle to feed the children on my own (23 January, 2001).

Rena's abandonment by her husband following her injury sheds light on three key sets of issues. Firstly, Rena's experience demonstrates the cultural assumption that disability automatically means a loss of capacity to work and a reduction in value, as a wife and mother. Rena's comments reveal that a wife's ability to work, and in this case, as in many others, to lead the family economically, is critical to the survival of the household as an economic and social unit (Ledgerwood, 1992; Ovesen et al., 1996). Rena's husband could not see how she could continue to play an economic role. Consequently, his attitude toward her changed. All he saw was limitations, restrictions and problems; she had lost her value as a wife, as an asset to support him. Feeling no pity for Rena and their children, he left. A new set of symbolic meanings was now associated with Rena's 'disabled' body and her husband assumed that these would seamlessly translate into a new material reality of poverty and shame for him and their family.

Secondly, Rena's experience reveals that marriage is based upon the fulfilment of gendered social roles, economic pragmatism and the symbolic value men acquire from their wives, particularly if they are beautiful. Disability unsettles the mutual social obligations that bind marriage, however fragile, together. When adults acquire a disability, it either pulls families closer or tears them apart (AFSC, 2000; Gartrell, 2004). Divorce is common following impairment; both men and women leave their spouses. Although there is no data on the incidence of abandonment following disability by gender, it is known that women living without male support are more likely to live in poverty (Ledgerwood, 1992; Gorman et al., 1999); disability would only amplify this tendency.

Thirdly, Rena uses the idiom of 'safety' *(sok)* to capture her socio-economic and cultural vulnerability, both prior to and following her accident (see also Hoban, 2003). Before her husband left, Rena lacked personal and cultural 'safety'; her husband, positioned as her protector, slept with other women; and on coming home, they fought and he was violent. Rena was 'unsafe', with few places to go to for support where her own transgression, rather than her husbands, would not be scrutinized. Many villagers identify a correlation between conflict in the home, poverty and a lack of safety. Although Rena no longer faces abuse and a lack of personal and emotional safety, her socio-economic vulnerability has been amplified by both her reduced capacity to engage in agricultural work and the loss of her husband's labour power. She has fallen from being middle class to poor and married to abandoned. Women, like Rena, experience vulnerability both within and outside of marriage. They use the idiom of 'safety' *(sok),* and its absence, to express the multiple sources of vulnerability which accompanies their lives as single, married and divorced women. Cultural attitudes toward gender and disability shape the structural inequalities women with disability face in their daily lives.

CULTURAL ATTITUDES TOWARDS GENDER AND DISABILITY

Cambodian society is hierarchically organised around age, which followed by gender, is the most important determinant of one's status (Ebihara, 1968; Ledgerwood, 1990; Gorman et al., 1999). At all levels of society, the status of men and women with disability is less than their able-bodied counterparts (Gartrell, 2004). Cambodian women, particularly those with disability grapple with forms of subjugation embedded within traditional gender ideals and new forms associated with development and contemporary society. Perceptions of gender identity are closely linked with notions of culture and tradition which place women at a lower status than men (Gorman et al., 1999; UNIFEM et al., 2004). Women always refer to their husbands as 'older' *(bong)* in recognition of their higher status. Men are valued simply because of their gender which in itself is evidence of greater karmic status and merit accumulated from past lives (Ebihara 1966; Gorman et al., 1999).

Men and women are ranked according to their karma within a single socio-religious hierarchy, and the virtues and vices of women can affect the status of men within this system. Disability is understood to be the result of karma, literally action-reaction (Harvey, 1987: 34), and is a form of repayment for de-meritous actions, thoughts and deeds performed in past lives. Disability, thus, symbolises poor karma and is equated with suffering in this life. To be born as a woman with a disability, or to acquire a disability, indicates extremely poor karmic status and reinforces the symbolic inequalities associated with both gender and disability.

Judy Ledgerwood (1994) explores the Khmer notion of the perfectly virtuous woman in one folktale which tells the story of how Khmer society should be ordered ideally, and at one time was. The tale illustrates the contradictory demands placed upon women: for example, women are meant to be shy, gentle and sweet, yet also hard headed business women. Ledgerwood (1994: 121-122) notes that:

> The story has much to teach us about how Khmer women are ideally to behave. They must know how to keep order in a household, how to cook delicious food, wash clothes, take care of babies. The virtuous woman is intelligent, advising and assisting her husband in his

[business] endeavours... is beautiful... generous... obedient... these various virtues (are) marks of high accumulations of merit from her previous lives... . Her karmic status as confirmed by her proper behaviour is sufficiently high that she and her spouse are rewarded in this lifetime.

The perfect woman is able-bodied, married, beautiful, and fulfils her role as wife, mother and economic contributor to the household. The ideal woman is active in the productive and reproductive spheres and has good karmic status, as indicated by her good character, beauty and physical ability. Attractiveness, including bodily integrity, is associated with virtue and goodness and is desirable in women. For example, women of high status must have "proper comportment and correct actions. They are to talk slowly and softly" (Ledgerwood, 1992: 4). Ledgerwood (1994, 1992) observes that Khmer men desire beautiful women who embellish their status (see also Asch and Fine, 1997); beauty is an embodied asset for the husband and the woman herself. Beauty gives social power. Women with disability consistently told me about their perceived failure to present themselves beautifully, to walk unassisted with ease and grace like other women at social events such as weddings and religious festivals. They even felt ugly in the spaces of their daily lives. They fail to display the bodily norms associated with beauty and desire.

In their research in the United States, Asch and Fine (1997: 245), speculate that men expect women's physical limitation to translate into limited emotional ability. Women's capacity for the emotional labour of caretaking is, thus, called into question, making them unattractive to men on two fronts: limited physical and emotional resources. In Cambodia, disability is believed to impair brain and nervous function, which in turn causes erratic emotions and a lack of awareness of the social norms of behaviour, including those associated with being a wife and mother. People with disability are seen as lesser people – the embodiment of poor character, diminished spirit and essence as a person (Gartrell, 2004). The assumption that disability causes emotional weakness shapes women's prospects for marriage and motherhood. Their capacity to address the emotional and physical needs of their spouses and children is considered uncertain by potential husbands.

MARRIAGE AND MOTHERHOOD

Even more important than notions of beauty and emotional capacity to cultural conceptions of women, is motherhood, an institution women with disability have long had difficulty entering. Women with disability have been deemed inadequate as sexual partners and mothers. However, as Morris (1993: 106) observes, motherhood provides a means for women with disability to assert and distance themselves from their disability and to strengthen their social and cultural capital. Affirmation of conformity to cultural ideals of gender diminishes the social differences associated with disability.

Sophy, a 22 year old mother of two, was the only women interviewed who had a disability at the time of marriage; the other two married women acquired disability following marriage. Villagers see Sophy as an exception and describe how her families' wealth and her beauty ensured her marriage. Initially, Sophy's parents were suspicious of her spouse-to-be, testing his honesty and questioning his intentions. Her mother's retelling of their courtship story illustrates her surprise that someone would fall in love with Sophy. Villagers commented that her husband must pity Sophy very much and their gossip implies that if he had known she had a disability, he would not have married her. Villages assume that Sophy is a burden to her husband and their relationship is the subject of considerable speculation and curiosity in the village (see also Sharp and Hanks, 1978; Asch and Fine, 1997). They tell a story of Sophy's husband being captivated by her beauty. Each day he would pass her house and see her sitting upstairs on the verandah. It was only after he had fallen in love with her that he realized she had a disability, and by then it was too late.

Sophy simulates the cultural ideal of the perfect woman; she is a wife and mother, beautiful, astute and restricted to the domestic sphere. Traditionally, women's spatial mobility was restricted to local and domestic spheres, and relatives accompanied women as independent travel "would not look good for the family" (fieldnotes, 5 December, 2000). Women have considerable social experience and influence, but limited independence. Sophy's movement patterns reflect this underlying cultural and social ideal. She rarely ventures far from home, and when she does, is always accompanied. She fulfils her domestic and mothering responsibilities and only requires the assistance of others to cart the water and prepare the firewood. Their domestic space is all on one floor enabling Sophy to move with ease. Both of Sophy's children were born by caesarean section in the district hospital. Sophy has acquired the status of marriage and motherhood and its associated self worth and esteem.

People with disability are seen as worthy of marrying one another, that is, marrying at their own level. In Daəm Dooŋ, Rot and Vanna, are one such example. They made offerings to the ancestors of each of their parents to sanctify their union, without the expense of marriage, a common practice for poorer families.[1] Villagers refer to both Rot and Vanna in laughable terms as literally as having insufficient water (*'mɨn krup tik'*), which loosely translates as an intellectual or learning disability.[2] Like Sophy and her husband, villager's gossip about Rot, Vanna and their child. They only lived with Rot's mother for several months before their union broke down. Rot was still cared for like a child by his own mother, and he in turn responded as a child - giving her, rather than Vanna - his wife - any money he earnt. Vanna became angry, and with their baby returned to live with her own mother. Publicly, Vanna and her mother reprimand Rot for failing to visit his baby daughter, but other villagers' are not surprised he does not know his role as father, after all, he has a disability. Villagers thought it appropriate for two people with mental disability to be together. Both Rot and Vanna are now supported by their mothers, extending their child like status despite now being parents themselves.

SEXUALITY

Virtuousness, virginity and marital fidelity are vital to a women's status and her sexuality is tightly controlled, firstly by her parents and then by her husband (Gorman et al., 1999: 30).

---

[1] *Saens* are a preferred option when the circumstances surrounding the union are questionable, such as non-consensual sex. They are considerably cheaper than weddings.

[2] The term is not listed in Headley (1977) but was defined by a local Khmer teacher as naïve, dumb, ignorant and uneducated. Rot was intellectually impaired, but Vanna was emotionally scarred. Her mother has been violent toward her since she was a child. The expression *mɨn krup tik* implies a lack of awareness and consciousness. Villagers use the phrase 'water in the heart' *(tik cət)* interchangeably with heart *(cət)*.

Several old Cambodian proverbs illustrate cultural attitudes toward women's sexuality. One compares a man to a diamond and a woman to a piece of white cloth. When they fall in the mud, the diamond can be washed clean, but the cotton remains dirty forever (Kuouch et al., 1992). Another compares a daughter to a jar of *prahok,* Cambodian fish sauce, with a very strong aroma. If the jar is broken, referring to the loss of virginity, the smell spreads, tarnishing the reputation of the family (CDPO, 1999). It is believed Cambodian women preserve the good name of the family. For example:

> Having a daughter is like having a toilet in front of the house. If they are good, everyone knows, but if it smells, word spreads quickly and the family's reputation is destroyed (6 February, 2001).

Women with disability, particularly mental disability, are at greater risk of non-consensual sex than non-disabled women. Several parents raised these concerns, and although they try to ensure the safety of their daughters with disability, it is not always possible to have someone at home to protect them (see Surtees, 2003). Although women with disability have been marginalized from voluntary sexuality and reproduction, it has not excluded them from sexual abuse and victimisation; girls with disability are an easy victim of abuse by male relatives. Women with disability are assumed by non-disabled people to be asexual or objects of sexual exploitation. Women with disability expressed concerns regarding their physical capacity to engage in sexual relations and childbirth indicating the need for greater awareness and dissemination of appropriate reproductive health information. Research focusing on these issues and women with disability's birthing experiences needs to be conducted.

VULNERABILITY IN MARRIAGE

Women in Daəm Dooŋ, as in Cambodia more generally, are concerned with the mistreatment to which they are vulnerable in marriage. Marital rape, domestic violence and abandonment are common and not specific to women with disability. Gossip and rumour are key sources of local knowledge about women with disability's experiences of marriage. Stories of abuse, vulnerability and economic exploitation perpetuate stereotypes and incite feelings of fear and reticence, which influence women's actions. The common view is that men only marry women with disability out of pity or to send them to beg; they are seen as unworthy to marry. Rarely are positive stories, such as Sophy and her husband told, and if known, they are less gossip worthy (see Elias and Scotson, 1994).

Manderson and Allotey's (2003) research on storytelling suggests that narratives of marginality, such as these stories, reinforce distinctive and oppositional identities, between women with and without disability, married and unmarried, for example, but also serve to strengthen commitment to wider society, in this case, to the institution of marriage. Although I did meet women who had chosen not to marry because they were fearful of being abandoned by husbands and left to raise children alone, the women interviewed remain committed, albeit ambivalent, to marriage as an institution. Marriage brings status and represents security but women with disability are aware of the risks marriage can also bring: abuse, rape and abandonment. They are more likely to be left by husbands than non-disabled women as Rena's experience illustrates (Gartrell, 2004). Women with disability are fearful for their futures both within and outside of marriage.

Sena, a 19 year old woman with a mobility impairment, would like to have children, but her mother is fearful of her marrying:

> I have heard stories of other women with disability, women with crutches, marrying and being taken by their husbands to beg....to earn money to look after them. I am fearful that Khmer men will treat her badly, especially since she has a disability. Sometimes when she is selling sweets, there are handsome young men who come to buy things. They see her face is beautiful...and fall in love with her....but when they see her walk...they are disappointed. When we look at her, there seems to be no hope, no ability to marry. Before a man did fall in love with her...but he was inferior...it was not a good match. I'm afraid that later on they will treat her badly or leave her (7th September, 2000).

Sena's mother is worried about her daughters' her long term socio-economic security and 'safety'. Sena has internalised Cambodian cultural notions of beauty and worth and judges herself as ugly, feeding her feelings of shame and social unease. When she was 15 years old, other young people in the village laughed at her when they saw her walk. Since this time she has felt shy and embarrassed and only visits familiar places around their house where villagers know her and she feels safe. Rarely does she attend village social events. Sena has no expectations for her future and although she would like to study hairdressing, her mother will not allow it believing that Sena does not have the ability. Sena faces multiple sources of vulnerability and disadvantage, which her mother's attitude perpetuates. Sena has no role models to guide her. Ultimately, Sena's mother, herself abandoned by her husband, will decide Sena's future husband, if she marries at all. For unmarried women, playing a key role in providing for one's family and parents' particularly as they age is an alternate, albeit less traditional, way of distanciation from disablement and creating a positive identity.

WOMEN ALONE

Women with disability who do not marry find themselves without positive cultural maps to attain dignity and status outside of marriage and motherhood. As Gorman and colleagues (1999) argues, women acquire status from being a wife and mother, and not from their role in work or education. Women with disabilities who do not marry however, have little choice but to engage in whatever work they can to support themselves, any dependents they may have or just to contribute to their households. Typically, women with disability have few employment options and have little choice but to engage in the lowest paid forms of work, such as running small businesses from home, to meet their daily needs (Gartrell, 2004). For some, not even this option is available if they are lack capital, live in an isolated location, or if other household members are not supportive.

Rattana is a 45 year old single woman who had polio as a child. She lives with her elderly father whom she supports by sewing and selling small goods at the front of their house. She has no siblings, and only one aunt who lives nearby. At home, Rattana cooks but relies on others to cart water, which she then stores near her cooking space. Rattana is too old to have children, and is denied this source of pride, social status, labour power, economic assistance, and carers for her old age. Rattana's value as a woman is diminished by her childlessness and single status, emphasising the importance of work and supportive social networks for her well-being.

Rattana has no one to rely upon and is 'without the strength of the body' to work in the most readily available forms of employment. She is left with few options but to run a small sewing business from home to meet her and her father's daily needs. Although she has acquired skills and psychological resources to assist her in the 'productive' sphere of village life, her life is very different from that of other village women around her. She must continually struggle to meet her and her father's basic needs in an environment full of barriers to her physical movement and socio-economic inclusion. In a culture which views women and disability as unworthy, women with disability struggle to find positive self-concepts and to avoid falling into depressive states lacking hope for the future, which only too quickly fulfil disabling social expectations and stereotypes.

Rattana draws a distinction between the heart and the body which enables her to salvage some hope and dignity. Rattana draws strength from her heart *(kɑmlaŋ c□t)* as her body is weak. Wendell (1996: 176) argues that detachment of the self from the impaired body is a sound strategy on which to base our sense of self, and therefore self esteem, on intellect and/or emotional experiences, activities and connections with others (see also Murphy, 1987). Rattana has a warm and friendly disposition. Her continued struggle to improve her living is well regarded by her neighbours, who pity her, helping where they can, for instance, going to the market for her. It is difficult for Rattana even to enter the market in her wheelchair, because of narrow and congested isles, blocked entrances and rough, often muddy surfaces. When Rattana's neighbours see her helping other women with disability, sharing her sewing skills with them, they comment that she has a good heart. This supportive social network is a vital source of material assistance, but more importantly, is the means through which she gains social acceptance, self confidence and feelings of hope.

CONCLUSION

Rena's experience raised three key sets of issues which are critical to shaping the lives of women with disability and particularly their experiences both within and outside of marriage. Firstly, negative cultural beliefs associating disability with lack of utility shapes the attitudes of potential spouses and society more generally. Secondly, marriage is based upon the physical and emotional labour required to fulfil gender roles, and women with disability are assumed not to have these capacities. And thirdly, the physical and emotional vulnerability of women with disability - whether single, married, divorced or abandoned - is determined by gendered socio-economic and cultural processes. Women with disability and their families make decisions to secure their future well-being based upon the risks associated with remaining single and marrying. Although some women with disability do manage to have satisfying marriages, such as Sophy and her husband, many are exposed to multiple and compounding sources of vulnerability as they struggle to meet their daily needs, to contribute to the families and care for dependents whilst retaining their dignity.

This research has found that disability challenges the foundations of Cambodian notions of the family as a unit of socio-economic security and provider of protection for women.

Marriage does not guarantee women's safety but exposes them to a different set of risks: marital rape, domestic violence, abandonment and single parenthood. Women with disability trigger fears in non-disabled people, particularly men, of endless responsibility, unreciprocated care, dependence and the false assumption that women with disability can not contribute to anyone else's well-being. Until the fears, anxieties and vulnerabilities that bodily difference arouses in non-disabled people are acknowledged, women with impairments will continue to live on the margins of society, struggling to access traditional and non-traditional forms of status and value. Whilst there is the freedom to be non-traditional, carving out new pathways to achieve status challenges women with disability to retain a strong internal sense of self in the face of stigma, discrimination, denial of opportunities and barriers. As single, married, divorced and abandoned women, women with disability encounter multiple sources of vulnerability which they negotiate as best as they can to maximize their safety in a society that is becoming increasingly socially polarized.

Motherhood is often regarded as synonymous with womanhood, and yet women with disability are largely invisible in discourses on motherhood. The interface between motherhood and disability has been poorly examined, and Prilleltensky (2004: 4) goes so far as to argue that motherhood is counter-indicated by disability. Rarely are women with disability thought of as sexual beings, mothers and carers for others. Rather, they are seen to be receivers of care, incompetent as mothers and unable to assume parental responsibility. Women with disability's capacity to choose to be mothers is shaped by these deep seated prejudices and their exclusion from motherhood must be understood as determined more by default than preference. Women with disability, those with and without children, have in the main been absent from discourses in feminism and the women's movement, disability studies and in more general discourses of social justice. Until their voices are heard, they will continue to experience significant vulnerability and structural disadvantage.

REFERENCES

American Friends Service Committee (AFSC), 2000, *My Heart is Not Disabled: People with Disabilities in Kampot Province*, Socio-Cultural Vulnerability and Coping Strategies (SCVCS) Research Project 4: Phnom Penh, Cambodia.

Asch, A., & Fine, M., 1992, 'Beyond Pedestals: Revisiting the Lives of Women With Disabilities', in M. Fine (ed.), *Disruptive Voices: The Possibilities of Feminist Research*, pp. 139-171. University of Michigan Press: Michigan.

Asch, A., & Fine, M., 1997, 'Nurturance, Sexuality and Women With Disabilities', in L.J. Davis (ed.), *The Disability Studies Reader*, pp. 241-259. Routledge: New York and London.

Asian Development Bank (ADB), 2005, *Country Strategy and Program 2005-2009: Cambodia.* ADB: Manila.

Annear, P., 1998, 'Health and Development in Cambodia', *Asian Studies Review,* 22(2): 193-221.

Cambodia, Ministry of Planning, 1997, *Socio-Economic Survey of Cambodia 1996. Volume II. Summary Results*, National Institute of Statistics, Ministry of Planning: Phnom Penh.

Cambodia, Ministry of Planning, 1999, *Socio-Economic Survey of Cambodia 1998*, National Institute of Statistics, Ministry of Planning: Phnom Penh.

Cambodia, Ministry of Planning and Ministry of Health, 2001, *Cambodia Demographic and Health Survey 2000*, National Institute of Statistics, Ministry of Planning/Ministry of Health: Phnom Penh.

Cambodia, Ministry of Planning, 2002, *Population and Poverty in Asia and the Pacific. Country Report: Cambodia*, Presentation of the Royal Government of Cambodia. Fifth Asian and Pacific Population Conference. Economic and Social Commission for Asia and the Pacific and United Nations Population Fund. 11-17 December 2002, Bangkok.

Cambodia, MOSALVA, 1996, *A National Strategy for MOSALVA and NGO's of the Rehabilitation Sector on Disability Issues and the Rehabilitation and Integration of Disabled People in Cambodia: Summary Report*, MOSALVA Taskforce on Disability Issues. MOSALVA: Phnom Penh.

Cambodia, Centre for Social Development, 2002, *National Poverty Reduction Strategy 2002-2000*, Centre for Social Development, Kingdom of Cambodia: Phnom Penh.

Cambodian Disabled People's Organisation, 1999, *Looking Back, Moving Forward. Proceedings of the First National Conference on Gender and Development in Cambodia*, Sept 7-9, 1999, Phnom Penh.

Department for International Development (DFID), 2000, *Disability, Poverty and Development*, DFID: London.

Disability Action Council (DAC) Secretariat, 2001, *Country Profile: Study on Persons with Disabilities (Cambodia)*, Supported by JICA-Cambodia: Phnom Penh.

Ebihara, M., 1966, 'Interrelations Between Buddhism and Social Systems in Cambodian Peasant Culture', in (Nash, M.), *Anthropological Studies in Theravada Buddhism*. Culture Report Series 13, pp. 175-196. South-East Asian Studies, Yale University Press: New Haven.

Ebihara, M., 1968, *Svaay, a Khmer Village in Cambodia*, unpublished doctoral thesis, University of Columbia, Ann Arbor: University Microfilm International [1971].

Elias, N., & Scotson, J.L., 1994, *The Established and The Outsiders: A sociological enquiry into community problems*, Sage Publications: London.

Elwan, A., 1999, *Poverty and Disability: A Survey of the Literature*, Social Protection Discussion Papers Series, No. 9932, Social Protection Unit, Human Development Network, The World Bank: Washington DC.

Estroff, S.E., 1993, *'Identity, Disability, and Schizophrenia. The Problem of Chronicity'*, in S. Lindenbaum and M. Lock (eds.), *Knowledge, Power and Practice: The Anthropology of Medicine and Everyday Life*, pp. 247-286. University of California Press: Berkeley.

Finkelstein, V., 1980, *Attitudes and Disabled People: Issues for Discussion*, World Rehabilitation Fund: New York.

Franklin, P., 1977, 'Impact of Disability on Family Structure', *Social Security Bulletin*, 40: 3-18.

Gartrell, A., 2004, *Flying on Hope: The Lived Experience of Disability in Rural Cambodia*, unpublished doctoral thesis, School of Geography, Anthropology and Environmental Studies, The University of Melbourne: Melboure, Australia.

Gender and Development Network, Cambodia, 2006, 'Gender in Poverty Reduction'. <www.ngoforum.org.kh/Documents/Sectorial%20Paper%20PRD2003/Gender .htm>

Gorman, S., Pon, D, & Sok, K., 1999, *Gender and Development in Cambodia: An Overview*, Working Paper 10, Cambodian Development Resource Institute: Phnom Penh.

Groce, N., & Scheer, J., 1990, 'Introduction', *Social Science and Medicine*, 30(8): v-vi.

Harvey, P., 1987, 'The Buddhist Perspective on Respect for Persons', *Buddhist Studies Review*, 4(1): 31-46.

Hoban, E., 2003, *'We're Safe and Happy Already: Traditional Birth Attendants and Safe Motherhood in a Cambodian Rural Commune*, unpublished doctoral thesis, The Key Centre for Women's Health in Society, Department of Public Health, The University of Melbourne: Melbourne, Australia.

Hughes, C., 2006, 'Cambodia', *IDS Bulletin*, 37(2): 67-78.

Ilagan, V.M., 2002, 'Persons with Disabilities: The Most Marginalized Among the World's Vulnerable', Disabled People's International, Asia Pacific Region. <www.worldenable. net/livelihoods/paperphilippines.htm>

Ingstad, B., & Whyte, S., 1995, *Disability and Culture*, University of California Press:Berkeley.

Kuoch, T., Miller, R., & Scully, M., 1992, 'Healing the Wounds of the Mahantdorí', in E, Cole, O, Espin, E, Rothblum, E. (eds), *Refugee Women and Their Mental Health. Journeys to Recovery: The Healing Process*, pp. 191-207. Haworth Press: New York.

Ledgerwood, J., 1992, A*nalysis of the Situation of Women in Cambodia. Research on Women in Khmer Society'*, Consultancy for UNICEF: Phnom Penh.

Ledgerwood, J., 1994, 'Gender Symbolism and Culture Change: Viewing the Virtuous Woman in the Khmer Story 'Mea Yoeng', in M. Ebihara, C. Mortland and J. Ledgerwood (eds.), *Cambodian Culture since 1975,* pp. 118-128. Cornell University Press: Ithaca and London.

Lonsdale, S., 1990, *Women and Disability: The Experience of Physical Disability Among Women*, Macmillan: London.

MacKinlay, L., 2004, *World Vision Cambodia Disability Research*, World Vision: Phnom Penh.

Manderson, L., & Allotey, P., 2003, 'Storytelling, Marginality, and Community in Australia: How Immigrants Position their Difference in Health Care Settings', *Medical Anthropology*, 22(1): 1-21.

Morris, J., 1993, 'Prejudice', in J. Swain, V, Finkelstein, S, French and M. Oliver (eds.), *Disabling Barriers - Enabling Environments*, pp 101-106. Sage Publications in association with the Open University Press: London, California and New Delhi.

Morris, J., (ed.) 1996, *Encounters with Strangers: Feminism and Disability*, The Women's Press Ltd: London.

Murphy, R., 1987, *The Body Silent*, M. Holt: New York.

Oliver, M., 1983, *Social Work with Disabled People*, MacMillan: Basingstoke.

Oliver, M., 1996, *Understanding Disability: From Theory to Practice*, MacMillan: London.

Ovesen, J., Trankell, I.B., & Ojëndal, J., 1996, *When Every Household is an Island. Social Organisation and Power Structures in Rural Cambodia*, Uppsala Research Reports in Cultural Anthropology, No 15: Stockholm, Sweden.

Prilleltensky, O., 2004, *Motherhood and Disability: Children and Choices,* Palgrave MacMillan: New York.

Shakespeare, T., 1994, 'Cultural Representations of Disabled People: Dustbins for Disavowal', *Disability and Society,* 9(3): 283-300.

Sharp, L., & Hanks, L.M., 1978, *Bang Chan: Social History of a Rural Community in Thailand,* Cornell University Press: Ithaca and London.

Stone, J., (ed.) 2005, *Culture and Disability: Providing Culturally Competent Services,* Multicultural Aspects of Counselling Series 21, Sage Publications: Thousand Oaks, California.

Surtees, R., 2003, 'Rape and Sexual Transgression in Cambodian Society', in L. Manderson and L.R. Bennett (eds.), *Violence Against Women in Asian Societies,* pp. 93-109. Routledge Curzon: London and New York.

Takamine, Y., 2004, *Disability Issues in East Asia: Review and Ways Forward,* working Paper Series No 2004-1, Human Development Sector Unit, East Asia and the Pacific Region, The World Bank: Washington, DC.

Thomson, R., 1997, 'Feminist Theory, the Body, and the Disabled Figure', in L.J. Davis (ed.), *The Disability Studies Reader,* pp. 79-292. Routledge: New York and London.

UNDP/Cambodia, 2001, *UNDP Development Report 2001,* UNDP: Phnom Penh.

UNDP, 2005, *World Development Report, Cambodia.* <http://hdr.undp.org/statistics/data/countries.cfm?c=KHM>

UNDP, 1995, *Human Development Report,* UNDP: New York.

UNICEF, 1990, *Cambodia: The Situation of Children and Women,* UNICEF: Phnom Penh.

UNIFEM, WB, ADB, UNDP and DFID/UK, 2004, *A Fair Share For Women. Cambodia Gender Assessment,* UNIFEM, WB, ADB, UNDP and DFID/UK: Phnom Penh.

van de Put, W., 1992, *Empty Hospitals, Thriving Business: Utilisation of Health Services and Health Seeking Behaviour in Two Cambodian Districts,* report for Medicins Sans Frontiers - Holland/Belgium. Medicins Sans Frontiers – Holland/Belgium: Phnom Penh.

Wendell, S., 1996, *The Rejected Body: Feminist Philosophical Reflections on Disability,* Routledge: New York.

INDEX

F

I

N

O

T